BIOMEDICAL CONTROVERSIES IN CATHOLIC IRELAND

Dr Don O'Leary is a historian and scientist. He worked in University College Cork from 1978 to 2017, providing technical support for scientific research, mainly in neuroscience. In parallel with this he studied history and was awarded a Ph.D. from the National University of Ireland in 1996. Most of his research is focused on the relationship between Catholicism and science, both internationally and in relation to Ireland. He is the author of *Vocationalism and Social Catholicism in Twentieth-Century Ireland* (Irish Academic Press, 2000), *Roman Catholicism and Modern Science* (Continuum/ Bloomsbury, 2006) and *Irish Catholicism and Science* (Cork University Press, 2012).

DON O'LEARY

A contemporary history of
divisive social issues

BIOMEDICAL CONTROVERSIES IN CATHOLIC IRELAND

ERYN PRESS

First published in 2020 by
Eryn Press
Cork
Ireland
erynpress.com

Paperback	ISBN: 978 1 78846 163 4
eBook – mobi format	ISBN: 978 1 78846 166 5
eBook – ePub format	ISBN: 978 1 78846 165 8
Amazon paperback edition	ISBN: 978 1 78846 164 1

Produced by Kazoo Independent Publishing Services
222 Beech Park, Lucan, Co. Dublin
kazoopublishing.com

Kazoo Independent Publishing Services is not the publisher of this work. All rights and responsibilities pertaining to this work remain with Eryn Press.

Kazoo offers independent authors a full range of publishing services. For further details visit kazoopublishing.com

Cover design by Andrew Brown
Printed in the EU

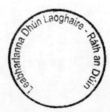

CONTENTS

———•———

———————•———————

Acknowledgements

I am grateful to my daughter, Dr Karen O'Leary, for her insightful comments, especially on points of scientific detail. I am indebted to Paula Elmore for her recommendations, and to Jane Rogers for copyediting the text. Thanks also to Kate O'Leary for her advice and support.

This book is dedicated to my family: Kate, Karen, Kevin and Laura; Sarah, Sid and Eryn; Claire and Conor.

Don O'Leary,
May 2020

Introduction

IN THE MID-1970S, ARTIFICIAL CONTRACEPTIVES WERE banned in the Republic of Ireland – even for married couples. Abortion and homosexual acts between consenting adults were both criminal offences under the terms of legislation passed during the reign of Queen Victoria.[1] There was a constitutional ban on divorce. Submissive politicians kissed the bishops' rings. The Church's reputation was not yet sullied by paedophile priests and brothers, cover-ups by bishops, forced adoptions of children born out of wedlock, and the exploitation of vulnerable women in Magdalene laundries. Medical science had not yet made it possible for a woman to give birth to her grandchild.[2] There was no internet or social media. Ireland was a very different country then.

The rapid advancement of science and technology has played an important role in social transformation, but there have been many other agents of change, such as the clerical scandals referred to above, the feminist movement, the mass media, and a more highly educated and independent-minded laity.[3] In view of all this, it may seem that Roman Catholicism is a spent force in Irish society, incapable of initiating or blocking social change. To see it this way would be to misunderstand social change in Ireland, especially in relation to the Catholic Church. Catholic opinions are crucially important, considering their majority status. Although the percentage of the population who are Catholic has fallen significantly in recent decades, it was still almost 80 per cent in the 2016 census.[4] Legislation and social change in the Republic of Ireland will be mainly determined by Catholic opinions for many years to come.

In this book Irish Catholic attitudes are examined in relation to contraception, abortion, human embryonic stem cell research, assisted human reproduction and assisted suicide. The timeframe is mainly from Pope Paul VI's encyclical on birth control, *Humanae Vitae* (1968), to Ireland's abortion referendum (2018). In view of the subject matter, some aspects of science, philosophy and Catholic doctrine will be explored. Philosophical debates about morality, and whether or not there is a rational basis for morality, will receive some attention but will not be examined at length.

Ethics, sometimes known as moral philosophy, may be regarded as a set of concepts and principles by which a state, community or organisation decides to regulate its behaviour. Distinctions are made between concepts such as right and wrong, good and evil, justice and criminality.[5] On what basis are ethical judgements made? A religious response would assert that a divine being has prescribed certain rules of moral behaviour. Conversely, immoral behaviour arises when these rules are not complied with.

Christian ethics is based on the Ten Commandments and the moral teachings of Jesus Christ. There are different traditions of Christian ethics, and variations within these traditions, which will not receive attention here. Even so, it is appropriate to make a few general observations to give at least some indication of the complexities and subjectivities that are encountered in attempts to avoid a plurality of moral perspectives. The assumptions of Christian ethics are not without major problems. For example, the existence of God is open to challenge – there are arguments for and against. If God does not exist, the moral laws supposedly expressing his will cannot be reasonably sustained. It is assumed that God is good, although it can be argued that the prevalence of suffering and evil calls this into question. If God is not good, why is disobedience to the divine authority wrong? It can be argued that, to act morally, we must do something because it is good, not merely because it is God's will. This introduces non-theological arguments. And how is God's will to be ascertained? There are so many different interpretations of the Bible and so many conflicting theological schools of thought – both within and between the various Christian churches – that God's will could be said to be beyond human discovery.[6]

In secular philosophical discourse the existence of God is very much open to question. Philosopher H. Tristram Engelhardt[7] argued that "the death of God" and the consequent loss of a religious perspective led inevitably to a plurality of competing moralities. What's more, he argued, there are no sound secular arguments that provide enough common ground to construct a single morality that commands consensus.

Therefore, morality and bioethics are cultural creations.[8] Philosopher Joel Marks took the implications of a godless universe to an extreme, arguing that without God there is no rational basis for morality – hence his provocative "amoral manifesto".[9] This philosophical stance is – as one would expect – anathema to practising Catholics and followers of other faiths. From an orthodox Roman Catholic perspective, it would have been condemned as relativism – the belief that there are no universal standards of right and wrong, good and evil, and that there is no objective knowledge. The concept of natural law or "law of reason" taught by the Church is the antithesis of relativism. It maintains that God endowed humans with the ability to understand what is morally right or wrong, independent of divine revelation. But this is not so straightforward. Theologians have frequently disagreed about the content and application of the natural law, especially in relation to sexual morality.[10]

Pope John Paul II, in his encyclical *Evangelium Vitae* (1995), upheld the concept of natural law, asserting that people of goodwill, despite experiencing "difficulties and uncertainties", would benefit from the moral insights it offered.[11] Apparently, such well-intentioned people were in a minority, the consequence being that liberal democracies had sacrificed "all forms of tradition and authority" to the cause of freedom. Objective and universal truths were repudiated as tolerance for a diversity of beliefs was eagerly embraced. Relativism stood "unopposed". In this dystopian world John Paul saw the violation of the most basic of human rights – the right to life. Abortion and euthanasia were frequently legalised under cover of democratic and pluralist values. The pope predicted that those democratic states that were devoid of sound moral values would eventually collapse amid social conflict.[12] Cardinal Cahal B. Daly (1917–2009) reasoned that there is an inverse relationship between moral restraints and legal restraints. If moral self-restraint and civic virtues declined unchecked there was then a tendency for the state to intervene in the lives of its citizens to preserve public order and social cohesion, to the point where personal freedoms were endangered.[13]

The Church declares itself supportive of democracy. The ideal democratic state, from its point of view, promotes social reforms that are supportive of morality.[14] State initiatives include legislation. Although citizens are not made virtuous by legislation, the bishops argue that some laws can create difficulties for moral behaviour by making immorality socially acceptable.[15] Catholics are urged to live in conformity with God's commandments, promulgated through the teaching authority of the Church. However, despite the "guidance of the Holy Spirit" and an "objective moral order", Catholics frequently disagree about distinctions between morality and immorality.[16] In states with Catholic majorities, such as the Republic of Ireland, the question arises as to whether or not Catholic moral beliefs should be upheld by state law. The Church's answer to this question is less than straightforward. In 1976 the Irish Catholic bishops collectively declared: "It is not the view of the Catholic hierarchy that, in the law of the State, the principles peculiar to our faith should be made binding on people who do not adhere to that faith."[17] In national referendums Catholics were, and are, expected to vote according to their conscience. This implies a considerable degree of individual freedom – but such freedom is very much curtailed by the obligation to vote according to conscience as informed by the authoritative teachings of the Church.[18] Catholic consciences are "subject to the Church's magisterium, whose task it is to expound authoritatively the entire moral law". The magisterium asserts that "there are absolute norms, which are binding in every instance and on all peoples."[19] A case in point is the prohibition against abortion, which is deemed never morally acceptable (except to save the life of the mother). Catholics who are faithful to the teachings of the Church cannot conform to an immoral state law or support it in any way,[20] not even in democratic states: "Morality is not a numbers game."[21]

The hierarchical Church does not claim unlimited powers of intervention in the social, economic and political dimensions of community life. The Second Vatican Council acknowledged the "rightful autonomy of earthly affairs".[22] The clergy are obligated to give spiritual guidance to the laity, but they are, in general, not experts in secular issues. It is the duty of the laity, with a "properly informed" conscience, "to impress the divine law on the affairs of the earthly city".[23] Yet this directive has its limitations: not everything immoral should be forbidden by the laws of the state. If an immoral practice is to be legally prohibited, is the law enforceable? Is it likely to command widespread compliance? Is its enforcement likely to cause harm to other aspects of social life? A case in point is the misguided Eighteenth Amendment to the Constitution of the USA and the National Prohibition Act 1920 that was passed to enforce it. The prohibition on the production, distribution, sale and consumption of alcohol proved to be unworkable. A major unintended consequence was that it stimulated the growth of organised crime on a vast scale and provoked widespread disrespect for the system of justice. A more pertinent case, in an Irish context, was the proposed amendments to Article 40.3.3 of the Constitution concerning abortion. On 25 November 1992 a majority voted in favour of the right to travel (Thirteenth Amendment) to another state and chose not to constitutionally prohibit access to information about services that were legally available abroad (Fourteenth Amendment). Restricting the rights of citizens in such circumstances would have done more harm than good and would, like the prohibition of alcohol in the USA, have proved unsustainable in the long term. The Irish Catholic bishops acknowledged that attempts to impose restrictions on travel or access to information would "lead to an unacceptable infringement of the personal liberty of citizens in a free society and would bring the law into disrepute".[24]

In its *Declaration on Procured Abortion* (18 November 1974) the Church acknowledges that civil law cannot address the entire domain of morality and that sometimes a great evil can only be avoided by tolerating a lesser one.[25] This raises the question: Which immoral acts or practices should be tolerated in civil law, and which should be prohibited? Is a majority vote always the best way of deciding what moral principles are enforced by law? How are the rights of minorities to be safeguarded in liberal democracies without infringing the rights of the majority? Minorities in Ireland include not only people of other religious faiths and none, but those Catholics who disagree with most of their co-religionists. In a liberal democracy such as Ireland there is broad support for the principle that the opinions of minorities should be facilitated, subject to the common good.

The laws of the state do not necessarily indicate the values held by the majority of its people. Toleration of a law does not necessarily mean approval in a moral sense. In other words, the values of the majority cannot be simply inferred from secular law.[26] This is not to argue that laws make no difference in altering morally relevant behaviour – it is to observe that laws and constitutional amendments, alone, have limited and unpredictable effects. For example, in an Irish context, it was argued by sociologist Ricca Edmondson that the Eighth Amendment to the Constitution, prohibiting abortion, did little to address the underlying causes. The point has been made that countries (such as the Netherlands) with far less stringent laws against abortion probably had proportionately fewer abortions than those originating from Ireland, where about five thousand women travelled to Britain each year for terminations of pregnancy.[27] Promoting respect for girls and women, and providing protection and support for those who find themselves pregnant in difficult circumstances, is potentially far more effective than the outcomes of referendums and Acts of parliament.

The Catholic Church teaches that the common good is best served when all members of society are protected. But what does "the common good" mean? The Church defined it as "the sum total of those conditions of social life which enable men [*sic*] to achieve a fuller measure of perfection with greater ease. It consists especially in safeguarding the rights and duties of the human person."[28] The common good has also been referred to in terms such as "public morality" and "justice", the meanings of which are often contentious in relation to specific issues.[29] There is, therefore, a lack of precision about what "the common good" actually means. Despite this lack of clarity, it can be observed that the common good and minority freedoms are interlinked – it is in the best interests of society to facilitate the freedom of individuals and social groups to the maximum, provided that there is due regard for the rights of others.[30] Patrick Hannon, then professor of theology at St Patrick's College, Maynooth, observed in his *Church, State, Morality and Law* (1992) that some people view artificial contraception, divorce and homosexuality as immoral but oppose the idea that such immoral practices should be prohibited by the laws of the state.[31] The contention was that, in societies where there was a diversity of opinions on some moral issues (such as divorce), the law should not impose restrictions when there was no perceived conflict, by a minority, between morality and the freedom sought. As far back as November 1973 the Irish Catholic bishops conceded that the state was not obligated to prohibit everything that was immoral, such as the importation and sale of contraceptives.[32]

Artificial contraception has long ceased to be a contentious issue in Catholic Ireland. The same cannot be said for abortion, human embryonic stem cell research, surrogacy and assisted suicide. Bioethical issues, driven by advances in the life sciences, will continue to generate controversy from time to time. It is likely that new cases will arise in the courts that will eventually press legislators to do what is expected of them – to legislate. Even the best drafted legislation will need to be amended in response to unforeseeable legal and ethical problems. In the meantime, this book will give readers a sound knowledge of the historical background, ethical arguments and scientific advances that will continue to be so important for understanding future debates.

Glossary[33]

Abortifacient: A drug or substance that causes abortion.

AHR: Assisted human reproduction.

AID: Artificial insemination using spermatozoa from a donor or third party.

AIH: Artificial insemination using spermatozoa from the husband.

Asexual reproduction: Reproduction without sex.

Blastocyst (human): An early-stage embryo, four to five days post-fertilisation. It comprises an outer layer of cells, a fluid-filled cavity and an inner cell mass. Human embryonic stem cells are derived from the inner cell mass.

Cells: The structural and functional units of living organisms.

Chromosomes: Long strands of DNA that contain genes in a linear sequence. Human cells (except gametes) contain 22 matching pairs and one pair determining gender – 46 chromosomes in total.

Cloning (reproductive): The process of generating a genetic copy of an organism for the purpose of reproduction. Cloning can be done by somatic cell nuclear transfer (see term below) or by artificially splitting early-stage embryos.

Cloning (therapeutic): The process of generating embryos for the purpose of harvesting embryonic stem cells. The embryos are destroyed in the process.

CAHR: Commission on Assisted Human Reproduction (2000–2005), a government commission set up by the then Minister for Health and Children, Micheál Martin.

Cryopreservation: Storage of biological tissue at very low temperatures below freezing point.

Dáil Éireann: The lower house of parliament.

DAHR: Donor-assisted human reproduction; the use of gametes donated by a third party or third parties in assisted human reproduction.

DNA: Deoxyribonucleic acid; the genetic material of most living organisms. It plays a major role in the determination of hereditary traits and is a major constituent of chromosomes within cell nuclei.

DS: Down Syndrome (trisomy 21) is a genetic anomaly. A person with DS has an extra (third) copy of chromosome 21. In some cases there is an incomplete extra chromosome or not all cells in the body carry the extra chromosome.

Embryo (human): The first eight weeks of development after fertilisation of the ovum.

ECHR: European Court of Human Rights.

EU: European Union.

Gametes: Male and female reproductive cells: ova and spermatozoa.

"Fatal foetal abnormalities": There is no consensus on the meaning of this term; but there is no consensus either on alternative terms such as "lethal foetal abnormalities/anomalies" or "life-limiting conditions". The vast majority of foetuses with these conditions are stillborn or die very shortly after birth. In some exceptional cases people who were diagnosed with such conditions before birth survive for years with severe physical and/or cognitive impairments.

Foetus (human): Post-embryonic, from the end of the eighth week of development to birth.

Gene: A unit of heredity that is composed of DNA.

GSAHR: General Scheme of the Assisted Human Reproduction Bill 2017.

hASCs (human adult stem cells): Stem cells that are not embryonic and can be sourced from various parts of the body, e.g. bone marrow, umbilical cord blood.

hESCs (human embryonic stem cells): Stem cells derived from the inner cell mass of embryos.

HPV: human papillomavirus.

Implantation: The embedding of the embryo, at the blastocyst stage of development, in the inner lining of the womb, about eight days post-fertilisation.

iPSCs (induced pluripotent stem cells): Adult cells, such as dermal fibroblasts, that are reprogrammed, under laboratory conditions, to a stem-like state. These stem cells can then be further manipulated to develop into a range of specialised cells such as neurons (see "pluripotent stem cells" below).

In vitro: "In glass" – i.e. under laboratory conditions.

In vivo: "In the body".

IVF: *In vitro* fertilisation – i.e. fertilisation outside the body, in a laboratory environment.

JCH: Joint Committee on Health (Oireachtas).

Life-limiting conditions: See "fatal foetal abnormalities" above.

Multipotent stem cells: Cells that can generate specialised cells for a specific tissue or organ.

NMH: National Maternity Hospital (Dublin).

Oireachtas: The legislature of Ireland. The Oireachtas is comprised of the President of Ireland and two houses of parliament – Dáil Éireann and Seanad Éireann.

Ovum (plural ova): Female mature reproductive cell/egg cell.

PLAC: Pro-Life Amendment Campaign.

PLC: Pro Life Campaign.

PLDPA: Protection of Life During Pregnancy Act 2013.

Pluripotent stem cells: Cells that can give rise to all cell types in the foetus and in the adult that are capable of self-renewal. These cells are not capable of generating an organism.

Pre-embryo: The validity of this term is sometimes disputed. It can be used to mean from fertilisation to implantation, or from fertilisation to when the primitive streak (see below) is identifiable.

PGD: Pre-implantation genetic diagnosis; the removal of a cell from an early-stage embryo for genetic testing as part of the embryo selection process in assisted human reproduction.

Primitive streak: A structure that develops in the early stages of embryonic development – in humans at about 14 days post-fertilisation. The future nervous system will develop in association with this structure. Some bioethicists argue that experimentation on human embryos should not be permitted after the primitive streak has developed because they see the feature as an indication of the emergence of a unique human being.

Pro-choice and pro-life: These terms are not objectively definable. It has been argued that a person's outlook can be both pro-life and pro-choice. For example, one can favour termination of pregnancy in cases of rape and "fatal foetal abnormalities" but not in cases of "severe non-fatal" abnormalities or Down syndrome.[34] In the context of Irish discourse about abortion, pro-life opinion will be understood as supportive of the retention of the Eighth Amendment of the Constitution of Ireland. At its most extreme it will be understood as regarding pre-implantation embryos as human beings, deserving of full human rights. Pro-choice will be understood as support for repealing the Eighth Amendment and broadening the grounds for access to abortion in Ireland.

Somatic cells: Cells other than gametes (not ova or spermatozoa).

SCNT: Somatic cell nuclear transfer; a cloning procedure that entails transferring a somatic cell nucleus into an ovum whose nucleus has been removed.

Seanad Éireann: The upper house of parliament.

Spermatozoon (plural spermatozoa): Male mature reproductive cell.

Stem cells: Cells that can divide indefinitely to produce identical cells which can be used to generate specialised cells.

Surrogacy: The carrying of a child by a woman for another person/persons.

SVHG: St Vincent's Healthcare Group Limited.

Tánaiste: Deputy prime minister and deputy head of the government of Ireland.

Taoiseach: The prime minister and head of the government of Ireland.

TD: Teachta Dála; "deputy to the Dáil" – member of Dáil Éireann.

Totipotent stem cells: Cells that can generate all cell types and can give rise to embryos with the potential for full development and live birth.

UK: United Kingdom of Great Britain and Northern Ireland.

UN: United Nations.

UN HRC: United Nations Human Rights Committee.

USA: United States of America.

Uterus: Womb.

Zygote: A fertilised ovum, the first cell of the embryo.

Endpoints

Endnotes

———•———

1 ·Offences Against the Person Act 1861 <http://www.irishstatutebook.ie/eli/1861/act/100/enacted/en/print> accessed 4 June 2019. Sections 58–59 of the Act applied to abortion. Sections 61–63 addressed homosexuality. The law against homosexuality was amended in 1885 by the Criminal Law Amendment Act 1885, section 11 <http://www.irishstatutebook.ie/eli/1885/act/69/enacted/en/print> accessed 4 June 2019.

2 See, for example, Courtney Hutchison, "Labour of love: woman carries her daughter's baby", 15 February 2011, and Jonann Brady, "Surrogate grandma gives gift of triplets", 11 November 2008; both reported by ABC News <https://abcnews.go.com/Health/WomensHealth/surrogate-grandmother-woman-birth-grandson-61/story?id=12912270> accessed 6 June 2019.

3 For further detail and discussion see Don O'Leary, _Irish Catholicism and Science: From "Godless Colleges" to the "Celtic Tiger"_ (Cork: Cork University Press, 2012), pp. 235–9.

4 In the 2011 national census, 84.2% of the Republic of Ireland's population identified as Roman Catholic. When calculated for Irish nationals the figure was 89.7%. Central Statistics Office (CSO), _Census 2011, Profile 7: Religion, Ethnicity and Irish Travellers_ (Dublin: Stationery Office, October 2012), pp. 6, 10 <http://www.cso.ie/en/media/csoie/census/documents/census2011profile7/Profile,7,Education,Ethnicity,and,Irish,Traveller,entire,doc.pdf> accessed 20 March 2015. The number of Irish Catholics declined by 105,800 and of non-Irish Catholics by 26,500. CSO, _Census 2016 Summary Results – Part 1_, Chapter 8, p. 72 <http://www.cso.ie/en/media/csoie/releasespublications/documents/population/2017/Chapter_8_Religion.pdf> accessed 13 April 2017.

5 This explanation is based on Antony Flew (ed.), _A Dictionary of Philosophy_ (London: Pan Books, 1984), pp. 112–13.

6 The same point is applicable to non-Christian religions. For example, Muslims frequently disagree about moral norms and the interpretation of the Koran.

7 Professor Engelhardt (1941–2018) co-founded the _Journal of Medicine and Philosophy_ in 1976 with Dr Edmund Pellegrino. He served as senior editor from 1976 to 2018.

8 H. Tristram Engelhardt, Jr, "Confronting Moral Pluralism in Posttraditional Western Societies: Bioethics Critically Reassessed", _Journal of Medicine and_

Philosophy, vol. 36, issue 3 (2011), pp. 243–60 <https://academic.oup.com/ jmp/article-abstract/36/3/243/894157> accessed 11 July 2011. For the point that morality is a creation of culture, see also Jesse Prinz, "Morality is a Culturally Conditioned Response", *Philosophy Now*, issue 82 (November– December 2011). <http://www.philosophynow.org/issue82/Morality_is_a_ Culturally_Conditioned_Response> accessed 10 December 2011. Volume 43, no. 6 of the *Journal of Medicine and Philosophy* (December 2018) is devoted to a critical analysis of the "death of God" thesis expounded by Engelhardt in relation to bioethics.

9   Joel Marks, "An Amoral Manifesto (1)", *Philosophy Now*, issue 80 (August– September 2011) <http://www.philosophynow.org/issue80/An_Amoral_ Manifesto_Part_I> accessed 29 August 2011; and "Confessions of an ex-moralist", *New York Times*, 21 August 2011 <http://opinionator.blogs. nytimes.com/2011/08/21/confessions-of-an-ex-moralist/?hp> accessed 29 August 2011.

10   Pádraig Corkery, *Bioethics and the Catholic Moral Tradition* (Dublin: Veritas, 2010), pp. 31–5.

11   Pope John Paul II, *Evangelium Vitae* (London: Catholic Truth Society, 1995), paragraph 2. See also paragraphs 62, 65, 70, 72.

12   *Evangelium Vitae*, paragraphs 19–20, 70. See also Pope John Paul II, *Centesimus Annus* (1 May 1991), paragraphs 46–47, in Joseph G. Donders (ed.) *John Paul II: The Encyclicals in Everyday Language* (Maryknoll, NY: Orbis, 1996), pp. 193–4.

13   Cardinal Cahal B. Daly, Introduction, in *The Bishops and the Law on Public Morality*, July 2005 <http://www.armagharchdiocese.org/2008/05/01/july-the-bishops-and-the-law-on-public-morality/> accessed 2 November 2014.

14   Sacred Congregation for the Doctrine of the Faith, *Declaration on Procured Abortion* (*Quaestio de abortu*), 18 November 1974, paragraph 23, in Austin Flannery (ed.), *Vatican Council II: More Postconciliar Documents* (Collegeville, Minn.: Liturgical Press, 1982 (1st edn)), p. 449.

15   Daly, op. cit.

16   Words in quotation marks from Sacred Congregation for the Clergy, *General Catechetical Directory* (*Ad norman decreti*), 11 April 1971, paragraph 63, in Flannery (1982), pp. 565–6.

17   Statement of the Irish Catholic Bishops' Conference (1976), quoted in Patrick Hannon, "The Conscience of the Voter and Law-maker", *Doctrine and Life*, vol. 42 (May–June 1992), p. 245.

18   *Pastoral Constitution on the Church in the Modern World* (*Gaudium et spes*), 7 December 1965, pararaph 43, in Austin Flannery (ed.), *Vatican Council II: The Conciliar and Post Conciliar Documents* (Dublin: Dominican Publications, 1992 (revised edn)), p. 944.

19   *General Catechetical Directory*, paragraph 63, in Flannery (1982), p. 566.

20   Sacred Congregation for the Doctrine of the Faith, *Declaration on Procured*

Abortion (*Quaestio de abortu*), 18 November 1974, paragraphs 22 and 26, in Flannery (1982), pp. 449–450.

21 "Homily of Bishop Brennan, Ferns Diocese at Knock Shrine, Sunday 7 July 2013" (press release, 8 July 2013), <http://www.catholicbishops. ie/2013/07/08/homily-bishop-brennan-ferns-diocese-knock-shrine-sunday-7-july-2013/> accessed 14 December 2013.

22 *Pastoral Constitution on the Church in the Modern World*, paragraph 36, in Flannery (ed.), *Vatican Council II* (1992), p. 935.

23 Ibid., paragraph 43, in Flannery (1992), p. 944.

24 Daly, Introduction, *The Bishops and the Law on Public Morality*.

25 *Declaration on Procured Abortion*, paragraph 20, in Flannery (1982), p. 448.

26 Ricca Edmondson, "Moral Debate and Social Change", *Doctrine and Life*, vol. 42 (May–June 1992), pp. 233–234.

27 See ibid., p. 235; Simon Lee, "Abortion Law: the Tragic Choices", *Doctrine and Life*, vol. 42 (May–June 1992), p. 295; and Louis McRedmond, "Vatican II Perspectives", *Doctrine and Life*, vol. 42 (May–June 1992), p. 301.

28 Declaration on Religious Liberty (*Dignitatis Humanae*, 7 December 1965), paragraph 6, in Flannery (1992), p. 803. See also *Pastoral Constitution on the Church in the Modern World*, paragraph 26, in Flannery (1992), p. 927.

29 See Hannon, "The Conscience of the Voter and Law-maker", pp. 248–50.

30 Declaration on Religious Liberty, paragraph 7, in Flannery (1992), p. 805; and Patrick Hannon, *Church, State, Morality and Law* (Dublin: Gill and Macmillan, 1992), pp. 94–5.

31 Hannon, *Church, State, Morality and Law*, pp. 2, 7.

32 "Hierarchy enters the contraceptive controversy: State not bound by Church's moral law, say bishops", *Irish Times*, 26 November 1973, p. 1; quoted in both Sandra McAvoy, "The Catholic Church and Fertility Control in Ireland: The Making of a Dystopian Regime" in Aideen Quilty, Sinéad Kennedy and Catherine Conlon (eds), *The Abortion Papers Ireland* Vol. 2, (Cork: Attic Press, 2015), p. 53; and Chrystel Hug, *The Politics of Sexual Morality in Ireland* (London: Macmillan Press, 1999), pp. 100–1.

Glossary

33 Sources of information for nomenclature include: Commission on Assisted Human Reproduction, *Report of the Commission on Assisted Human Reproduction* (Dublin: Stationery Office, 2005); Irish Council for Bioethics, *Ethical, Scientific and Legal Issues Concerning Stem Cell Research: Opinion* (Dublin: Irish Council for Bioethics, 2008); and the *Oxford Concise Science Dictionary* (Oxford: Oxford University Press, 1996 (3rd edn)).

34   See, for example, Chris Fitzpatrick, "In the media everyone is pro-choice or
     pro-life. I am both", *Irish Times*, 16 September 2017 <https://www.irishtimes.
     com/life-and-style/health-family/in-the-media-everyone-is-pro-choice-or-
     pro-life-i-am-both-1.3222318> accessed 23 September 2017.

CHAPTER ONE

———————•———————

Papal Pronouncements

Faithful Dissent

IN THE EARLY DECADES OF THE TWENTIETH century the need for artificial means of contraception became broadly accepted by the Protestant churches.[1] A proposal to condemn contraception as immoral was rejected by Anglicans at the Lambeth Conference of 1930. At the Lambeth Conference of 1958, Anglicans accepted that artificial contraceptive methods were, in certain circumstances, morally permissible in family planning.[2] The attitude of the Roman Catholic Church was, in contrast, harsh and extremely restrictive. When Pope Pius XI issued his encyclical *Casti Connubii* on 31 December 1930 he used intemperate language to condemn artificial contraception. Terms such as "criminal abuse", "shameful and intrinsically vicious", "horrible crime" and "moral ruin" conveyed the pope's displeasure.[3] The encyclical was widely distributed and was generally seen as authoritative by Roman Catholics worldwide.[4] However, in the mid-twentieth century the institutional church's influence over the laity diminished as opinions about sexual morality changed. Scientific and technical developments in relation to human reproductive biology played a major role in this.

In 1960 the first contraceptive pill was marketed in the USA and within a few years it became one of the main pharmaceutical products sold worldwide.[5] The pill proved to be a highly effective and convenient means of birth control and it raised the standards by which other contraceptives were judged. It deeply influenced the liberalisation of attitudes towards sex.[6] Pressure grew from within the Roman Catholic Church to review its teaching. That it might approve of the contraceptive pill did not seem highly improbable at the time. In 1951 Pope Pius XII had expressed approval of the rhythm method, which was based on calculating the infertile days of the menstrual cycle. But the rhythm method was notoriously unreliable. The pope indicated that any scientific improvement in the method would be well received by the Church. Many Catholics believed that the pill was an appropriate response to their needs. They saw no moral distinction between using hormones to control the menstrual cycle and using mucous tests to ascertain its infertile phase.[7]

Pope John XXIII responded to demands for an examination of the contraceptive issue by setting up a small commission, which met for the first time in 1963. In 1965 Pope Paul VI increased the commission's membership. Members of the Pontifical Commission on Population, Family and Birth did not reach unanimous agreement on their recommendations. There was very strong support in the commission for a change in the Church's teaching on contraception. Members who argued that artificial contraception was morally permissible for married couples expressed their opinions through the medium of a majority report, which was sent to the pope in June 1966, and leaked to the press in 1967.[8] Opinions expressed in the majority report, together with the less restrictive atmosphere prevailing in the Church in the aftermath of the Second Vatican Council, generated optimism among those who wanted change. Despite this, Pope Paul rejected the advice in the majority report.

In *Humanae Vitae* (25 July 1968), he reiterated the traditional teaching of the Church, maintaining that it was not morally permissible to use artificial contraceptive methods. In paragraph 12 of the encyclical he declared that there could be no separation between the unitive (sexual) and procreative (reproductive) aspects of sexual intercourse, which in Catholic moral teaching was permitted only within marriage.[9] Catholic couples were permitted to practise birth control by taking advantage of the infertile days of the menstrual cycle. The moral distinction between natural and artificial means of birth control was retained. Catholics could "rightly use a facility provided them by nature" – as distinct from "means which directly exclude conception" and "obstruct the natural development of the generative process".[10] It did not matter that in both cases the intention was the same.

The pope asserted that the teaching of the Church was "indisputable," and that Roman Catholics were not permitted freedom of choice in this matter.[11] But *Humanae Vitae* did not settle the question. A storm of protest arose within the Church as optimism turned to bitter disappointment. Many priests disagreed with the contents of the papal document and some were compelled to leave their posts when they spoke out against it.[12] In Ireland, a case in point is Fr James Good, who served as professor of theology at University College Cork. He resigned his position after being censured by Bishop Cornelius Lucey for his outspoken criticism of the encyclical.[13] Millions of married Catholics throughout the world refused to comply with the papal directive and some even left the Church in protest. Surveys of Catholic opinion indicated, consistently, that over 80 per cent of married couples did not feel bound by the restrictions of *Humanae Vitae*.[14] The assertion that there is a moral distinction between natural and artificial means of contraception did not win consensus within the Catholic Church.

The credibility of the institutional church was severely damaged. The pope no longer seemed quite so infallible. Comparisons were made between the Church's judgement on birth control and the censorship it had imposed on Galileo over three centuries earlier.[15] Millions of Catholics who regarded themselves as loyal members of the Church chose to disobey a clear directive from the papacy.[16] The consequences of such a development were enormous. Many Catholics believed that the papacy was wrong on this aspect of sexual morality and therefore were less inclined to accept its guidance on other moral matters.[17]

The controversy about *Humanae Vitae* was particularly intense in some countries, such as the Netherlands and the US. Irish critics were not in the avant-garde of theological discourse. Still, differences of opinion about the encyclical were expressed by Irish Catholics.[18] In the late 1960s the Catholic laity was becoming more highly educated, more self-confident, and less deferential to the clergy. There was a greater exposure to foreign influences. Many Irish Catholics hoped that the Church would change its teaching on birth control. There was also a legal obstacle to overcome. Two items of legislation supported the Church's prohibitive stance: the Censorship of Publications Act 1929 prohibited the publication, distribution and sale of literature advocating birth control practices; and Section 17 of the Criminal Law (Amendment) Act 1935 prohibited the importation, manufacturing and sale of contraceptive devices. These legislative measures were becoming less sustainable as secular and liberal attitudes exerted a greater influence on Irish society. In December 1973 the Supreme Court ruled in the McGee case that the prohibition of the importation of contraceptives under the 1935 Act was unconstitutional. This required the enactment of new legislation.[19]

In May 1975 the Irish Catholic hierarchy, mindful of the tenets of *Humanae Vitae*, issued a pastoral letter, *Human Life is Sacred*, denouncing the "contraceptive mentality" that they associated with unchristian attitudes. They claimed that those who were prominent in the campaign for contraception were also in favour of abortion, and that some pills and "appliances", such as intra-uterine devices, acted "primarily" as abortifacients.[20] The "contraceptive mentality" did eventually prevail, despite the strong views of the bishops. In July 1979 the Family Planning Act provided for contraceptives to be made available to married couples in pharmacies on medical prescription. After 1979 the law became less restrictive. Legislation passed in 1985 and in 1992 liberalised the law on family planning and removed legal restrictions on the availability of contraceptive devices.[21]

In *Humanae Vitae* Pope Paul VI stated that the Church's moral teaching on marriage was based on "the natural law as illuminated and enriched by divine Revelation".[22] The Church taught that any rational person who studied a moral issue, without prejudice, was capable of discovering the natural law which offered general principles for addressing the problem at hand. The version of natural law adopted by the Roman Catholic Church was elaborated by St Thomas Aquinas in the thirteenth century. The Thomistic tradition of natural law was vulnerable to criticism under a number of headings.[23] Developments in the natural sciences and social sciences had utterly transformed perspectives on human nature. And yet the Church clung tenaciously to a discredited medieval worldview. This was to profoundly influence its response to future developments in the biological sciences.[24]

Gifts of God or Gifts of Science?

Pope Paul VI did not address the issue of assisted human reproduction (AHR) in *Humanae Vitae*. Options for treating infertility were then very limited. Assisted or artificial insemination had been used to treat infertility for many years before the publication of *Humanae Vitae*.[25] In this procedure male reproductive cells (spermatozoa) are transferred to a woman's vagina near the cervix or to the uterus by means other than sexual intercourse. Assisted insemination using a husband's semen was frequently referred to using the acronym AIH. When the husband was unable to produce sufficient spermatozoa, assisted insemination by a third-party donor (AID) was sometimes resorted to. Pope Pius XII made known his views on assisted insemination on 29 September 1949 when he addressed the fourth International Convention of Catholic Doctors at Castelgandolfo. On that occasion he ruled out artificial insemination – even within marriage and when no third-party donor was involved. Artificial methods were not to be ruled out simply because they were artificial or new; some technical methods were morally permissible if the intention was to "facilitate" or "enable the natural act".[26] Pius reaffirmed his judgement on 29 October 1951.[27] The Roman Catholic Church, frequently associated with a repressive attitude towards sex, insisted on sexual intercourse for reproduction. It was morally permissible to assist or enhance the act – but not to replace it. This theological stance was elevated to a higher authoritative level when it was reiterated in *Humanae Vitae* in 1968 (although the encyclical addressed birth control, not AHR). The papal insistence on the "inseparable connection" between sexual intercourse and reproduction expressed in paragraph 12 of the encyclical applied equally to contraception and to the AHR technologies.

Scientists took little notice of paragraph 24 of *Humanae Vitae*, which called on them to pursue research consistent with Catholic ethics. The first birth due to *in vitro* ("in glass") fertilisation (IVF) occurred ten years after the publication of the encyclical. This landmark event in AHR generated an increased awareness of the problem of infertility worldwide. IVF was the outcome of ten years of research by two British scientists, Patrick Steptoe and Robert Edwards. In this medical procedure, egg cells (ova) were removed from the body of a woman unable to conceive normally and were fertilised externally in a laboratory apparatus. In some cases, two or three of the resultant embryos were then transferred to the woman's uterus.[28] Usually only one embryo survived and adhered to the uterine wall. After 1978, thousands of couples who were experiencing infertility turned to IVF to have children.[29]

In Ireland, conformist Catholic opinions about AHR were expressed in periodicals such as *Doctrine and Life*, *The Furrow* and *Position Papers*. Catholic authors were aware that progress in science and technology had been so rapid that ethical thinking had failed to keep pace with it. An ethical vacuum emerged and Catholic moralists feared that it would become greater with every new development in science and technology. It was feared that human life and dignity would be devalued in a society that failed to rigorously apply Christian ethics to the biomedical sciences.[30] The task of devising a comprehensive system of Christian ethics to keep pace with developments in the biomedical sciences was seen as quite arduous and was not well served by the excessively disciplinary tendencies of the Vatican. There was probably some discontent with the teaching authority of the Church in this context. The Dominican priest, Fergal O'Connor, was highly critical of the harsh disciplinary measures taken by the Vatican against the eminent Swiss theologian, Hans Küng, who had dared to question papal infallibility.[31] O'Connor, widely known for his outspoken views on a wide range of social and political issues, argued that Pope John Paul II's call for basic freedoms to be granted to citizens of communist countries lacked credibility when the ecclesiastical authorities in Rome showed so little compassion and tolerance for Catholics whose views were not in accordance with what was sanctioned by the institutional church.[32]

There were some points of disagreement and uncertainty among Catholic moralists about the moral implications of reproductive medicine, and also about anticipated future developments. The technique of assisted insemination was not new and was widely applied as a solution to male infertility. A contributor to *Doctrine and Life*, Fr William Cosgrave, observed that there was considerable support from Catholic moralists for AIH as a means of avoiding childlessness. There was very little support for AID, or for egg transfer by donor – the female equivalent of AID. Donation of gametes (reproductive cells – ova and spermatozoa) by a third party was viewed as a violation of the marriage covenant and was therefore seen as morally objectionable. Similar opinions were expressed about IVF. Many Catholic moralists were in agreement with the use of IVF when spermatozoa and ova were not sourced from a third party.[33] Moral objections were also raised against surrogacy, especially where third-party donation of gametes occurred. In the 1980s, surrogacy generated controversies about the meaning of motherhood, the role of gestation, the welfare of women, and the importance of the bond between mother and child.[34]

IVF procedures frequently generated embryos that were surplus to requirements. These "spare" embryos were frozen, for later use in research (not in Ireland), or discarded. Cosgrave believed that most Christian moralists objected to the freezing of embryos on the basis that it was contrary to human dignity. There was greater opposition to discarding these embryos or destroying them in research projects. Still, some moralists argued that research on these embryos was acceptable because they could not be stored indefinitely and would eventually have to be terminated. Furthermore, some authors were sceptical about the idea that the embryo should be regarded as a person. In putting forward his observations, Cosgrave relied very much on the published works of Catholic moralists who seemed to be pushing out the boundaries of theology as far as possible to seek accommodation with the latest scientific advances.[35]

A contributor to *Doctrine and Life*, Killian Dwyer, took issue with Fr Cosgrave, pointing out that AIH had been condemned several times by the ecclesiastical authorities in Rome. Dwyer argued that Catholics who referred to the works of dissenting theologians in this matter were acting contrary to the teaching authority of the Church. A point of central importance to Dwyer was that it was immoral to separate the conception of a child from sexual intercourse.[36]

Meanwhile, in Britain, there was optimism about the potential of science and technology to overcome problems of infertility, especially following the first human IVF birth in 1978. However, this optimism was moderated by deep concerns about how to devise and implement good ethical standards. Against this backdrop, in 1982 the British government set up the Committee of Inquiry into Human Fertilisation and Embryology, chaired by Dame Mary Warnock, to consider the legal, ethical and social implications of recent and potential advances in the biomedical sciences relating to AHR. On 26 June 1984 the committee formally submitted its findings under the title *Report of the Committee of Inquiry into Human Fertilisation and Embryology*, commonly referred to as the Warnock Report.

Some of the committee's recommendations were incompatible with Catholic moral teaching. These included the provision of AID and egg donation to infertile couples, subject to active regulation and monitoring by a new statutory licensing authority.[37] Some women with healthy ovaries were unable to benefit from assisted insemination techniques because of blocked or diseased fallopian tubes, thus preventing ova from reaching the womb. In some of these cases, surgery solved the problem. In other cases, IVF offered the only hope of overcoming infertility. The committee recommended that IVF should be made available under licensing and inspection conditions similar to those for AID.[38]

The committee advocated that an embryo should be given "some protection in law" but that it should not be granted the same legal status as a child or adult.[39] The majority of the committee members approved of the recommendation that legislation should permit research to be carried out on embryos created through IVF up to the end of the fourteenth day after fertilisation.[40] This latter recommendation in particular was incompatible with Catholic moral teaching but was not yet a contentious issue in Catholic Ireland.[41] Abortion, in contrast, had already generated heated controversy.

In 1981 prohibitive legislation was already in place (sections 58 and 59 of the Offences Against the Person Act (1861)). Despite this, there was some public concern that legislative prohibition without constitutional underpinning was not strong enough. There was a movement from restrictive to liberal legislation in Britain, most western European states, and the US. Liberal trends in Ireland raised concerns that legislation alone might prove inadequate to maintaining the ban on abortion.[42] Abortion rates were increasing in the West and thousands of Irish women made their way to Britain each year for the purpose of procuring an abortion. In April 1981 the Pro-Life Amendment Campaign (PLAC) was formed to lobby for an amendment to the Constitution of Ireland (1937) that would put in place a legal prohibition against abortion. The anti-abortion campaign was successful. On 7 September 1983 the electorate voted for a constitutional ban on abortion.

It was anticipated that the Eighth Amendment to the Constitution would consolidate the illegality of abortion. Although this objective commanded broad consensus, many of those who voted against the amendment were not in favour of abortion. The wording of the amendment had been drafted under the Fianna Fáil government led by Charles Haughey. When the Fine Gael–Labour coalition came to power in 1982 it came under strong political pressure to press on with the constitutional initiative. The Taoiseach, Garret FitzGerald, despite his reservations, decided to accept the wording.[43] The new Article 40.3.3 stated: "The State acknowledges the right to life of the unborn and, with due regard to the equal right to life of the mother, guarantees in its laws to respect, and as far as practicable, by its laws to defend and vindicate that right." The outcome of the 1983 referendum was seen by some contemporary observers as a reaction against liberal trends that had become apparent in Irish society since the 1960s. Such a reaction was probably reinforced by recollections of Pope John Paul II's visit to Ireland in 1979, when he spoke out against liberal values.[44]

Concerns lingered about the possibility of legalised abortion in Ireland because, despite Article 40.3.3, Ireland, as a member state of the European Economic Community (EEC, later the European Union) was obligated to respond to rulings of the European Courts of Justice and Human Rights.[45] The Fianna Fáil–Progressive Democrats coalition government negotiated a protocol in the Maastricht Treaty (7 February 1992) to assuage public unease that abortion might be imposed against the will of the people. The protocol declared that: "Nothing in the Treaty on European Union ... shall affect the application in Ireland of Article 40.3.3° of the Constitution of Ireland."[46] This protocol was consistent with the principle of subsidiarity in an EEC context – that is, that some matters are best left to the member states themselves to resolve.

The case against abortion in Ireland, then, seemed legally secure and settled. But all was not what it seemed. Doubts about the Eighth Amendment expressed by FitzGerald and others were vindicated in 1992 when a landmark Supreme Court judgment (*Attorney General v X* – the X Case) established the right of a pregnant woman to an abortion if there was a substantial risk to her life, including the risk of suicide, and when such risk could only be averted by the termination of her pregnancy. The issue of threatened suicide as grounds for abortion was especially controversial. The anti-abortion lobby was adamant that the X Case had to be overturned. The Irish Catholic bishops expressed their dismay about the Supreme Court judgment and urged legislators to take immediate action.[47] Referendums were held in 1992 and again in 2002 to exclude the risk of suicide as a basis for lawful abortion. In both cases the proposed reforms were rejected by the electorate. Despite this, the consensus against a liberal abortion regime seemed to be relatively clear, notwithstanding the persistent legal ambiguity about the word "unborn" which was to have such profound consequences in later years.

In the 1980s the moral ramifications of IVF seemed far more complex than the issue of abortion, even when there was no third-party donor of sperm or egg. Although IVF was not an issue of contention in Ireland in the mid-1980s, there was some awareness that advances in the biomedical sciences would raise new and very complex questions for Christian ethicists. Rev. Donal Murray, Auxiliary Bishop of the Archdiocese of Dublin since 1982, observed that many concerned and conscientious Christians would find it difficult to reach agreement on such issues as genetic engineering and contraception. In his pamphlet *Christian Morality and In Vitro Fertilisation* (1985), he expressed opposition to the recommendations of the Warnock Report. Bishop Murray's opinions can be taken as representative of the Irish Catholic hierarchy. In later years, as Bishop of Limerick (1996–2009), he served as chairman of the Irish Catholic Bishops' Consultative Group for Bioethics.

Murray referred to a widespread understanding that the embryo was not regarded as a person because the word "person" was associated with consciousness, self-sufficiency and autonomy. This was contrary to Catholic theology, which saw the relationship between Christ and an individual human being starting at conception. Murray then expressed the opinion that "the child conceived by IVF is a 'product'" – an opinion that was to be expressed from time to time by other Catholic writers in future years. It is likely that Murray had some inkling of how offensive this would be to couples who turned to IVF as a last resort to overcome infertility, so he immediately stated that seeing the child as a "product" did not mean that he/she would be ill-treated or not "welcomed" by the parents. Despite this he maintained that creating "something" through the use of science and technology was "fundamentally different" from the conception of a child through sexual intercourse. While the child conceived through sexual intercourse was "a gift of God", it was difficult to see the process of creating a child through science and technology in the same light – where human control rather than God's benevolence would play a central role. With the steady progress of science, techniques would, ultimately, "work on every occasion".[48] Implicit in these observations is a concern that the benefits of science and technology would surpass God's benevolence. Murray envisaged that science would advance to the point where gender and other characteristics could be selected. Improvements in diagnostic techniques would facilitate terminations of pregnancy in the early stages of development to prevent the birth of children with physical defects.

Childless couples who placed their hopes on IVF would find little comfort in what Murray had to say on the issue of infertility. He was aware of this, but was adamant that "good consequences" could not transform something that was immoral into something that was moral. Murray did not completely rule out the use of science and technology to overcome infertility. He argued that, in cases where a woman's fallopian tubes were blocked, it was morally permissible for medical scientists to remove an ovum from the ovary of a patient and transfer it beyond the blocked area. Sexual intercourse could then take place with some possibility of fertilisation.

Murray argued that the best solution to the problem of blocked fallopian tubes was its prevention. He referred to paragraph 10 of the *Response to the Warnock Report* (1985) published by the Catholic Bishops' Joint Committee on Bioethical Issues, quoting the bishops of England and Wales to make the point that this medical condition was preventable in about 90 per cent of cases. It was thought that the three main causes of tubal occlusions were previous abortions, the use of intra-uterine devices (IUDs) for contraception, and sexually transmitted diseases.[49] The implication was that Catholic morality was far more potent than science and technology in addressing this medical problem.

Britain's Committee of Inquiry into Human Fertilisation and Embryology, chaired by Mary Warnock, had anticipated future possible developments in the biomedical sciences, for example: the creation of human–animal hybrids; the creation of artificial wombs (ectogenesis); the transfer of human embryos to the wombs of non-human species; reproductive cloning; gene therapy to prevent some genetic diseases; and the development of a biopsy technique to detect abnormalities in early-stage embryos created through IVF so that these would not be transferred to the mother's womb.[50] Although these developments were either remote possibilities or had not yet occurred, ethicists felt that they should be proactive rather than merely reactive.

After 1978, clinical units offering IVF were set up in several countries, including Australia (1980), the USA (1981), Sweden and France (1982). Demands grew for a similar service in Ireland. In May 1985 the Institute of Obstetricians and Gynaecologists of the Royal College of Physicians of Ireland (representing the vast majority of consultants in that specialist field of medicine) voted to accept guidelines for IVF.[51] These guidelines were adopted "verbatim" by the Medical Council of Ireland and were later published in *A Guide to Ethical Conduct and Behaviour and Fitness to Practice* (1989). Professor Robert Harrison of St James's Hospital (Dublin) carried out IVF procedures on three women at Sir Patrick Dun's Hospital (Dublin) in May/June 1985, none of which resulted in a live birth. Information leaked to the press and, due to the controversy that arose, a moratorium was called on further IVF procedures so that the issue could be discussed further. Harrison did not explicitly point to the Catholic Church as the source of the controversy in this instance, but he did at least imply that the "great influence" of the Church was an impediment to reproductive medicine in Ireland.

The main source of opposition to Harrison's pioneering work in Ireland almost certainly came from the Catholic hierarchy. A meeting of "interested parties" was held at St Patrick's College, Maynooth, from 30 August to 1 September 1985.[52] The conference title was *New Developments in Human Reproduction – Vision and Choices*. An exchange of views took place between scientists, doctors, nurses, philosophers, theologians, clergy and lawyers. Leading Irish gynaecologists advocated setting up a government-funded national IVF clinic in Dublin. This was in response to the increasing incidence of infertility and the sharp decrease in the number of children being offered for adoption in Ireland. A range of techniques was considered. The greatest interest was in IVF.

This elicited a theologically conservative response. With *Humanae Vitae's* strictures on artificial contraception evidently in mind, it was asserted that the unitive and procreative aspects of sexual intercourse could not be separated in favour of the unitive. To be morally consistent, it was then argued, the same separation could not be permitted for procreative purposes either.[53]

The second main argument against IVF was that it was "intrinsically expressive of a relationship of dominance rather than of companionship … the relationship is intrinsically expressive of a relationship of production and the equality of the child to its parents as a gift of God is not expressed." There was some difficulty in seeing a child created through IVF as a "gift of God". One of the conference speakers, Dr John Finnis, referred to Pope John Paul II's apostolic exhortation, *Reconciliatio et Paenitentia* (1984) to make the point that "a dissenting moral theology" that had been accepted by many priests was rejected by the ecclesiastical authorities in Rome. However, the author of the report on the conference proceedings, Vivian Boland (OP), was not convinced that IVF could be decisively rejected on grounds of Catholic theology. There was a counterargument to be acknowledged. Catholic moral theology supported the position that it was morally permissible for a couple to avail of medical intervention to make sexual intercourse possible. On this basis, it was argued that IVF could be viewed as "simply a more sophisticated technical help for the full accomplishment" of the conjugal act.[54]

Theological opinion was weighted heavily against IVF. There was also a constitutional dimension to consider – or so it seemed. It was observed that some biomedical procedures might be incompatible with Article 41 of the Constitution of Ireland, which upheld the family unit as "the necessary basis of social order and as indispensable to the welfare of the Nation and the State". There was some speculation that AID and surrogacy might be regarded as unconstitutional because of the participation of third parties in procreative initiatives.

The conference was attended by Mary Warnock, whose opinions, in view of the recommendations of the Warnock Report, could not have been expected to harmonise with Catholic moral teaching. Warnock did not take issue with the contention that a fertilised human ovum was "human life". But she did disagree with the view that a pre-fourteen-day-old embryo was a child. She also rejected the Church's code of morality based on "natural law" and did not see any useful role for arguments based on religious ideas that were "not open to debate".[55]

The Warnock Report was of course concerned with putting forward recommendations for legislative measures only in the UK relating to IVF and other biomedical procedures. Nevertheless, there was some disquiet at the conference that its recommendation about research on human embryos might be implemented, possibly because of the fear that the Irish electorate, influenced by ideas inconsistent with Catholic moral principles, might exert pressure on members of the Oireachtas to enact similar legislation.

Harrison described the proceedings of the conference as "very contentious and polarized". Despite opposition from the Catholic Church, he was granted permission to resume the practice of IVF by the Department of Health, the Medical Council and the board of management of St James's Hospital.[56] Harrison, the leading figure in bringing fertility services to Ireland, founded the Human Assisted Reproduction Unit (HARI) at the Rotunda Hospital in 1989. As director of this unit he oversaw the birth of about 4,000 babies using AHR technologies – which sometimes gave rise to public controversy.[57] Harrison and his colleagues were criticised for "playing God and making babies". He in turn was critical of a religious ethos that accepted infertility simply as "God's will" without considering medical intervention. Irish couples were travelling to Britain for fertility treatment, and Harrison was adamant that this was avoidable.[58]

Several months after the conference at Maynooth, the Irish Catholic bishops issued their findings against IVF. In March 1986 they observed that many people did not understand why the hierarchy expressed opposition to IVF when the Church held parenthood in high esteem. The reason for such opposition, they maintained, was serious moral impediments. There was a low success rate associated with IVF. Reference was made to medical practices abroad, but the main concern was with Britain. The Irish Catholic bishops claimed that multiple ovulations were induced to counteract the poor results of the IVF process, leading ultimately to large numbers of "spare embryos". Some of these embryos were used for research. The bishops claimed that a high proportion of IVF embryos were malformed, screened out and discarded. They were adamant that these practices were in violation of what was best in medical ethics, which was respect for human life. They invoked the principle that no human being should be treated merely as a means to an end. Reference was made to the recommendation in paragraph 11.30 of the Warnock Report, which provided for research on supernumerary embryos created through IVF.[59] The bishops also reiterated their opposition to the marginalisation of sexual intercourse and their objection to what they saw as the immoral intrusive role of science and technology in generating human life. They believed that IVF dehumanised procreation. The best response to the growing problem of infertility was to address its main preventable causes, which were the use of IUDs, abortion, and sexually transmitted diseases.[60]

Many medical problems were associated with IVF. Marital relationships frequently suffered severe stress. Women had to endure the adverse side effects of drugs that led to visual problems, dizziness, migraine and weight gain. Hyperstimulation of the ovaries sometimes led to ovarian cysts and other problems requiring hospitalisation. In a few cases women died due to ovarian stimulation. Other risks included ectopic pregnancies, spontaneous abortion, multiple births and low birth weight. The Catholic bishops could have reasonably argued against IVF on the basis of women's welfare. They failed to do so. Their main concerns were emphasising the importance of sexual intercourse within marriage as the only morally acceptable means of procreation, and defending the rights of the unborn.[61] The omission of support for the welfare of women in *In Vitro Fertilisation: Statement of Bishops' Commission for Doctrine of the Irish Episcopal Conference* (1986) did not serve the best interests of the Catholic Church in Ireland.

Directives from Rome and Maynooth

Catholic moral principles seemed to dictate decisively against *in vitro* fertilisation and some of its associated biomedical procedures. Despite this, there was still considerable uncertainty about the moral status of IVF – not only in Catholic Ireland but also in Catholicism internationally. The Congregation for the Doctrine of the Faith received enquiries from episcopal conferences, individual bishops, theologians, scientists and medical doctors about the ethical implications of biomedical procedures, especially relating to early-stage human embryos. On 22 February 1987 the Congregation, under the prefecture of Cardinal Joseph Ratzinger (the future Pope Benedict XVI), responded with its *Instruction on Respect for Human Life in Its Origin and on the Dignity of Procreation (Donum Vitae)*.[62] The Congregation reiterated a number of moral principles which proved to be very restrictive for those loyal Catholics who would otherwise have turned to the new biomedical technologies to overcome childlessness.

Human life was to be respected and protected from conception onwards. A fertilised egg – a zygote – was to be treated as if it was a person with full human rights.[63] It was deemed immoral to discard embryos or to destroy them in the course of research. To do so was comparable, in a moral sense, to the practice of induced abortion. The Congregation saw a connection between IVF and the destruction of embryos. The freezing of embryos was unacceptable because it was deemed offensive to human dignity and exposed embryos to dangers of manipulation. The creation of embryos by asexual means (i.e. without sex) through splitting in the very early stages of development ("twin fission") or cloning was also found to be immoral. Every child had the right to be conceived, carried in the womb, and born within marriage. In every marriage the wife and husband could only become parents through each other. Conception was to be brought about "through the specific and exclusive acts of husband and wife". Procreation exclusively in marriage was essential for the wellbeing of civil society.[64]

The Congregation referred to paragraph 12 of *Humanae Vitae* to reiterate the theological principle that there is an "inseparable connection" between the unitive and procreative aspects of sexual intercourse.[65] The creation of human life through artificial means was seen as accepting the "domination of technology over the origin and destiny of the human person". A child conceived as a result of biomedical intervention could be regarded as "an object of scientific technology", which was morally objectionable because it was offensive to human dignity. The Congregation objected to what it saw as the excessive power of biologists and medical doctors.[66] It called on legislatures to control the application of biomedical techniques to safeguard the welfare of society.[67] In the Republic of Ireland, successive governments were unmoved by the Congregation's exhortation to legislate. There was an extreme reluctance to address a range of very complex ethical issues which were fraught with political risks.

Fr Patrick Hannon, professor of moral theology at St Patrick's College, Maynooth, observed that there were various responses to the Congregation's *Instruction* both inside and outside the Roman Catholic Church. Those who disagreed with the inseparability of the unitive and procreative aspects of sexual intercourse in *Humanae Vitae* took issue with its reiteration in the *Instruction*. Furthermore, Hannon observed, the *Instruction* was ranked in importance "somewhat below an encyclical". The moral judgements of the *Instruction* were not declared infallible. If IVF and egg transfer were to be regarded as immoral, there was still a need to demonstrate such a finding.[68] However, the persuasive powers of the Church had greatly diminished in the late twentieth century. The majority of Catholics persisted in their refusal to accept the teaching of the institutional church on artificial contraception. Many priests, theologians, and even some bishops were not convinced by the Vatican's stance. Yet there was a general tendency not to express open disagreement because of fear of punitive action by the ecclesiastical authorities, and loyalty to Rome.[69]

Those in the upper echelons of the hierarchy were aware of the alienation of many Catholics from the institutional church arising from the strictures of *Humanae Vitae.* The Catholic Archbishop of Dublin, Dr Desmond Connell, was very mindful of this when he spoke at St Patrick's College, Maynooth on 2 March 1999. His speech received extensive coverage in the *Irish Times.* The archbishop believed that dissent on the issue of contraception was a root cause of "à la carte Catholicism".

Connell told his audience that reproductive technologies had given rise to unhappy and resentful children. The meaning of the term "unwanted child" was clear enough, but its converse – the "wanted child" – was not sufficiently understood. What could possibly be wrong with wanting a child? Surely such an attitude was eminently consistent with social responsibility and more likely to promote harmonious family relationships? Not from the archbishop's point of view! The wanted child was the child that was planned, "produced by the decision of the parents", which began to "look more and more like a technological product". This was clearly so in cases of IVF and surrogacy. Children were "no longer welcomed as a gift but produced as it were to order".[70] This altered the relationship between parents and children. Parental attitudes were tainted by a sense of "consumer ownership" and the child conceived with the aid of technology did not belong to the family "in a personal sense". The attitudes of these parents were conveyed "unconsciously" to the child, who came to resent "a parentage based on power". Connell declared that no child could find contentment in life "as a product". He maintained that such a child would not find "meaning in a life produced by technology".[71] The archbishop did not refer to any evidence from the social sciences to substantiate his provocative assertions. His theological worldview was deeply offensive to couples who had struggled to overcome nature's obstacles in seeking a child-centred life. It also failed to consider that technology for AHR could be seen as God-given.[72]

The practice of contraception, it seemed, had dragged Irish society down to levels of decadence sometimes associated with ancient Rome. Archbishop Connell maintained that by breaking the bond between sexual intercourse and procreation, contraception had set in train "the sexual revolution", which in turn had led to broken families, promiscuity, divorce, and a greater tolerance of abortion. Contraception had "dishonoured" women, and, by obstructing conception, was even seen as "disrespectful towards God as the author of life". It did not seem to matter that, in many instances, unplanned pregnancies generated poverty and hardship, imposed undue strain on marital relationships, and frequently proved detrimental to the health of mothers. Connell concluded his speech by reminding priests of their duty to uphold the teaching of the Church on issues of sexual morality. They would not be martyred for such evangelical initiatives. Instead, they would have to endure "ridicule, dissent, and betrayal".[73] Connell's provocative opinions elicited critical responses, especially from women who were no longer willing to comply with ecclesiastical pronouncements on matters of family planning and sexual morality.[74]

Endnotes

———————•———————

1   Leslie C. Griffin, "The Catholic Bishops vs. the Contraceptive Mandate", *Religions*, vol. 6 (2015), p. 1412.

2   Owen Chadwick, "Great Britain and Europe" in John McManners (ed.), *The Oxford Illustrated History of Christianity* (Oxford: Oxford University Press, 1992), pp. 378–9.

3   Pope Pius XI, *Casti Connubii* (31 December 1930), commentary by Fr Vincent McNabb (London: Sheed & Ward, 1933), pp. 25–6.

4   Sharon M. Leon, *An Image of God: The Catholic Struggle with Eugenics* (Chicago: University of Chicago Press, 2013), p. 94.

5   Lara V. Marks, *Sexual Chemistry: A History of the Contraceptive Pill* (New Haven: Yale University Press, 2001), pp. 1–3.

6   At this time the rapid growth of human populations throughout the world, and the intensification of the Cold War, were seen as grave threats to the future of humankind. John Rock, an American Catholic obstetrician–gynaecologist who carried out some of the early clinical trials on the first contraceptive pill, declared that the greatest threat to world peace and good living standards was "not atomic energy but sexual energy". He saw the contraceptive pill as, potentially, a powerful instrument against war and starvation. Ibid., p. 13.

7   Marks, op. cit., p. 218.

8   George Weigel, *Witness to Hope: The Biography of John Paul II* (New York: Cliff Street Books, 2001), pp. 206–7.

9   Pope Paul VI, *Humanae Vitae* (25 July 1968), paragraph 12, in Austin Flannery (ed.), *Vatican Council II: More Postconciliar Documents* (Collegeville, Minn.: Liturgical Press, 1982 (1st edn)).

10 Ibid., paragraph 16.

11 Ibid., paragraph 4.

12 Eamon Duffy, *Saints and Sinners: A History of the Popes* (New Haven: Yale University Press, and S4C, 1997), p. 281.

13 John A. Murphy, *The College: A History of Queen's/University College Cork* (Cork: Cork University Press, 1995), p. 281; and Louise Fuller, *Irish Catholicism Since 1950: The Undoing of a Culture* (Dublin: Gill and Macmillan, 2002), p. 199.

14 Richard P. McBrien, *Lives of the Popes: The Pontiffs from St Peter to John Paul II* (New York: HarperCollins, 2000), p. 380.

15 Marks, *Sexual Chemistry*, pp. 217, 219, 229.

16 Edward Stourton, *Absolute Truth: The Catholic Church in the World Today* (London: Viking, 1998), pp. 56–9.

17 Robert Blair Kaiser, *The Encyclical that Never Was: The Story of the Commission on Population, Family and Birth, 1964–1966* (London: Sheed & Ward, 1987), p. 272. See also Seán Fagan, *Does Morality Change?* (Dublin: Columba Press, 2003), p. 12.

18 Fuller, *Irish Catholicism Since 1950*, pp. 195–212; and Dermot Keogh, *Twentieth-Century Ireland: Nation and State* (Dublin: Gill and Macmillan, 1994), pp. 266–7.

19 Fuller, *Irish Catholicism*, p. 209; and Keogh, *Twentieth-Century Ireland*, p. 326.

20 The Archbishops and Bishops of Ireland, *Human Life is Sacred: Pastoral Letter of the Archbishops and Bishops of Ireland to the clergy, religious and faithful* (May 1975), paragraph 112. It seems that the Holy See anticipated as early as 1974 that rapid advances in the biomedical sciences would lead to the production of abortion-inducing pharmaceuticals that could be self-administered, and that these would become widely available. Pills that prevented the implantation of fertilised ova were regarded as abortifacients. See *Catholic Press and Information Office, The Catholic Church and Abortion* (Dublin: Veritas, 1994), p. 14.

21 Fuller, *Irish Catholicism*, pp. 243, 246.

22 Pope Paul VI, *Humanae Vitae*, paragraph 4; see also paragraph 11.

23 For a critique of natural law theory see Desmond M. Clarke, *Church and State: Essays in Political Philosophy* (Cork: Cork University Press, 1985), pp. 47–68. For an understanding of natural law different from that of the institutional Church, especially concerning the issue of artificial contraception, see Seán Fagan, "Do We Still Need Natural Law?", *Doctrine and Life*, vol. 47, no. 7 (September 1997), pp. 407–16.

24 The Irish Catholic bishops exercised poor judgement in relating science to theology when they stated in their pastoral letter *Human Life is Sacred* (paragraph 19) that "modern genetic science makes it more difficult to deny that the human soul is present from the moment of conception." But genetics had nothing to say about the immortal soul – belief in the immortal soul is outside the subject-matter of science.

25 Teresa Iglesias, *IVF and Justice: Moral, Social and Legal Issues Related to Human In Vitro Fertilisation* (London: Linacre Centre, 1990), p. 143.

26 Pope Pius XII, "The Holy Father Condemns Artificial Insemination", translation of an address to the fourth International Convention of Catholic Doctors, 29 September 1949, *Linacre Quarterly*, vol. 16, no. 4 (October 1949), pp. 1–6.

27 Gerald Kelly, "The Teaching of Pope Pius XII on Artificial Insemination", *Linacre Quarterly*, vol. 23, no. 1 (February 1956), pp. 6–7, 17 <https://epublications.marquette.edu/cgi/viewcontent.cgi?referer=https://www.google.

ie/&+httpsredir=1&article=3780&context=lnq> accessed 2 April 2018.

28 In Ireland, the ethical guidelines of the Medical Council in the 1990s required that all embryos created through IVF had to be transferred to the woman's reproductive system. The maximum number transferable to the uterus was three. Any others were transferred to the cervix, where they were extremely unlikely to implant. This ruled out the freezing of embryos, research on embryos, and the "official" discarding of surplus embryos. Deirdre Madden, "The Status of Human Embryos in Irish Medical Practice", in Elisabeth Hildt and Dietmar Mieth (eds), *In Vitro Fertilisation in the 1990s: Towards a Medical, Social and Ethical Evaluation* (Aldershot, UK: Ashgate, 1998), p. 223.

29 See Jill Allison, *Motherhood and Infertility in Ireland: Understanding the Presence of Absence* (Cork: Cork University Press, 2013), p. 149 and note 1, p. 247. By 2005 about 8,000 couples were attending Irish fertility clinics each year, many for IVF treatments. About 1,000 babies were born due to assisted human reproduction techniques (not all from IVF). See also "Assisting new life", *Irish Times*, 8 June 1998 <https://www.irishtimes.com/news/health/assisting-new-life-1.160919> accessed 27 March 2018.

30 A.R. Dennis, "Ethical Dilemmas and the Modern Doctor", *Doctrine and Life*, vol. 30, no. 1 (January 1980), pp. 6–15.

31 Hans Küng's status as a Catholic theologian was revoked by Pope John Paul II in 1979.

32 Fergal O'Connor, "The Church, Society and Abortion: A Comment", *Doctrine and Life*, vol. 30, no. 3 (March 1980), pp. 157–8.

33 William Cosgrave, "Recent Moral Thinking on Human Genetic Engineering", *Doctrine and Life*, vol. 34, no. 8 (October 1984), pp. 442–4.

34 For a detailed discussion on surrogacy, see Deirdre Madden, *Medicine, Ethics and the Law* (Haywards Heath, UK: Bloomsbury Professional, 2016 (3rd edn)), pp. 273–328.

35 Reference was made to John Mahoney's *Seeking the Spirit: Essays in Moral and Pastoral Theology* (1981), Richard McCormick's *Notes on Moral Theology 1965 through 1980* (1981), and Bernhard Häring's *Ethics of Manipulation: Issues in Medicine, Behaviour Control and Genetics* (1975). Cosgrave, "Recent Moral Thinking on Human Genetic Engineering", pp. 443–8. Bernhard Häring, a German Redemptorist, served as a theological adviser to Pope Paul VI. Interviewed by the author Robert Blair Kaiser in January 1964, he saw no reason – in a moral sense – why women could not avail of the contraceptive pill. Kaiser, *The Encyclical that Never Was*, pp. 43–4. Richard A. McCormick played a very important role in the development of Catholic moral theology after the Second Vatican Council. His opinions about biomedical ethics differed considerably from those of the teaching authority of the Church. See James F. *Childress*, "Reproductive Interventions: Theology, Ethics, and Public Policy", in Charles E. Curran (ed.), *Moral Theology: Challenges for the Future, Essays in Honour of Richard A. McCormick*

(New York: Paulist Press, 1990), pp. 285–309.

36   Killian Dwyer, "Artificial Human Reproduction", *Doctrine and Life*, vol. 34, no. 10 (December 1984), pp. 587–90.

37   Department of Health and Social Security (United Kingdom of Great Britain and Northern Ireland), *Report of the Committee of Inquiry into Human Fertilisation and Embryology* (London: HMSO, 1984), paragraphs 4.16, 6.6 and 13.3.

38   Ibid., paragraph 5.10.

39   Ibid., paragraph 11.17.

40   Ibid., paragraph 11.30.

41   Terminating early-stage embryos, either for scientific research purposes or through disposal, was, in the context of abortion, viewed as "a grave sin". See *Sacred Congregation for the Doctrine of the Faith, Declaration on Procured Abortion (Quaestio de abortu)*, 18 November 1974); in Flannery, *Vatican Council II: More Post Conciliar Documents*, pp. 445–6 and note 19, p. 452.

42   Cornelius O'Leary and Tom Hesketh, "The Irish Abortion and Divorce Referendum Campaigns", *Irish Political Studies*, vol. 3 (1988), pp. 43–62.

43   Louise Fuller, *Irish Catholicism since 1950: The Undoing of a Culture* (Dublin: Gill and Macmillan, 2002), p. 240; O'Leary and Hesketh, "The Irish Abortion and Divorce Referendum Campaigns", pp. 51–3; and J.P. O'Carroll, "Bishops, Knights – and Pawns? Traditional Thought and the Irish Abortion Referendum Debate of 1983", *Irish Political Studies*, vol. 6 (1991), p. 55.

44   Fuller, *Irish Catholicism*, p. 240.

45   See Lisa Smyth, "Ireland's Abortion Ban: Honour, shame and the possibility of a moral revolution", in Aideen Quilty, Sinéad Kennedy, and Catherine Conlon (eds), *The Abortion Papers* Vol. 2 (Cork: Cork University Press, 2015), p. 169.

46   "Protocol annexed to the Treaty on European Union and to the treaties establishing the European Communities", *Treaty on European Union* (Maastricht, 7 February 1992) <http://europa.eu/eu-law/decision-making/treaties/pdf/treaty_on_european_union/treaty_on_european_union_en.pdf> accessed 17 March 2016.

47   Irish Catholic Bishops' Conference, "The Sacredness of Human Life", issued after meetings on 9–11 March 1992; *Doctrine and Life*, vol. 42 (May–June 1992), pp. 345–6.

48   Donal Murray, *Christian Morality and In Vitro Fertilisation: A Question of Morality* (Dublin: Veritas Publications, 1985), pp. 21–2. The text of this pamphlet was used for a paper delivered at the Glenstal Ecumenical Conference, 26 June 1985.

49   Ibid., p. 23.

50   *Report of the Committee of Inquiry into Human Fertilisation and Embryology*, Chapter 12, "Possible Future Developments in Research".

51   These guidelines were drafted by Professor W.T. Thompson from Belfast,

who was at the time serving on the UK's IVF Voluntary Licensing Authority – later to become the Human Fertilisation and Embryology Authority. A sub-committee of the Institute of Obstetricians and Gynaecologists was set up to monitor and give advice on developments in reproductive medicine. It comprised clinicians, paramedicals, ethicists and legal experts. Robert F. Harrison, "The Development of IVF Practice in Ireland – A personal view", *Human Fertility*, vol. 15, no. 1, pp. 4–5.

52　Words in quotation marks from Harrison, p. 5.

53　Vivian Boland, "New Developments in Human Reproduction", *Doctrine and Life*, vol. 35, no. 8 (October 1985), pp. 465–6.

54　Ibid., pp. 466–7.

55　Ibid., pp. 467–8.

56　Harrison, "The development of IVF practice in Ireland", p. 5.

57　"Pioneer of IVF dies", *Irish Medical Times*, vol. 51, no. 5 (10 February 2017), p. 8, <https://search-proquest-com.ucc.idm.oclc.org/docview/1868279005/fulltext/1D2ACF73AB1943D2PQ/20?accountid=14504> accessed 8 April 2018.

58　Gemma O' Doherty, "30 years of miracle babies", Independent.ie, 26 July 2008 <https://www.independent.ie/lifestyle/30-years-of-miracle-babies-26464754.html> accessed 10 April 2018. It is very likely that the Catholic Church impeded the expansion of fertility services in Ireland. Journalist Anne Dempsey reported that an attempt to set up a "sperm bank" in Galway in the late 1980s was vetoed: "Banking on fatherhood", *Irish Times*, 8 July 1996 <https://search-proquest-com.ucc.idm.oclc.org/docview/310085653/8C8F1CECDE2A421DPQ/51?accountid=14504> accessed 28 March 2018.

59　The Irish bishops also referred to paragraph 11.22 of the Warnock Report, which stated that "no embryo which has been used for research should be transferred to a woman".

60　*In Vitro Fertilisation: Statement of Bishops' Commission for Doctrine of the Irish Episcopal Conference*, published in *The Furrow*, vol. 37, no. 3 (March 1986), pp. 197–200. For a summary of this document see "'In Vitro' Fertilisation: Irish Bishops' Commission on Doctrine", *Doctrine and Life*, vol. 36, no. 5 (May–June 1986), pp. 263–4.

61　Susan Ryan-Sheridan, *Women and the New Reproductive Technologies in Ireland* (Cork: Cork University Press, 1994), pp. 13–20, 38–40.

62　For a more extensive examination of the *Instruction on Respect for Human Life in Its Origin and on the Dignity of Procreation* see Don O'Leary, *Roman Catholicism and Modern Science: A History* (New York: Continuum, 2006), pp. 224–8. See also "Respect for Human Embryos and Artificial Human Procreation: Summary of the Recent Vatican Document", *Doctrine and Life*, vol. 37, no. 4 (April 1987), pp. 205–12. Reference is made to the *Instruction/Donum Vitae* in *Catechism of the Catholic Church* (Dublin:

Veritas, 1995), paragraphs 2375–8.

63 Congregation for the Doctrine of the Faith, *Instruction on Respect for Human Life in Its Origin and on the Dignity of Procreation* (*Donum Vitae*), 22 February 1987 (Dublin: Veritas, 1987), p. 4.

64 Ibid., pp. 6–7.

65 Ibid., pp. 8–9.

66 Ibid., pp. 9–10.

67 Ibid., pp. 11–12.

68 Patrick Hannon, "*In Vitro* Fertilisation", *The Furrow*, vol. 38, no. 12 (December 1987), pp. 744–5.

69 Seán Fagan, "*Humanae Vitae* 30 Years On", *Doctrine and Life*, vol. 49, no. 1 (January 1999), pp. 51–4.

70 Cardinal Connell's idea of children being seen as products or commodities in the context of assisted human reproduction was probably not unusual in the higher echelons of the Church. See Magdalena Radkowska-Walkowicz, "How the Political Becomes Private: In vitro fertilization and the Catholic Church in Poland", *Journal of Religion and Health*, vol. 57 (2018), pp. 979–93.

71 Carol Coulter, "Catholic archbishop outlines changes in relationships from family planning: 'Contraceptive culture' has led to unhappy, resentful children", *Irish Times*, 3 March 1999, p. 6. The full text of Archbishop Connell's speech, "Child resents a parentage based on power", was published on the *Irish Times* website, 8 March 1999 <http://www.irishtimes.com/news/child-resents-a-parentage-based-on-power-1.160394> accessed 9 April 2016.

72 For opinions about technology being God-given, see Allison, *Motherhood and Infertility in Ireland*, p. 177. For criticism of the idea of a child conceived through IVF as an object of technology, see also Pádraig Corkery, *Bioethics and the Catholic Moral Tradition* (Dublin: Veritas, 2010), p. 54; and Deirdre Madden, "Is there a Right to a Child of One's Own?", *Medico-Legal Journal of Ireland*, vol. 5 (1), 1999, pp. 8–13.

73 Coulter, "Catholic archbishop outlines changes in relationships".

74 Orla McDonnell and Jill Allison, "From Biopolitics to Bioethics: Church, state, medicine and assisted reproductive technology in Ireland", *Sociology of Health & Illness*, vol. 28, no. 6 (2006), pp. 822–4.

CHAPTER TWO

———•———

Stem Cell Research and Assisted Human

Reproduction

2000–2005

To Assist or Not to Assist?

THE BIRTH OF THE FIRST CLONED MAMMAL, Dolly the sheep, in July 1996, generated much controversy about the ethics of scientific research. In a process known as somatic cell nuclear transfer (SCNT), the nucleus was removed from an ovum and replaced with the nucleus from a somatic cell (i.e. not an ovum or spermatozoon) of the animal selected for cloning. The process rarely worked, but when it did, the ovum, with its implanted nucleus, reacted as if it was fertilised, giving rise to an embryo. This embryo, if not defective and if transferred to a suitable uterine environment, would grow into an organism almost completely genetically identical to the implanted nucleus.[1] The outcome of the SCNT procedure at the Roslin Institute near Edinburgh indicated that, with further scientific research, humans could be cloned. There was of course widespread opposition internationally to such an idea. The Vatican, through its Pontifical Academy for Life, expressed condemnation of reproductive cloning in its document *Reflections on Cloning* (1997) on the basis that it was offensive to human dignity, was incompatible with the principle of equality, and would be detrimental to the wellbeing of human clones.[2]

Cloning techniques applied to mammalian cells were not generally used to reproduce the organism. Generally, the purpose was to create embryos as sources of stem cells for scientific research. These five- or six-day-old embryos were destroyed in the course of extracting stem cells from them. Human embryonic stem cell lines were derived from unused blastocysts (early-stage embryos) which had been created for couples availing of IVF therapy.

Not all human stem cells are embryonic. Stem cells can be derived from other sources, such as the umbilical cords of newborn babies, and from a number of adult tissues such as bone marrow. Yet human embryonic stem cells (hESCs) were far more suited to research needs because they had greater potential in producing different types of cells. There were formidable technical problems in identifying, extracting and culturing human adult stem cells (hASCs). But hASCs were not without their particular advantages. First, there were no moral objections to their use because embryos were not destroyed to obtain them. Second, hASCs were less likely to give rise to tumours than were hESCs.[3]

It was hoped that, ultimately, it would be possible to use stem cells for clinical purposes, to generate a broad range of specialised cells, tissues and organs. The advantage of generating stem cells by SCNT was that it enabled the use of a patient's own genetic material. Therefore, these stem cells would not be recognised as foreign matter by the immune system, thus avoiding the complications of lifelong immunosuppressant therapy. But creating human hESCs through SCNT was extremely difficult. Therefore, in countries that permitted research using human hESCs, such as the USA, South Korea and Britain, scientists relied on supernumerary embryos from IVF procedures to source these cells.

In Ireland the Oireachtas had failed to pass legislation addressing the extremely complex ethical, legal and social implications of new biomedical techniques. Senator Mary Henry's Regulation of Assisted Human Reproduction Bill (1999) was defeated in the Seanad.[4] Ireland did not compare favourably with other European states in matters concerned with the regulation of assisted human reproduction (AHR), and there was a growing awareness of this. IVF, the freezing (cryopreservation) and storage of gametes and embryos, and the use of donor gametes, featured in services available to Irish couples with impaired fertility, enabling many of them to have children. The birth of the first Irish baby arising from IVF treatment occurred in 1987.[5] Medical procedures were regulated by Medical Council Guidelines and applied only to registered medical practitioners. Very few research scientists were answerable to the Medical Council.[6]

The Fianna Fáil–Progressive Democrat coalition government decided to seek expert advice before taking any legislative initiatives. The abortion referendum of 1983 and its consequences indicated that addressing issues relating to AHR would be politically risky and carry little prospect of any political dividends. In March 2000 Micheál Martin, Minister for Health and Children, established the Commission on Assisted Human Reproduction (CAHR) with the following terms of reference: "to prepare a report on the possible approaches to the regulation of all aspects of assisted human reproduction and the social, ethical and legal factors to be taken into account in determining public policy in the area". It was intended that the report would also serve "as the basis for informed public debate before the finalisation of any policy proposals".[7]

In addition to legislation, the commission was also to consider the role of professional regulation on the basis of medical ethics. The twenty-one-member commission included physical and social scientists, medical consultants, paramedical professionals, administrators and legal experts.[8] In the context of deciding the scope of its research the commission understood the term "assisted human reproduction" to mean procedures that required the manipulation and use of gametes and embryos.[9] The commission was obligated to consult widely and this included talking to philosophers and theologians.[10] However, there seems to have been relatively little theological input into the commission's working group sessions.[11] The commission did not include any Catholic moral theologian. Even so, members' attention was drawn to Catholic moral teaching.

The Irish Catholic hierarchy made its views known through its Bishops' Committee for Bioethics, which submitted a detailed document to the CAHR under the title *Assisted Human Reproduction: Facts and Ethical Issues* (2000). It also issued submissions through the Irish Episcopal Conference.[12] The bishops were concerned that the government should act to protect the right to life of the unborn, and to safeguard the status of the family based on marriage. The Irish Episcopal Conference observed that there was a distinction to be made between reproductive and "therapeutic" cloning. The conference recommended that reproductive cloning should be prohibited by law because of concerns about risks and safety; because human procreation would be reduced to "the level of a manufacturing process", which would be detrimental to human dignity; and because it would fundamentally change the very meaning of parenthood.[13] In relation to health and safety, there was strong scientific evidence to indicate that there would be an extremely high frequency of spontaneous abortions, severe to fatal postnatal health problems, and increased risks to mothers.[14] This observation offered an overwhelming argument against reproductive cloning.

Therapeutic cloning was a process of generating embryos for the purpose of creating hESCs. It was radically different from reproductive cloning in its objectives and it offered the prospect of very important research data. Scientists anticipated that this type of cloning would eventually lead to the effective treatment of a broad range of diseases such as Alzheimer's and Parkinson's. But the bishops pointed out that there was nothing therapeutic about "therapeutic cloning" because the embryo was sacrificed in the process.[15] The possibility of improving or preserving the health of patients could not be used as justification because it was immoral to treat a human embryo as a means to an end. The bishops then argued for the use of hASCs as a morally acceptable alternative to hESCs. Bone marrow is an important source of hASCs. These cells had for years been used quite successfully in the treatment of leukaemia. Human ESCs, in contrast, had no successful clinical benefit associated with them and scientific research indicated strongly that hESCs were far more likely than hASCs to give rise to tumours. There was also the additional disadvantage that extracting hESCs from embryos was more difficult than sourcing hASCs from bone marrow samples.[16]

The Irish Episcopal Conference recommended that the creation of embryos specifically for research purposes should be banned because it was unethical. It also recommended that cloning human embryos for "therapeutic" purposes should be legally prohibited. It then addressed the ethical aspect of donating human gametes and embryos. Every child had a right to know its origins and to know the identity of its parents. This right was to take precedence over any assurances of confidentiality given to the donors. Every child had a right to be born into a family. The separation of biological parenthood from social parenthood created problems of identity for the child and should be avoided when it was possible to do so. The Irish Episcopal Conference saw no ethical difficulties in storing gametes for research purposes provided that the donors had given consent. It saw no insuperable ethical difficulty with the storage of gametes for procreative purposes in some medical circumstances, where consent was given – for example in cases of patients about to undergo radiotherapy or chemotherapy.

The storage of embryos was more complex in an ethical sense and more difficult to resolve within the limits of orthodox Catholic moral practices. The basic principle governing the relationship between parents and their embryos was one of guardianship – not one of ownership. This had serious implications for the moral evaluation of IVF. Generally, fertility treatment led to the creation of more embryos that could be safely used in one treatment cycle. If the first treatment cycle was unsuccessful, the additional embryos, preserved at low temperatures, could be used in a subsequent treatment; or they could be used if the couple wished to have another child. It was frequently the case that embryos were placed in storage indefinitely because couples had either changed their minds or their circumstances had changed. The Irish Episcopal Conference observed that, in other jurisdictions, legislation made provision for a number of alternatives. The embryos could be disposed of, used for research, or donated to other couples – all of which were deemed to be unethical. The bishops believed that unwanted embryos in storage would eventually be disposed of and for this reason they saw "insuperable ethical problems" arising from the production and storage of spare embryos. They recommended that if the storage and disposal of human spermatozoa and ova were to be permitted, it should be regulated on the basis of "appropriate" legislation. Measures should be taken in assisted human reproduction (AHR) procedures to avoid the creation of more human embryos than could be safely transferred to a mother's womb in any one treatment cycle. All fertilised ova should be used for "normal implantation" (note: implantation occurs when the embryo embeds itself in the wall of the uterus, where it continues to develop), and there should be a prohibition on the storage of human embryos.[17]

In the concluding paragraphs of its submission the Irish Episcopal Conference addressed the complex issues of AHR in the context of the allocation of relatively scarce resources in the health services. Should AHR be viewed as a healthcare service? If so, then citizens could claim it as an entitlement. This presented a major difficulty when viewed against the backdrop of limited resources in the healthcare services and patients on waiting lists for life-saving treatments. Yet, a formidable counterargument was that if AHR was not publicly funded it would become accessible only to the wealthy, which was not deemed satisfactory either. Therefore, the bishops recommended that if the state was to allocate resources to treat infertility, "serious attention" needed to be given to identifying its causes, including those relating to lifestyle, rather than relying excessively on "the facilitation of circumventive procedures".[18]

On 12 February 2003 the Irish Catholic bishops published a summary of the recommendations they had submitted to the CAHR. To disseminate their opinions and recommendations more widely and in greater detail they published a booklet, *Assisted Human Reproduction – Facts and Ethical Issues*, on the internet.[19] Their findings were based on moral principles under the following headings: the right to life and bodily integrity; the right to an identity of origin; and the essential meaning of human sexuality – which dictated against the excessive intrusion of technology in procreation.[20]

The bishops observed that, unlike Britain and Northern Ireland, no laws were in place governing IVF – although some safeguards were in place. The Irish Medical Council's *Guide to Ethical Conduct and Behaviour* (1998) stated that "any fertilised ovum must be used for normal implantation and must not be deliberately destroyed."[21] Nevertheless, the bishops observed that, before the publication of the *Guide to Ethical Conduct and Behaviour*, claims had been made that surplus embryos were placed in the cervix rather than in the uterus, and these claims had not been denied.[22] It was so difficult in practice to provide IVF services effectively that it led inevitably to the death of many human embryos.[23]

The bishops examined a number of other procedures for AHR, including assisted insemination by donor (AID), assisted insemination by husband (AIH), gamete intra-fallopian transfer and intra-cytoplasmic sperm injection. All were found to be mildly to seriously ethically problematic. The bishops acknowledged in principle that couples contending with infertility had a right to benefit from medical intervention. But such a right was not an absolute right and needed to be considered in the light of other considerations, such as the respect for life, a child's right to know his or her origin; and the prudent use of limited healthcare resources.[24] In the concluding paragraph of their submission to the CAHR the bishops observed that infertility seemed to be on the increase. They emphasised the importance of prevention rather than undertaking heavy expenditures which would "essentially circumvent rather than cure infertility". They pointed to two possible causes worthy of investigation: first, changed patterns of sexual behaviour, including contraception; and, second, changed patterns of work and associated levels of stress.[25]

The bishops did not resort to heavy theological language in their submission to the CAHR. They intended to communicate their views to Irish society as a whole, not just to Catholics. Their ethical principles, therefore, were not only based on Catholic moral principles, but were also informed by principles concerning fundamental human rights.[26]

Church versus State

The Fianna Fáil–Progressive Democrat coalition government was in no rush to engage with complex ethical issues that might inflict political damage. The government's proposal to amend the Constitution on the matter of abortion was rejected by a narrow margin on 6 March 2002.[27] This seems to have influenced members of the government to adopt an attitude of extreme caution on ethical issues that were even more complex. They could, to some degree, procrastinate while the CAHR proceeded with its lengthy and arduous task. But the public funding of scientific research in the EU put pressure on government ministers to indicate their attitude towards human embryonic stem cell (hESC) research. The European Commission proposed that the moratorium on hESC research should be lifted. This was in the context of funding for scientific research under the Sixth EU Research Framework Programme (2003–2006). On 6 November 2003 the Fine Gael leader, Enda Kenny, asked Mary Harney, Tánaiste and Minister for Enterprise, Trade and Employment, about the government's position on the matter. Harney replied that the moratorium would expire at the end of December 2003. If no decision was reached by the Council of Ministers on 27 November, research could proceed without any EU controls in states that deemed it ethically acceptable. Harney was due to attend a meeting of the Council of Ministers on 27 November. The matter in question, as she saw it, was whether hESC research should proceed with controls or without them.[28] The Irish Catholic bishops saw it quite differently.

The Catholic hierarchy was determined to impress upon the government and the people its deep concerns about future funding of scientific research entailing the destruction of human embryos. On 29 October 2003 Cardinal Desmond Connell (Archbishop of Dublin), Dr Joseph Duffy (Bishop of Clogher), and Dr Patrick Walsh (Bishop of Down and Connor) met the Taoiseach, Bertie Ahern, as representatives of the Irish Bishops' Conference. On 6 November Bishop Joseph Duffy wrote to the Taoiseach on behalf of the hierarchy. This letter, indicating the points made by the bishops to the Taoiseach, was published on 13 November. The bishops asserted that the destruction of human embryos could not be justified, not even if scientific research led to therapeutic benefits. They believed that the Irish government should take a leading role in pressing the EU to give increased funding to adult stem cell research. They pointed out that the clinical use of hASCs, through bone marrow transplants, had yielded good results for many years.

The bishops welcomed the stated desire of the Taoiseach to prevent the use of hESCs for scientific research in Ireland. Attention was also drawn to the Taoiseach's "stated desire to safeguard the protection of human embryos at European level". The bishops noted an apparent contradiction here with government policy, which seemed to be neutral on the matter. It was widely understood that an Irish delegation to the European Commission had "made it clear on several occasions that it would not oppose the Commission proposal allowing for EU funding of destructive embryo research". The bishops asserted that neutrality on such an important issue was not an option. They pressed the Taoiseach to change government policy. Philippe Busquin, European Commissioner for Research and Development, the other delegations in the Council of Ministers, and especially the Italian presidency, should be informed that the Irish government was opposed to joint funding for scientific research that entailed the destruction of human embryos.

The Catholic hierarchy acknowledged the Irish government's concern that a failure to adopt the European Commission's proposal might lead to unregulated research which could otherwise be avoided. Even so, a worse outcome from their point of view was that a formal decision by the Council of Ministers would explicitly give consent to the sacrifice of human embryos for stem cell research – giving it greater legitimacy. This in turn would put those trying to negotiate strict controls in the next research budget at a severe disadvantage.

The bishops believed that it was possible for the Irish government to negotiate amendments to the European Commission's proposal. If Ireland adopted a clear policy in favour of protecting "life from its beginnings" this would be of "crucial significance" because of an awareness of the anti-abortion clause in the Constitution. Indeed, a failure of the Irish government to act clearly in defence of human embryos would strengthen the negotiating position of those who regarded them as expendable in the cause of advancing medical science.[29] Evidently, the bishops intended appealing directly to Irish public opinion to add greater weight to their arguments.

The issue of stem cell research was raised in the Seanad on 19 November 2003. Mary Harney attended to explain government policy on the matter. In June 2002 nearly €2.3 billion had been set aside by the EU for research in the life sciences, including stem cell research – both adult and embryonic. However, on 30 September 2002 a number of European states, including Ireland, had expressed dissatisfaction with the lack of clear guidelines and safeguards concerning hESC research. Because of this the Council of Ministers agreed to a proposal by the European Commission to impose a moratorium until 31 December 2003. Harney made it clear that research on hESCs would be confined to those derived from supernumerary embryos created from IVF treatments. There were also additional restrictions. Scientists would need to thoroughly examine the potential of hASCs before considering hESCs; and, in the latter case, they would have to share stem cell lines.

The funding was already in place. The only decisions to be made were those concerned with guidelines and safeguards. Harney made it clear that the principle of subsidiarity applied in this matter. In this context, subsidiarity meant that the EU would not give financial support to a research project using hESCs in a state that deemed it illegal or unethical.[30] It was clear that hESC research could not be imposed on Ireland against its will. Yet the absence of research on hESCs was not as clear-cut as it seemed. Harney stated that current medical practice in IVF procedures in Ireland resulted in surplus embryos. These could be frozen but would only remain viable for three to five years.[31] In her concluding statements Harney emphasised that, contrary to opinions in some quarters, there was nothing in the European Commission's proposal that would lead to the passing of legislation permitting hESC research in Ireland.[32]

In the ensuing debate, concern was expressed that the Oireachtas was not being consulted by the government on such an important ethical issue. Senator Terry Leyden (Fianna Fáil) quoted at length Bishop Duffy's letter to the Taoiseach to emphasise the concerns of the Catholic bishops. He argued that government policy was not consistent with the Irish Constitution's provisions for the protection of the unborn. It was unusual that the matter was being dealt with by the Minister for Enterprise, Trade, and Employment rather than by the Minister for Health and Children.[33] Indeed, it seemed exceptionally inappropriate that hESC research was being discussed in the EU under the headings of competitiveness and trade. This gave credence to the view that human embryos were being treated as commodities.

Harney reiterated that the purpose of a forthcoming meeting in Europe was for the member states of the EU to reach agreement on guidelines and regulations for research – the decision about funding hESC research had already been taken. Additionally, she was not acting unilaterally on behalf of Ireland. She had consulted the Minister for Health and Children initially. Her department was addressing this controversial issue because the science research budget had been within the remit of the competitiveness council since the term of the previous government. The minister then addressed the constitutional issue. She argued that there was no judicial clarity about the status of embryos outside the womb and that, therefore, no one could state definitively what the Constitution had to say on the matter.[34]

Harney referred to a document indicating that the Catholic University of Louvain did not rule out the acceptability of hESC research if certain rigorous ethical and scientific guidelines were adhered to. The senators were not impressed and a number of critical observations were made. It would be most unusual for a university to publicly take an institutional stance on a controversial ethical issue. It was speculated that the source was an editorial in a publication. But this was beside the point – which was that the Catholic University of Louvain did not represent the Roman Catholic Church. The Catholic bishops of Ireland were among those who did![35]

Senator David Norris exclaimed that he had "heard a great deal about Catholicism" – which, in this context, probably meant too much. He argued that an embryo was not "a full human being". Why not? Norris declared: "it has no central nervous system and no consciousness ... I have never seen anybody attempt to take one to a pantomime or the zoo or to secure voting rights for it. The argument is absolutely ludicrous."[36] Despite this, it seemed (as pointed out by Senator Martin Mansergh) that the majority of the electorate would support the position adopted by the Roman Catholic Church.[37] It is reasonable to assume that Harney was aware of the potential political fallout – hence her ill-judged reference to the Catholic University of Louvain to find some support for government policy on the basis of Catholic ethics.[38]

There seemed to be a lack of ethical consistency in Ireland's position on hESC research. It was prohibited in Ireland and yet Irish money would fund such research in countries where it was permitted. How could such a stance be defended? The beleaguered minister argued that Ireland's position was eminently defensible when the principle of subsidiarity was considered. Nations pooled sovereignty in designated areas of governance but retained independence in carefully chosen matters which were held to be of great importance in an ethical sense. If such an ideal was sacrificed then Ireland would be vulnerable to receiving dictation on ethical issues from its European neighbours.[39] This would clearly cause deep resentment.

The bishops had lost considerable influence in Irish society, not least because their responses to a succession of revelations about the sexual abuse of children by priests and brothers was widely seen as pathetic and scandalous. Still, they possessed the potential to inflict some damage on a government that would fail to take due account of Catholic ethical principles. The vote concerning hESC research in the EU was due to be taken by the Council of Ministers in Brussels on 27 November. Ireland's vote was due to be cast by Mary Harney. On Sunday 23 November, Cardinal Desmond Connell appealed publicly to Mary Harney and Bertie Ahern to ensure that Ireland took a stance in defence of human life by voting against the EU proposal. The issue, as he presented it, was whether or not to allow the EU to fund hESC research which would require the sacrifice of human embryos.[40] Connell obviously intended to apply maximum political pressure by publishing his appeal. This was also the *modus operandi* of Bishop Joseph Duffy of Clogher, whose sermon on the topic, delivered at St Macartan's Cathedral in Monaghan, was published the following day. Duffy stated that the government was to vote on an EU proposal "to fund stem cell research involving destruction of human embryos". He then said that "the Government is free to vote either way."[41]

Connell and Duffy had presented a misleading account of the government's position. The EU proposal did not address the question of whether or not to fund hESC research. This misinterpretation of government policy by the bishops served to enhance the political impact of their statements. To add further political clout to their stance, Duffy claimed that government policy on the issue of hESC research was in conflict with the wishes of the "vast majority" of the electorate and was contrary to the will of the Oireachtas, which had been unanimously expressed by an all-party committee. He pointed out that Fianna Fáil's own MEPs had voted against the proposal in the European Parliament the previous week.[42]

The issue of stem cell research was raised in the Dáil on 25 November 2003. Mary Harney stated that if no guidelines and controls were agreed, the only restrictions that would apply would be those already in place in many of the member states of the EU.[43] The former Fine Gael leader, John Bruton, argued for ethical consistency across the EU: ethics was not dependent on location, changing as one travelled from one state to another. This failed to take account of the critical importance of subsidiarity in the EU. Harney responded vigorously, observing that most member states of the EU regarded abortion as ethical.[44] The implications of such an observation were clear. Bruton failed to put forward an effective counterargument. Harney rejected the claim that the Dáil had not been adequately consulted about hESC research. She pointed out that Fine Gael did have ample opportunity to put forward a parliamentary motion but had not done so.[45]

The Council of Ministers of the EU failed to agree on guidelines for the funding of stem cell research at their meeting, which had been rescheduled for 3 December. The Irish Catholic bishops, at their General Meeting in Maynooth, made reference to this failure in a press release on 10 December, and took the opportunity to express "great concern" about "the consequential lack of clarity" on the issue. The bishops declared their determination to oppose any proposals that would involve funding the destruction of human embryos.[46] Their assumed occupancy of the high moral ground on this matter was very much at the expense of the Fianna Fáil–Progressive Democrat coalition government – and especially of Mary Harney. Press releases by the bishops failed to give due attention to the complex political background of the decision-making process in the EU and created the impression that there was a simple moral choice to be made by the government – the choice between good and evil. The publication of private correspondence between the Taoiseach and Cardinal Desmond Connell on 24 December, following requests for information under the Freedom of Information Act, indicated that this was not the case.

It was revealed that a copy of the text of Connell's press release dated 23 November, with a covering letter expressing hope for a "good outcome", had been sent to the Taoiseach. Ahern responded four days later, pointing out that the cardinal misunderstood the government's position on hESC research. Ahern stated that the issue being voted on was concerned with guidelines and controls for funding scientific research projects; it was not to decide whether funding should be provided for stem cell research. That decision had already been taken in the process of setting up the Sixth Framework Research Programme. The cardinal's stance seemed self-contradictory to Ahern. Ahern argued that a failure to agree on guidelines would lead to a considerably less restrictive system of research funding.[47] This in turn did not seem compatible with the ethical concerns expressed by Connell.

Discord in Irish Catholicism

The Irish Catholic bishops were acutely aware that many Roman Catholics held opinions that were contrary to church teaching. In July 2004 they published their views about this under the heading "Notification on Recent Developments in Moral Theology and Their Implications for the Church and Society". The bishops observed that there had been a continuous "development" of the Church's moral teaching over the centuries. This represented "a constant deepening of knowledge" under the guidance of the Holy Spirit, which was filtered through the teaching authority for dissemination to the faithful multitudes, who were to accept it with "humility and gratitude".[48] In the era pre-dating the Second Vatican Council something had gone seriously amiss because moral theology had succumbed to "rigorist legalism" and was in dire need of renewal.[49] It does not seem to have occurred to the bishops that such a problem might have been largely due to the excessive strictures imposed on theologians by the ecclesiastical authorities. Or perhaps the Holy Spirit was less than diligent in transmitting divine inspiration? This of course was not contemplated. With the teaching authority of the Church above reproach, the process of elimination led definitively to the theologians.

The Second Vatican Council had attempted to stimulate renewal in moral theology. The *Catechism of the Catholic Church* was presented as the "comprehensive summary of the Church's teaching on morality".[50] Evidently, it was not comprehensive enough for all Roman Catholics, many of whom did not see humility as a virtue and had become distinctly ungrateful when subjected to ecclesiastical directives. Disciplinary measures were taken against liberal theologians pressing for a renewal of moral theology,[51] stifling attempts to counteract the increasing divergence between the institutional church and the Catholic laity on a range of moral issues. The Irish Catholic bishops singled out Fr Seán Fagan's *Does Morality Change?* (1997) as a misguided attempt to make progress in moral theology.[52] Fagan had expressed cautious approval of IVF and was critical of the Church's insistence that the procreative and unitive aspects of sexual intercourse must be present in every such act.[53] Fagan's opinions were closer to public opinion than those of the bishops.

The CAHR took measures to ascertain public opinion towards AHR a few months after its inception.[54] AHR was defined with reference to two types of intervention – assisted insemination and IVF.[55] The commission employed the services of a market research organisation to undertake a survey to ascertain attitudes amongst the general public towards AHR and related issues. Sixty-eight per cent of respondents approved of AHR as an appropriate response to the problem of infertility, with only 14 per cent expressing outright disagreement. Eighty-five per cent favoured AHR for married couples, and 63 per cent agreed with it for couples in stable relationships. Forty-five per cent agreed with third-party donation of gametes in AHR and 35 per cent disagreed. Forty-five per cent expressed support for medical research on embryos provided that it was likely to lead to more effective treatment of genetic diseases.[56] These findings, and others, and taking into account the fact that about 88 per cent of the population was Roman Catholic, indicate that many Catholics were exercising individual judgement very much independent of what the bishops were seeking to inculcate.

The CAHR put forward forty recommendations in its report. Some of its proposals were in agreement with Catholic teaching, such as number 35, which prohibited human reproductive cloning; and number 37, which prescribed against the creation of interspecies human embryos. The CAHR observed that a range of AHR services were already being provided under the guidelines of the Irish Medical Council. The CAHR regarded these guidelines alone as insufficient and accordingly proposed a legislative basis for the regulation of AHR.[57] Its first recommendation was that legislation should be enacted to set up a regulatory body to control AHR services in the state.

A number of recommendations were sharply at variance with Catholic ethical principles as promulgated by the hierarchy. These included the following:

10. Appropriate guidelines should be put in place by the regulatory body to govern the options available for excess frozen embryos. These would include voluntary donation of excess healthy embryos to other recipients, voluntary donation for research or allowing them to perish.

16. The embryo formed by IVF should not attract legal protection until placed in the human body, at which stage it should attract the same level of protection as the embryo formed *in vivo*.

17. Services should be available without discrimination on the grounds of gender, marital status or sexual orientation subject to consideration of the best interests of any children that may be born.

30. Surrogacy should be permitted and should be subject to

regulation by the regulatory body.

34. Embryo research, including embryonic stem cell research ... under stringently controlled conditions, should be permitted on surplus embryos that are donated specifically for research. This should be permitted up to fourteen days following fertilisation ... The generation of embryos through IVF specifically for research purposes should be prohibited.

36. Regenerative medicine should be permitted under regulation.[58]

40. Pre-implantation genetic diagnosis (PGD) should be allowed, under regulation, to reduce the risk of serious genetic disorders.[59]

The Oireachtas Joint Committee on Health and Children discussed the *Report of the Commission on Assisted Human Reproduction* (March 2005) at its meeting on 21 July 2005. The meeting was attended by senior civil servants from the Department of Health and Children.[60] The Joint Committee comprised politicians from both houses of the Oireachtas. Members of the committee were led to believe that they were to conclude their work by April 2006. Liam Twomey, an independent TD, referred to the CAHR's report to make the point that the joint committee was considerably restricted in what it could achieve because of the ambiguity of Article 40.3.3 of the Constitution, which upheld the right to life of the "unborn". Only a Supreme Court judgment, or a constitutional amendment (which would require a referendum), could provide clarification. In the absence of such clarification little progress could be made on many of the recommendations of the commission's report, especially those that were likely to provoke disagreement. In response to Twomey, Brian Mullen, principal officer at the Department of Health and Children, acknowledged that the department had not "given any serious consideration" to this constitutional issue.[61]

The Joint Committee discussed the *Report of the Commission on Assisted Human Reproduction* again on 15 September 2005. The meeting was attended by several members of the CAHR, who had been invited to answer questions.[62] There was a lack of accurate and verifiable statistical information about AHR services in Ireland, but a number of estimates were put forward for consideration. About 1,000 babies were born each year as a result of AHR services. The success rate was between 25 and 30 per cent, which meant that about 6,000 to 8,000 people each year were using the services.[63] There was still no legislation concerning informed consent procedures, safety of patients or quality of services provided.

There were no regulations about what to do with supernumerary embryos. Embryos did not remain viable indefinitely when stored at very low temperatures: there was considerable uncertainty about the upper limit of viability, but a general guideline was for storage up to five years.[64]

Other issues needed to be addressed. Would the state enable people on low incomes, who would otherwise not be in a position to afford such services, to avail of AHR?[65] Was it ethical to use PGD to screen out embryos with genetic abnormalities? The indications were that demand for PGD would increase. Some Irish couples had travelled to the United Kingdom, Spain and Belgium for PGD to reduce the risk of having a child with a genetic abnormality.[66]

There was no evidence that any clinic in Ireland provided a service for surrogacy, but anecdotal evidence indicated that some Irish couples had availed of surrogacy services abroad. Surrogacy was a very complex issue with legal, ethical, social and psychological dimensions. Should surrogate mothers be paid? If so, how much? Should a child have the right to know the identity of its surrogate mother? A British report indicated that difficulties could arise when a surrogate mother changed her mind about handing over the child to the commissioning couple, as had happened in a small percentage of cases.[67] Achieving consensus on issues such as stem cell research, PGD and surrogacy was most unlikely. However, as observed by Senator Mary Henry (a medical practitioner), there was widespread agreement on the need to establish some system of regulation.[68]

The Catholic hierarchy set about a detailed examination of the *Report of the Commission on Assisted Human Reproduction* shortly after its publication. A press release by Diarmuid Martin, Archbishop of Dublin, was issued through the Catholic Communications Office (an agency of the Irish Catholic Bishops' Conference) on 12 May 2005 to indicate the preliminary findings of the Catholic bishops. Predictably enough, they found that it contravened Catholic moral teaching on marriage and on the protection, from conception, of human life. The press release indicated that a detailed response would be issued at a later date and that the Catholic Church would contribute to the public debate that needed to take place on a wide range of issues raised by the commission.[69] The Pro Life Campaign, a self-declared non-denominational lobby group, condemned the recommendations of the report as "extreme" and "unethical."[70]

An opinion poll commissioned by the Irish Council for Bioethics indicated that Irish society was deeply divided on bioethical issues, and that there was also a widespread lack of understanding. Five hundred adults were interviewed from 19 August to 3 September 2005. The survey found that 44 per cent believed that supernumerary embryos from IVF procedures should be used for medical research, 30 per cent were opposed, and 25 per cent did not know. Of those who stated their support for hESC research, 82 per cent maintained their position when informed that such research would entail the destruction of embryos; five per cent changed their opinion, and 13 per cent did not know. Fifty-four per cent believed that hESC research should receive financial support from the government; 20 per cent were opposed. Forty-two per cent were of the opinion that unborn children should be screened for genetic abnormalities to inform decisions about whether or not pregnancies should be terminated; 43 per cent disagreed.[71] From these opinion poll findings it seemed that many Roman Catholics either disagreed with the moral prescriptions of the hierarchy, or were not well informed about the official teachings of their church.

Endnotes

————•————

1   In this procedure there is a small genetic difference between the donor of the somatic cell nucleus and the embryo, arising from the fact that mitochondrial DNA (deoxyribonucleic acid) is passed on through the maternal line only, and therefore is present in the cytoplasm (more specifically in the mitochondria) of the ovum rather than in its nucleus.

2   For further information about this see Don O'Leary, *Roman Catholicism and Modern Science: A History* (New York and London: 2006), pp. 233–5.

3   This was indicated by scientific research on animal stem cells. Irish Council for Bioethics, *Ethical, Scientific and Legal Issues Concerning Stem Cell Research: Opinion* (Dublin: Irish Council for Bioethics, 2008), pp. 16-17.

4   Robert F. Harrison, "The Development of IVF Practice in Ireland – A personal view", *Human Fertility*, vol. 15, no. 1, pp. 7–8.

5   Paul Cullen, "Frozen embryos and the Constitution: what was at stake in this case", *Irish Times*, 16 November 2006, p. 4.

6   Commission on Assisted Human Reproduction, *Report of the Commission on Assisted Human Reproduction* (Dublin: Stationery Office, 2005), p. 1.

7   Ibid., pp. x, 1, 79.

8   The *Report of the Commission on Assisted Human Reproduction* (pp. i–ii) lists 25 members, but four were replacements for those who resigned in the period 2000–2002. The commission was supported by a secretariat of four staff.

9   *Report of the Commission on Assisted Human Reproduction*, p. x.

10 Ibid., Micheál Martin to Dervilla Donnelly, March 2000, in Appendix 1, p. 79.

11 Theological advice at Working Group meetings was given by Canon Kenneth Kearon, Director and Head of Ecumenical Studies Programme, Irish School of Ecumenics, Dublin; and Rev. Paul Tighe, Head of Department of Theology, Mater Dei Institute, Dublin. See *Report of the Commission on Assisted Human Reproduction*, p. iii.

12 In December 2001 the Irish Episcopal Conference made an additional and shorter submission, based on the earlier *Assisted Human Reproduction*, to the commission.

13 Irish Episcopal Conference, "Submission to the Government Commission on Assisted Human Reproduction by the Irish Episcopal Conference – December 2001", Catholic Communications Office <http://www. catholiccommunications.ie/Pressrel/ahrsubmission.html> accessed 12

October 2004. This document was republished as "Submission to the Commission on Human Reproduction" in *Doctrine and Life*, vol. 53, no. 3 (March 2003), pp. 181–7.

14   Philip Cohen and David Concar, "The awful truth", *New Scientist*, no. 2291 (19 May 2001), pp. 14–15 <www.newscientist.com> accessed 29 December 2006; and Claire Ainsworth *et al.*, "Human Cloning: If not today, tomorrow", *New Scientist*, vol. 177, no. 2377 (11 January 2003), pp. 8–11.

15   The bishops referred to the Declaration of Helsinki, revised text, 1975.

16   Irish Episcopal Conference, op. cit.

17   Ibid.

18   Ibid.

19   Irish Bishops' Conference, "Publication of Catholic Bishops' Submission to Government Commission on Assisted Human Reproduction", Catholic Communications Office, press release, 12 February 2003 <http://www. catholiccommunications.ie/Pressrel/12-february-2003.html> accessed 1 November 2004.

20   Bishops' Committee for Bioethics, *Assisted Human Reproduction: Facts and Ethical Issues* (Dublin: Veritas, 2000). This booklet was revised by the Bishops' Committee for Bioethics on 3 April 2003 and posted on the internet <http:// www.catholiccommunications.ie/pastlet/ahr.html> accessed 1 November 2004. References are to the revised internet edition. The three guiding ethical principles were explained in Chapter 1.

21   *Assisted Human Reproduction*, Chapter 2, section D; in reference to Irish Medical Council, *Guide to Ethical Conduct and Behaviour*, 26.4 (Dublin: Irish Medical Council, 1998).

22   Ethical guidelines of the Medical Council in the 1990s required that all embryos created through IVF had to be transferred to the woman's reproductive system. A maximum of three embryos were transferable to the uterus. Any others were transferred to the cervix, where they were extremely unlikely to implant. This ruled out the freezing of embryos, research on embryos, and the "official" discarding of surplus embryos. Deirdre Madden, "The Status of Human Embryos in Irish Medical Practice" in Elisabeth Hildt and Dietmar Mieth (eds), *In Vitro Fertilisation in the 1990s: Towards a Medical, Social and Ethical Evaluation* (Aldershot, UK: Ashgate, 1998), p. 223.

23   *Assisted Human Reproduction*, Chapter 3, section B. It was common practice to use more than one embryo in each IVF cycle, usually up to three. The bishops understood that the success rate in reference to pregnancies was close to 30% and, in terms of live births, somewhere between 15% and 20%. There was some evidence to indicate that success rates using frozen embryos were not significantly less. Natural-cycle IVF was far less ethically problematic than those procedures that relied on drugs to stimulate the ovaries to produce several ova. In natural-cycle IVF there was no drug-induced super-ovulation and, therefore, no possibility of surplus embryos. However, the bishops

acknowledged that natural-cycle IVF was "very tedious and unpredictable", with a much lower success rate than standard practice IVF. *Assisted Human Reproduction*, Chapter 2, section D.

24 Ibid., Chapter 4, paragraph 2.

25 Ibid., Chapter 4, paragraph 3.

26 Reference was made to the Universal Declaration of Human Rights (New York: United Nations Organisation, 1948), 3 and 16.

27 Louise Fuller, *Irish Catholicism since 1950: The Undoing of a Culture* (Dublin: Gill and Macmillan, 2002), p. 249.

28 Dáil Debates, vol. 573, col. 1234 (6 November 2003).

29 They bolstered this contention with an anecdote. Commissioner Philippe Busquin had attended a meeting of the Joint Bioethics Committee of the Bishops' Conferences of England and Wales, Ireland and Scotland on 2 October 2003. He suggested that, because the Irish government seemed ready to support the European Commission's proposal, it was less likely that other countries would oppose it in cases where there was little or no constitutional protection of the unborn in place. Irish Bishops' Conference, "News, 13 November 2003: Catholic Bishops' Letter to Taoiseach on Embryonic Stem Cell Research Made Public", Catholic Communications Office <http://www. catholiccommunications.ie/News/news-13november2003-lettertotaoiseach. html> accessed 12 October 2004.

30 Seanad Debates, vol. 174, no. 14, cols 1096–7 (19 November 2003).

31 Ibid., col. 1099.

32 Ibid., cols 1099–1100.

33 Ibid., cols 1104–1105. Several references were made to the teaching of the Roman Catholic Church throughout the debate.

34 Ibid., cols 1139–1141.

35 Ibid., cols 1098, 1115, 1120, 1122, 1128, 1135.

36 Ibid., col. 1124.

37 Ibid., col. 1135.

38 Harney stated (col. 1142) that she referred to the Catholic University of Louvain "to explain the difficult ethical complexities" and did not intend to create the impression that she was quoting it as an authoritative source on Catholic teaching. She was unable at the time to give precise details of the source of the document she quoted.

39 Ibid., cols 1141–1143.

40 Desmond Connell, "EU Funding for Embryonic Stem-Cell Research: Statement by Cardinal Desmond Connell: Sunday, 23rd November 2003 – immediate", internet document released by the Communications Office, Archdiocese of Dublin <www.dublindiocese.ie>.

41 Joseph Duffy, "The Diocese of Clogher; News: 24 November 2003" <http:// www.clogherdiocese.ie/news/news-24november2003-homilystmacartans-stemcellresearch.html> accessed 12 October 2004.

42 Ibid.

43 Dáil Debates, vol. 575, col. 424 (25 November 2003).

44 Ibid., cols 428–429.

45 Ibid., cols 431, 433.

46 Catholic Communications Office, "Catholic Bishops' Winter Meeting", 10 December 2003 <http://www.catholiccommunications.ie/Pressrel/10-december-2003.html> accessed 12 October 2004.

47 Arthur Beesley, "Taoiseach disputed cardinal's stance on stem cells" and "At odds on the stem-cell research issue", both articles in the *Irish Times*, 24 December 2003, pp.1, 6. Ireland was due to assume the presidency of the EU the following week. There seemed little prospect of agreement and Mary Harney stated that there was no possibility of her being able to bring about agreement on guidelines and controls during the term of the Irish presidency (*Irish Times*, p. 6). Church and state were in agreement on other issues, including opposition to human cloning and euthanasia, and support for an acknowledgement of Europe's Christian heritage in the proposed EU Constitution (*Irish Times*, p. 1). For an insight into Bertie Ahern's relationship with Cardinal Desmond Connell, and with his successor, Archbishop Diarmuid Martin, see Ronald Quinlan, "Letters reveal Taoiseach's efforts to defer to bishops", *Sunday Independent*, 4 February 2007, p. 6.

48 Irish Bishops' Conference, "Notification on Recent Developments in Moral Theology and Their Implications for the Church and Society", July 2004, paragraph 5 <http://www.catholiccommunications.ie> accessed 25 February 2007.

49 Ibid., paragraph 7.

50 Ibid., paragraph 7.

51 See O'Leary, *Roman Catholicism and Modern Science*, pp. 190, 202.

52 Irish Bishops' Conference, "Notification on Recent Developments in Moral Theology", paragraph 8.

53 Seán Fagan, *Does Morality Change?* (Dublin: Columba Press, 2003). The edition of Fagan's book referred to by the Irish Bishops' Conference was jointly published by Gill and Macmillan (Dublin) and the Liturgical Press (Collegeville) in 1997.

54 In October 2001, though the medium of the national press, the CAHR invited interested organisations and individuals to submit their views. It received over 1,700 submissions in response. It hosted a public conference at Dublin Castle on 6 February 2003, at which attendance exceeded 250. *Report of the Commission on Assisted Human Reproduction*, p. 38.

55 *Report of the Commission on Assisted Human Reproduction*, p. x.

56 Ibid., pp. 39–41.

57 Ibid., p. 67.

58 This referred to therapeutic cloning, which required the use of SCNT to generate embryonic stem cells for the treatment of pathological conditions.

Details about regenerative medicine relating to recommendation number 36 are given on pages 61–2 of the commission's report.

59 *Report of the Commission on Assisted Human Reproduction*, List of Recommendations, pp. xv–xvii. Only two members of the commission expressed disagreement with the recommendations: Gerry Whyte, Associate Professor of Law at Trinity College Dublin, did not agree with those recommendations that permitted the deliberate destruction of embryos; Christine O'Rourke, Advisory Counsel at the Office of the Attorney General, disagreed with the recommendations on surrogacy. Ibid., pp. 73–7.

60 These were principal officer Brian Mullen and two assistant principal officers, Liam McCormack and Peter Hanrahan.

61 *Joint Committee on Health and Children*, 29JHC 1, no. 60, 21 July 2005 (Dublin: Stationery Office), cols 1928–1930.

62 Members of the CAHR who attended the meeting and responded to questions from the Joint Committee were Professor Dervilla Donnelly, Professor Marina Lynch, Dr Miriam McCarthy, Dr Mary Wingfield, Professor Gerry White, Professor Andrew Greene, Dr Aonghus Nolan and Dr Deirdre Madden.

63 *Joint Committee on Health and Children*, 29 JHC 1, no. 61, 15 September 2005 (Dublin: Stationery Office), cols 1941–1942.

64 Ibid., col. 1956.

65 Ibid., col. 1947.

66 Ibid., cols 1964–1965.

67 Ibid., cols 1961–1964.

68 Ibid., col. 1948.

69 Catholic Communications Office, "Press Release, 12 May 2005: Comments of Archbishop Diarmuid Martin on the Report of the Commission on Assisted Human Reproduction" <http://www.catholiccommunications. ie/Pressrel/12-may-2005.html> accessed 20 May 2005. One of the eleven items on the agenda of the bishops' three-day June General Meeting at Maynooth was a discussion on their preliminary response to the *Report of the Commission on Assisted Human Reproduction*. Details were given by the Catholic Communications Office, "Press Release, 16 June 2005: Irish Bishops' Conference, June General Meeting 2005" <http://www. catholiccommunications.ie/Pressrel/16-june-2005.html> accessed 28 June 2005.

70 "CAHR recommendations 'extreme and unethical' – PLC", *Catholic Herald and Standard*, no. 6200 (20 May 2005), p. 6. Fr Kevin Doran, a lecturer at Milltown Institute in Dublin, was also critical of the report.

71 Irish Council for Bioethics, *Public Attitudes Towards Bioethics: Irish Council for Bioethics Research Report September 2005* <http://www.bioethics.ie/ publications/index.html> accessed 5 March 2007, pp. 5, 9, 12, 34, 35, 38. See also William Reville, "Is it time to ensure that ethics match the science?",

Irish Times, 9 February 2006, p. 15; and Dick Ahlstrom, "Over 50% favour embryo research, says poll", *Irish Times*, 17 November 2005.

CHAPTER THREE

———•———

Frozen Embryos and Stem Cell Research

2005–2006

The European Dimension

The Fianna Fáil–Progressive Democrat coalition government probably anticipated that, in the course of a heated controversy, public opinion would shift decisively against human embryonic stem cell research. Despite the great potential of such research, government ministers were not emboldened to undertake any changes in policy. Micheál Martin, Minister for Enterprise, Trade and Employment, reiterated the government's support for the principle of ethical subsidiarity on 4 October 2005. He had replaced Mary Harney as the government minister with responsibility for Irish policy concerned with EU funding of human embryonic stem cell (hESC) research. Martin informed the Dáil that the European Commission, when presenting its proposals for the Seventh Framework Programme (2007–2013), had declared its intention not to change its policies concerning "fundamental ethical principles" relating to scientific research. Stem cell research was taking place in Ireland, but the stem cells were from adult sources.[1]

Public discourse about hESCs took place against the backdrop of a troubled relationship between church and state arising from the sexual abuse of children by priests and members of religious orders who had been in positions of trust, especially in the educational system. A number of senior Fianna Fáil and Progressive Democrat politicians expressed opinions which varied somewhat in their criticisms of the Roman Catholic Church in Ireland. The Taoiseach, Bertie Ahern, defended the relationship of church and state, praising the Church's role in education, and in society generally. But he also expressed measured criticism of the Church's failure to respond vigorously and appropriately to allegations of the sexual abuse of children. Liz O'Donnell, a senior Progressive Democrat politician and TD, saw matters differently and criticised the "cosy" relationship between church and state. Micheál Martin denied that there was any evidence of "undue deference" towards the Church. Mary Harney expressed support for her party colleague, Liz O'Donnell. Her opinion was implicitly supportive of Martin's position on the issue of stem cell research. She observed that the government had steadfastly adhered to a policy at EU level that was opposed by the Catholic hierarchy.[2]

In April 2006 the European Commission published its proposals for the Seventh Framework Research Programme. On 25 April Gay Mitchell, Fine Gael TD and MEP, pointed out that Italy, Austria, Germany, Luxembourg, Malta, Slovakia, and Poland disagreed with the pooled funding from EU states for hESC research. Micheál Martin replied that some member states, including Ireland, had not yet adopted "definitive positions". Under the sixth programme, which was near its end, a rigorous ethical review process was in place for funding hESC research. More than 90 per cent of stem cell projects were reliant on postnatal sources. Only eight projects that used hESCs had been approved for public funding and Ireland was not involved in any of those projects. The principle of ethical subsidiarity, applied in the sixth programme, was to be maintained in the seventh European framework programme of scientific research.[3]

In May 2006 the issue of stem cell research was again discussed at European level in relation to the seventh framework programme. It was in this context that Gay Mitchell argued that funding sourced from Irish taxpayers should not be used for research based on hESCs when such research could not be undertaken in Ireland.[4] The European Parliament was due to vote on the funding of stem cell research on 15 June. It was anticipated that this would lead to a broader debate on the issue within the European Commission, and at discussions of the European Council of Ministers. On the day before the parliamentary vote the Irish Catholic bishops issued a press release reiterating their stance against hESC research and observing that Ireland, at European level, had failed to take a leading role in opposing the destruction of human embryos.[5]

Italy, Austria, Germany, Luxembourg, Malta, Slovakia, and Poland had together formed a "blocking minority" to EU proposals for funding hESC research. However, after the election of Romano Prodi as Prime Minister of Italy, his government declared its intention to liberalise the state's embryo research laws, and Italian opposition to hESC research was withdrawn. The minority opposition was no longer a blocking opposition. European Catholic bishops expressed their disapproval of EU proposals. In Ireland, it seemed that some government backbenchers were worried that Irish support for the funding of hESC research, in those EU states where it was legal, would alienate a substantial sector of the electorate.[6]

Micheál Martin was criticised by pro-life lobby groups for his support of EU funding for hESC research. His invocation of the principle of ethical subsidiarity was challenged by the journalist David Quinn in the *Irish Catholic*. Martin had stated on national television a few days earlier that Ireland should not attempt to exercise undue pressure on other EU countries on the matter, otherwise Ireland might have to contend with demands for policy changes concerning abortion and other sensitive social issues. Quinn argued that abortion was irrelevant in this case because it was not within the scope of the EU in terms of legislation. Also, he maintained, Ireland had special protection against any such initiative under the provisions of the Maastricht Treaty. Quinn observed that the vote on hESC research had narrowly passed in the European Parliament, and that the majority of Irish MEPs had voted against it.[7] Evidently, it was embarrassing to Fianna Fáil that, in stark contrast to government policy, its four MEPs – Eoin Ryan, Liam Aylward, Seán Ó Neachtain and Brian Crowley – had voted against the funding of hESC research (in EU states where it was legal).[8] Such a development must surely have impressed upon the leadership of Fianna Fáil the hazardous nature of undertaking legislative initiatives in the field of bioethics.

The EU was deeply divided on the issue of hESC research. This was clearly indicated by the vote in the European Parliament – 284 votes for, 249 votes against, and 32 abstentions. The European Parliament voted to prohibit financial support, under the seventh framework programme, for the deliberate creation of human embryos for research purposes. Financial support would also be limited by the legal restrictions on stem cell research imposed by individual EU member states. The EU would not directly support the destruction of embryos, but it would fund hESC research arising from such destruction. From an orthodox Catholic point of view such a policy was morally deficient. The "thick-headed" and "blind secularism" of European leaders was denounced in *L'Osservatore Romano* and was seen as incompatible with "the religious convictions of the majority of its people..."[9]

On 24 July 2006 the Competitiveness Council of the European Council of Ministers gave its approval to the funding of hESC research, subject to strict regulations and ethical principles.[10] The European Commission issued a declaration supportive of the Council of Ministers on this issue. The Commission of the Bishops' Conferences of the European Community responded by stating that the Catholic Church recognised the importance of promoting economic development in the EU based on knowledge, research and innovation. However, the European bishops were critical of the EU because, although the destruction of embryos would not be directly funded, hESC research would, from their point of view, promote such destruction in some of the member states. Additionally, they contended that EU policy on the issue contravened Article 1 of its Charter of Fundamental Rights, which states: "Human dignity is inviolable. It must be respected and protected."[11]

EU policy on funding hESC research was cautious and restrictive in the face of opposition from some member states. The European Catholic bishops, not least in Ireland, had expressed their resolute opposition. Fianna Fáil MEPs had voted against government policy on the issue. And there were, apparently, rumblings of discontent in the Fianna Fáil party generally about the stance of Micheál Martin. All this would have typically sharpened a politician's instincts to be evasive or ambivalent. Asked if he would support hESC research in Ireland, the minister replied: "If it could be shown that embryo stem cell research could lead to cures, then I would be open to it, at least in terms of supernumerary embryos produced by in vitro fertilisation." He rejected the assertion that, because Ireland makes contributions to EU funds, the state had a right to determine how this money was spent in other member states of the union.[12]

The Catholic bishops in Ireland had in May 2005 indicated their intention to give a detailed response to the *Report of the Commission on Assisted Human Reproduction*. They did so in 2006 with the publication of their booklet *Towards a Creative Response to Infertility*. Their criticisms of the report were based on principles concerning human sexuality, the family, human dignity and the right to life. The Church expected the state to legislate for the common good, which required safeguarding the rights of every individual and respecting the rights of the family. The bishops acknowledged that their collective vision of the world was very much informed by theology and the Bible. However, they believed that the natural ability of people to discern right from wrong without recourse to religious beliefs was also important. There was a secular dimension, based on the concept of human rights, which they believed added strength to their moral prescriptions for society.[13] Most of the text of the bishops' booklet was concerned with commenting on each of the forty recommendations of the CAHR.

The bishops were careful to impress upon the laity that they approved of scientific research in the service of humankind subject to ethical principles. Thus they advocated, for example, the use of adult stem cells in place of hESCs.[14] There would always be a temptation to take advantage of supernumerary embryos generated by IVF as sources of hESCs. Alternative ways of treating infertility seemed particularly attractive to the Church. The bishops advocated that the state should allocate resources to identifying and treating the causes of infertility – "including social or life-style causes".[15] They recommended "Natural Procreative Technologies" (known as "NaPro Technology") as an "effective" treatment of infertility, both male and female. NaPro Technology was "not so much a particular treatment, as an approach to treatment" which included elements of "fertility awareness", drug therapy and surgery.[16] Reference was made to Thomas W. Hilgers' *Medical Applications of Natural Family Planning* (1991), published by the Pope Paul VI Institute Press, to explain how NaPro Technology worked. The explanation was rather nebulous. In order to treat infertility, NaPro Technology "cooperates with the procreative mechanisms in producing a form of treatment which corrects the condition, maintains the human ecology and sustains the procreative potential".

The bishops believed that an essential feature of NaPro Technology was the identification of the fertile phase of the menstrual cycle, relying on "a variation of the ovulation method CrM NFP" to optimise the chances of achieving a pregnancy for couples with low fertility.[17] Drug therapy or surgery could be used to remedy some problems when these were identified. Treatment was to be offered only to married couples. The bishops concluded by "strongly" recommending that financial support should be provided to explore "the potential of natural procreative therapies" and to promote the further development of NaPro Technology services.[18]

The response of medical practitioners was generally sceptical.[19] Furthermore, there seems to have been very little demand for the procedure. It is most unlikely that the government gave serious consideration to the bishops' proposals, which seemed to be inspired by unrealistic expectations of therapeutic benefits. The ability of the Irish Catholic bishops to influence government policy on biomedical ethical issues was not what it had once been.

There was, of course, a distinction to be drawn between the pronouncements of bishops and the opinions of Irish Catholics in general. The government was in no rush to proceed with drafting legislation on complex bioethical issues when there was a considerable risk of finding itself at odds with a large sector of the electorate. Not surprisingly, it had great patience with the deliberations of the Joint Committee on Health and Children. At its meeting on 4 July 2006 opposition members of the committee were clearly frustrated by the delaying tactics of Fianna Fáil. There was a perception that government politicians were trying to delay putting forward proposals for legislation on assisted human reproduction services before the general election, due the following year. The complexities of assisted human reproduction and cognate issues facilitated a government strategy of insisting on an endless round of consultations and discussions. From a Fianna Fáil perspective, opposition politicians in the Joint Committee were trying to use the *Report of the Commission on Assisted Human Reproduction* to embarrass the government.[20] But there was little cause for concern because the government majority on the committee ensured that this would not happen. Fianna Fáil's delaying tactics were bolstered by a case in the High Court concerning the fate of frozen embryos. Reports in the press indicated that the Joint Committee would not publish its recommendations before the High Court delivered its judgment.[21] The proceedings and outcome of this High Court case will be examined next.

Roche v. Roche: High Court Judgment

The High Court case of *Mary Roche v. Thomas Roche and Others* highlighted the pressing need for legislation and a comprehensive set of guidelines for the regulation of assisted human reproduction services in the Republic of Ireland. It brought into sharp focus a number of contentious issues concerning the legal status of early-stage embryos and the rights and duties of parents. The case also drew public attention to the different attitudes of church and state towards "the unborn". It received extensive coverage in the print and broadcast media, especially in July 2006.

Mary Roche and her husband Thomas had separated a few months before their case was brought to court. Their first child, a son, had been conceived by natural means in 1997. Fertility problems arose afterwards, and the couple attended the Sims Clinic in Dublin for IVF treatment in 2002. Mary Roche subsequently became pregnant and gave birth to a daughter. Three embryos created through IVF had not been used and were preserved under frozen conditions at the Sims Clinic. After the couple separated Mary Roche sought to have the three remaining embryos implanted. Her husband refused to give his consent.

The question of consent was of critical importance. Was consent actually given? What precisely was consented to? If consent had been given, could it be withdrawn? Documents signed by the couple and the IVF clinic were less than clear on these points. Mr Justice Brian McGovern presided. The plaintiff was represented by senior counsel (SC) Gerard Hogan. The defendants included Thomas Roche, two doctors, and the Sims Clinic. Thomas Roche was represented by John Rogers SC. There was also a third party to the proceedings because the state had a particular interest in the case. The Attorney General was a notice party and was represented by Donal O'Donnell SC. The case was not merely concerned with settling an issue of private contractual law. There was also a constitutional dimension because of Article 40.3.3 of the Constitution. McGovern decided to proceed with the private contractual aspect of the case first.

Hogan argued that when the first three embryos were implanted, leading to pregnancy, the wife's consent alone was sufficient for that specific medical procedure to be carried out. Therefore, only her permission was required for the same procedure to be repeated. He asserted that the initial consent given by the husband was "irrevocable". He also argued on the basis of the constitutional protection of the unborn. The best means of protection was implantation in the woman's womb.[22] His client, Mary Roche, told the court that her estranged husband was the father of the frozen embryos and that it was his duty to care for his children. Her husband had signed a contract taking responsibility for the outcome of IVF treatment. This included financial support for any children who might be born from the implantation of the three remaining embryos.[23]

Thomas Roche told the court that he believed the three embryos in question were only to be implanted if the IVF treatment was not initially successful. When his wife became pregnant in February 2002 no further discussions took place about another child. Therefore, he claimed, he now had a right not to have any more children with his wife, from whom he was now separated. Even so, he conceded that the contract he signed at the Sims Clinic in January 2002 meant that he would be the legal father of any "resulting child", and that no clause in the document allowed him to withdraw his consent. But John Rogers argued that the consent document was applicable only to fertilisation. If the court decided that implantation was to be covered by the document of consent, Thomas Roche should have a right to withdraw his consent. Otherwise his wife would have control over how many children she would have, leaving her husband with no say in the matter.[24]

The opinion of the Attorney General was that Thomas Roche could not withdraw his consent, regardless of the couple's separation. However, Rogers referred to a joint consent document signed by the couple which indicated that the three embryos in storage could not be defrosted without the consent of husband and wife. Events could arise, such as separation, which provided good reasons for withdrawal of consent. Furthermore, Rogers argued, it was not the policy in other states to compel a man to be a father against his will.[25] This point elicited support outside the courtroom when Liam O'Gogain, chairman of the support group Parental Equality, expressed the opinion that a case would be most unlikely to reach the High Court if a man insisted his former partner have their children against her will.[26]

The *Roche v. Roche* case was without precedent in Ireland, but not in other states. In Britain, Natalie Evans had sought permission to use her frozen embryos without the consent of her former partner, Howard Johnston. The case was heard in March 2007 in the European Court of Human Rights (ECHR). Johnston's objection to the use of the embryos was sustained. Still, the Irish case was seen as fundamentally different because of the constitutional dimension.[27]

In Ireland, more than one thousand births had occurred due to IVF. Increasing recourse to IVF was part of a wider trend in the EU. More women were delaying having children. In Ireland, career advancement and high house prices were seen as important contributory factors. With many couples delaying having children, female infertility was becoming increasingly frequent.[28] And in view of the thousands of couples seeking judicial separation and divorce every year it was virtually certain that a court case similar to the above would arise.[29]

There were two important issues to be addressed beyond considerations of contractual law: the status of the embryo; and parental rights. From an orthodox Catholic point of view the verdict was clear enough. David Quinn saw it as a case of a mother wishing for another child and her husband wishing not to become a father again. But he was already the father of the embryos. And the embryos were undeniably human. In terms of making the correct ethical choice, that settled the issue for Quinn. The rights of the embryo superseded parental rights.[30] If this assertion was upheld in Irish law it would have had dire consequences. If fatherhood could be imposed on Thomas Roche, then, in contrary circumstances, motherhood could be imposed on Mary Roche.[31] This was both ethically and politically untenable.

Pro-life ethics supported Mary Roche's legal action, although it was doubtful if the Constitution did so. Did the term "unborn" apply to early-stage embryos stored in laboratories? It was dubious in a constitutional sense and Quinn anticipated that a court ruling might create an "open season on embryos". He could not rely on the government to put matters right. Micheál Martin was reported to have agreed in principle to hESC research using supernumerary embryos from IVF procedures; and Quinn believed that if a government minister had expressed such an opinion ten or twenty years earlier he would have incurred "severe damage to his reputation". He was almost certainly correct. The same cannot be said for the conclusion he drew from his observation. Quinn believed that the reason Martin remained "almost entirely unscathed" was due to a greatly reduced concern about the destruction of "early" human life in Irish society.[32] This opinion was unsubstantiated. The *Report of the Commission on Assisted Human Reproduction* indicated that many people were not well informed about the issues involved and had not adopted firm opinions on a range of bioethical issues. Many of those who were well informed probably held nuanced views, mindful of the ethical complexities involved.

As legal proceedings continued with *Roche v. Roche*, another case came to light which gave an insight into the legal interpretation of "unborn". A woman, referred to as "D", had taken a case to the ECHR against Ireland. The case was first heard in September 2005. She claimed that the state had violated her human rights because Irish law denied her access to abortion in circumstances of "lethal foetal abnormality".[33] She was pregnant with twins. In her fourteenth week of pregnancy an ultrasound scan indicated that one foetus had died at about eight weeks. Amniocentesis confirmed a severe congenital abnormality (trisomy 18/ Edwards syndrome) in the second foetus. The prognosis was that the second foetus, if born alive, was most likely to die within a few days. The woman did not wish to let nature take its course and travelled to Britain to procure an abortion in January 2002.

The state challenged D's claim, arguing that she had not exhausted all the legal options open to her. What were her options? She did not meet the X Case criteria. Was abortion illegal in Ireland? The answer was yes – but not absolutely yes. The state argued, regarding Article 40.3.3 of the Constitution, that the X Case "demonstrated the potential for judicial development", notwithstanding the fact that the foetus in the X Case was viable. The courts were not likely to interpret Article 40.3.3 with "remorseless logic" in cases of "lethal genetic abnormality". If there was no significant possibility of the surviving foetus being born alive, there was "at least a tenable argument" that it was not "unborn" in an Irish constitutional sense. Even if it were judged to be "unborn", it could be argued in the Irish courts that "its right to life was not actually engaged" because "it had no prospect of life outside the womb."[34] The state was aware that some foetuses with trisomy 18 were born alive and that the median survival age was approximately six days. The diagnosis in this case was "fatal".[35]

The state contended that if the woman had won her case in Ireland she would have been able to procure an abortion in Ireland. In support of this point it pointed out that the three masters of the three largest maternity hospitals in the Republic had publicly stated, during the abortion referendum debate of 2002, that they would be willing to facilitate abortion in cases of lethal abnormality if there were no legal impediment. The ECHR found in favour of the state.[36]

On 18 July 2006, shortly after the ECHR judgment, Mr Justice McGovern ruled in favour of the husband in the *Roche v. Roche* case. He found that there was no contractual agreement between the husband and wife about what was to be done with the three embryos in the circumstances that had arisen. The purpose of freezing the embryos was to use them if the first implantation failed. The consent forms signed by the couple were defective because they lacked clarity on a number of important points. There was no provision made for contingencies that might arise, such as separation, divorce or death. If the court had found that the documents signed by the couple committed both of them to the implantation of the three remaining embryos, it would not have been deemed necessary to undertake an examination of the status of the embryos.[37] McGovern stated that, in the light of his judgment on consent, interconnected matters of public and constitutional law, including issues relating to family law and the status of embryos, would now have to be examined.[38] This evoked a sense of a case just beginning rather than ending.[39] It was now necessary to hear arguments for and against the proposition that the deep-frozen embryos were "unborn" in a constitutional sense. If the embryos were found to have a right to life, it would have to be decided if this was greater than the rights of the father. If the right to life took priority, the embryos could be implanted in their mother.[40] After hearing six days of testimony from experts, McGovern adjourned the case until the beginning of the new law term in October.[41]

The question of when human life begins seemed to be of central importance to the outcome of the case. From a "pro-life" perspective it was simple. Life began at fertilisation. Any other answer, such as life beginning at implantation, development beyond the possibility of twinning, when the primitive streak formed, the emergence of heartbeat, or the detection of brainwaves, seemed arbitrary and motivated by utilitarian and commercial motives. There was a considerable advantage of "logical simplicity" in the pro-life stance. And yet counsel for the Attorney General insisted that the High Court would not be called upon to identify the point at which human life begins.[42]

Constitutional protection for the rights of the embryo no longer seemed so secure. Archbishop Diarmuid Martin was concerned that a judge might make a decision on the constitutional importance of the human embryo in "an almost total legislative vacuum" and without much public debate. He expressed surprise that there was now a possibility that the Constitution might be interpreted to mean that a foetus would not be protected in Irish law if there was an indication that it would not survive long after birth.[43] Seán Brady, Archbishop of Armagh and Primate of All Ireland, stated that he did not understand how the erosion of protection for human embryos had occurred. The voice of the Roman Catholic Church needed to be heard.[44] Some government ministers probably did listen but, evidently, were not persuaded. There were more pressing concerns.

In the EU, science and enterprise ministers were due to vote on a €50 billion European science programme. Deep divisions persisted among the member states about the funding of hESC research. There was concern in Irish government circles that disagreement on this issue might cause delays in the implementation of the entire programme, estimated to be worth hundreds of millions of euro for science in Ireland. The Irish government delegation to the EU, led by Micheál Martin, maintained support for the principle of ethical subsidiarity, which seemed the best approach to attaining consensus. It was understood that the Irish government continued to support the policy of "pooled funding" for EU programmes and opposed the idea that individual EU states should be given the option of determining exactly what their financial contributions would or would not be used for.[45]

The funding of science in the context of EU politics took priority over the ethical concerns expressed by the Irish Catholic bishops. Developments within Ireland were to cause more discontent in Irish ecclesiastical circles. Judge Brian McGovern had already ruled on the issue of whether or not there was a legally binding contract in favour of Mary Roche. He found that no consent, express or implied, existed which would have granted her the right to have the three embryos implanted in her womb against the wishes of her estranged husband. The second issue was one of public interest, pertaining to the Constitution. It was on this issue that Judge McGovern delivered his High Court judgment on 15 November 2006.

McGovern addressed the question of whether or not the embryos in question were "unborn" in the context of Article 40.3.3 of the Constitution. Expert testimony had already confirmed that there was an absence of consensus in the medical and scientific communities about the moral status of early-stage human embryos. McGovern asserted that it was not within the competence of the High Court to give a decision about when human life begins. Scientific and medical expertise could describe in extensive detail the development of embryos and foetuses but could not determine when a human organism became a "human being". There were conflicting philosophical and religious opinions on the issue, but it was not the function of the judiciary to arbitrate here either.

It was the function of the law courts to interpret the law, not to uphold morality or a particular religious opinion. The interpretation of the law could not be satisfactorily concluded without reference to history. What had the people intended when the Eighth Amendment to the Constitution (1983) had given rise to Article 40.3.3? The historical record confirmed that Article 40.3.3 was associated with the issue of abortion. The intention had been to secure the prohibition against abortion as expressed in sections 58 and 59 of the Offences Against the Person Act 1861. Abortion was to be forbidden except in cases where there was a substantial risk to the life of the mother. The association of Article 40.3.3 with abortion indicated that the word "unborn" referred to a foetus or an embryo that had implanted in the uterus. In other words, an embryo created through IVF was not "unborn" because it was not in the uterus and therefore did not have the potential to be born. If IVF embryos were not "unborn" in a constitutional sense, then they did not have the protection of law. Limited protection was to be found in the *Medical Council's Guide to Ethical Conduct and Behaviour* (sixth edition, 2004). The Medical Council declared that "the deliberate and intentional destruction of *in vitro* human life already formed is professional misconduct" and that "any fertilised ovum must be used for normal implantation and must not be deliberately destroyed."[46] Medical doctors had good reason to fear a ruling of professional misconduct from the governing body of their profession. However, the ethical guidelines did not have the force of law.

McGovern acknowledged that what was legally permissible was not necessarily morally acceptable. In view of the absence of any legal sanctions, McGovern found that the status of embryos outside the womb was "precarious". It was the responsibility of the Oireachtas, or the people in a referendum, to decide what measures should be taken to establish the legal status of IVF embryos.[47]

It now seemed that hESC research was legally permissible in Ireland, and that it was not illegal to import hESC lines created outside the jurisdiction. This provoked criticism from pro-life supporters. Archbishop Diarmuid Martin expressed concern about what he saw as the apparent unreliability of constitutional protection for human life in its earliest stages of development.[48] The Pro Life Campaign argued that the rights of the embryo should not be adversely affected simply because it was outside rather than inside the womb.[49]

The pressing need for legislation was highlighted yet again, but the government showed little inclination of acting with any sense of urgency. It now seemed unlikely that it would introduce any legislative proposals for parliamentary debate before the next general election, which was due in summer 2007;[50] notwithstanding Mary Harney's press statement of 15 November 2006. She informed the public that she had already instructed officials at her department, Health and Children, "to begin preparing for legislation", mindful of the *Report of the Commission on Assisted Human Reproduction* and the outcome of the deliberations of the Oireachtas Joint Committee on Health and Children. Due consideration would also be given to the High Court judgment.[51]

Proceedings at a Joint Committee meeting, a few weeks after the McGovern judgment, indicated that some time was being given to IVF and related issues at the Department of Health and Children. On 12 December three officials from the department attended a session of the Joint Committee for discussions. They were Fergal Goodman, principal officer; Colette Bonner, deputy chief medical officer; and Liam McCormack, assistant principal officer. Goodman briefed the committee on the state of progress or – more accurately – the lack of it. Fiona

O'Malley asked if the heads of a Bill had been prepared.[52] Goodman replied that he and his colleagues understood that the minister did not wish them to "move directly to preparation of the legislation".[53] A range of competing and interlocking issues needed to be examined.[54] A number of important questions were under consideration in the department. What issues would impact on the remit of other departments? How should AHR services be regulated? Was a regulatory authority the best way of regulating AHR services? If a regulatory authority was set up, then to what extent should some issues be addressed under primary legislation and others directly by the Minister for Health and Children, or by the regulatory authority? What status would be granted to human embryos for the purpose of legislation? What guidelines or regulations should be applied to address the thorny question of supernumerary embryos created during IVF treatments? If donor programmes were permitted, this would raise issues of legal parentage and adoption.[55] If the state permitted the provision of AHR services, would this apply only to married heterosexual couples? If so, what were the implications for existing equal status legislation?[56]

An important point made by McCormack and Goodman was that developments in science and technology could create unforeseen difficulties for those who were in the process of drafting legislation. For example, a definition of "embryo" with reference only to the process of fertilisation could be challenged, as it had been in Britain, on the basis that there were other ways of creating embryos – for example, cloning by SCNT, which was used to create Dolly the sheep.[57]

Goodman informed the Joint Committee that the Department of Health was examining legislation and regulatory mechanisms in other jurisdictions. It was important not only to examine the text of legislation, but also to ascertain how it worked in practice. What worked well abroad might not work well in Ireland. Therefore, when considering policy options, it was necessary to undertake a study of how new legislation and regulatory protocols would impact on existing Irish legislation. Work had only advanced as far as "the initial phase". Outline policy proposals and options still needed to be developed. No specific legislative proposals were under consideration. Therefore, Goodman and his colleagues were not in a position to inform the committee about the nature of the proposed legislation or how extensive it would be.[58]

The question of regulating AHR clinics featured prominently in the Joint Committee's discussions. Was it possible to deal expeditiously with the regulation of AHR clinics and leave other issues to be addressed sometime in the future?[59] Liam McCormack questioned the prudence of proceeding with what he termed piecemeal legislation. If, for example, the donation of gametes (ova and spermatozoa) or embryos was permitted, this would impact on other legislation such as that relating to legal parentage. It did not seem possible to deal with specific ethical issues in isolation.[60] This policy position, taken at face value, seemed reasonable. But, from the political perspective of Liz McManus (Labour), "an easy way to avoid doing anything is to decide to do everything at once."[61] Her cynicism was well founded.

Frustration and disappointment were not the exclusive burdens of the political opposition in the Joint Committee. Fiona O'Malley, a member of the Progressive Democrats – the minor party in government – did not refrain from expressing her dissatisfaction.[62] She observed that rapid progress could be made if there was the political will to do so. Conversely, the absence of political will could obstruct progress indefinitely. There were no grounds for optimism that the government was about to push forward with legislation on AHR with a due sense of urgency.

Endnotes

1   Dáil Debates, vol. 606, no. 3, col. 1451 (4 October 2005); see also vol. 613, no. 4, col. 1793 (1 February 2006).
2   Patsy McGarry, Mark Brennock and Barry Roche, "Aherne elaborates on his defence of church", *Irish Times*, 12 November 2005.
3   Dáil Debates, vol. 618, no. 1, cols 306–307 (25 April 2006).
4   Ibid., vol. 620, no. 3, cols 767–768 (25 May 2006).
5   Catholic Communications Office, "Press Release 14 June 2006: Bishops express concern in advance of EU Parliament vote on funding of research on human embryos" <http://www.catholiccommunications.ie/Pressrel/14-june-2006.html> accessed 15 June 2006; and Fiona Gartland, "Bishops call over adult stem cell research", *Irish Times*, 15 June 2006, p. 7.
6   "Stem-cell research could get green light", *Catholic Herald and Standard*, 16 June 2006, p. 6.
7   David Quinn, "Minister in stem cell funding row", *Irish Catholic*, 22 June 2006, p. 1.
8   See Michael Kelly, "Church approves most stem cell research: How your MEP voted", *Irish Catholic*, 22 June 2006, p. 6.
9   Carol Glatz, "Vatican deplores EU's 'thick-headed' cloning vote", *Catholic Herald and Standard*, 23 June 2006, p. 4.
10 European Commission, "Research, funding: Seventh Framework Programme nears fruition" <http://ec.europa.eu/research/biosociety/news_events/news_seventh_framework_programme_fruition_en.htm> accessed 6 March 2007.
11 Commission of the Bishops' Conferences of the European Community, "Risk of Promoting the Destruction of Human Embryos", 26 July 2006 <http://www.zenit.org/english/visualizza.phtml?sid=93173> accessed 6 March 2007.
12 "Minister backs embryo research in Ireland", *Catholic Herald and Standard*, 30 June 2006, p. 6.
13 Irish Catholic Bishops' Conference, *Towards a Creative Response to Infertility: A Detailed Response of the Irish Catholic Bishops' Conference to the Report of the Commission on Assisted Human Reproduction* (Dublin: Veritas, 2006), Introduction.
14 Ibid., p. 32.
15 Ibid., p. 43.
16 Ibid., p. 44.
17 CrM NFP is the Creighton Model of Natural Family Planning, promoted

by the Pope Paul VI Institute in the USA. The institute was cofounded by Dr Thomas W. Hilgers and his wife Susan Hilgers. Research was carried out at St. Louis University and Creighton University. "About the Institute," Pope Paul VI Institute, 2006, <https://web.archive.org/web/20061121190654/http://www.popepaulvi.com/about.htm> accessed 7 April 2020.

18 Irish Catholic Bishops' Conference, *Towards a Creative Response to Infertility*, pp. 44–5.

19 Jill Allison, *Motherhood and Infertility in Ireland: Understanding the Presence of Absence* (Cork: Cork University Press, 2013), p. 113.

20 Joint Committee on Health and Children, 29JHC 1, no. 95, 4 July 2006 (Dublin: Stationery Office), cols 3094–3096, 3100–3105.

21 Olivia Kelly, "IVF report delayed pending court embryo case outcome", *Irish Times*, 7 July 2006, p. 4; and T.P. O'Mahony, "Status of the unborn has yet to be determined by Supreme Court", *Irish Examiner*, 19 July 2006, p. 7.

22 Carol Coulter, "Parties in frozen embryos row to hear how case will proceed", *Irish Times*, 4 July 2006, p. 1; and Mary Carolan, "Embryo case 'to raise question' of when life begins", *Irish Times*, 4 July 2006, p. 4.

23 Mary Carolan, "Woman expects husband to maintain any children", *Irish Times*, 6 July 2006, p. 4.

24 Mary Carolan, "Man wants no more children with his wife", *Irish Times*, 6 July 2006, p. 4.

25 Mary Carolan, "Counsel rejects AG's 'dramatic' position in embryos case", *Irish Times*, 7 July 2006, p. 4.

26 Siobhan Maguire and Dearbhail McDonald, "Playing with time", *Sunday Times*, 9 July 2006, p. 12.

27 Ibid.

28 Ibid.

29 The divorce rate rose to over 3,400 (in a population of slightly over four million) in 2005, nearly 2% over the rate in 2004. In the same period judicial separations dropped from 1,258 to 973. Seán McCárthaigh, "Number of couples divorcing rises 2% to more than 3,400", *Irish Examiner*, 19 July 2006, p. 8.

30 David Quinn, "'Spare' embryos are human. The courts must protect them", *Sunday Times*, 9 July 2006, p. 16.

31 In the Evans v. Johnston case at the ECHR, the right of Johnston not to be a father of a child born to Evans was defended with reference to the point that motherhood could not be forced on Evans. Deirdre Madden, *Medicine, Ethics and the Law* (Haywards Heath, UK: Bloomsbury Professional, 2016 (3rd edn)), pp. 257–8.

32 Quinn, "'Spare' embryos are human".

33 *Report of the Expert Group on the Judgment in A, B and C v. Ireland*, section 3.6.1.

34 ECHR, *D v. Ireland* (application number 26499/02), paragraph 69.

35 Ibid., paragraph 3. A case similar to "D" (*D (A Minor)*) came to the attention of the ECHR at a later date; ECHR, Grand Chamber judgment, *A, B and C v. Ireland* (application number 25579/05), 16 December 2010, paragraph 134.

36 Carol Coulter, "Widening the grounds for abortion" (p. 16) and "Foetus may not always be an unborn, argues State" (p. 1), both articles in the *Irish Times*, 14 July 2006.

37 Carol Coulter, "Case shows IVF consent forms must be clearer and broader", *Irish Times*, 19 July 2006, p. 4. See also Carol Coulter and Alison Healy, "New court hearing in embryos case opens tomorrow", *Irish Times*, 19 July 2006, p. 1.

38 "Husband's case on embryos upheld", *Irish Times*, 19 July 2006, p. 4.

39 Alison Healy, "Sense of a case just beginning, not ending", *Irish Times*, 19 July 2006, p. 4. See also Caroline O'Doherty, "Now the big question: should a frozen embryo be protected by the Constitution?", *Irish Examiner*, 19 July 2006, p. 1. There was some awareness in Ireland about similar debates elsewhere. In the USA, President George Bush vetoed a bill that was intended to extend federal funding for embryonic stem cell research. Funding was allowed only for stem cell lines created before 9 August 2001. The biotech industrial sector and scientists had pressed hard for the bill, arguing that access to more embryos for additional stem cell lines was critically important to push hESC research to its full biomedical potential. Denis Staunton, "Bush blocks federal funds for embryonic stem cell research", *Irish Times*, 20 July 2006, p. 11.

40 Caroline O'Doherty, "Father's consent forms did not address break-up", *Irish Examiner*, 19 July 2006, p. 6.

41 Expert evidence was given by: James Clinch, a retired obstetrician and gynaecologist, and a former master of the Coombe Hospital (Dublin); Eleonora Porcu, an Italian doctor with expertise in IVF research; Martin Clynes, professor of biotechnology at Dublin City University; Günter Rager, director of the Institute of Anatomy and Embryology at the University of Freiburg; Aonghus Nolan, a clinical embryologist who had served as a member of the CAHR; Mary Wingfield, a consultant gynaecologist, fertility specialist, and director of the Merrion Fertility Clinic in Dublin; and Maybeth Jamieson, a clinical embryologist at the Glasgow Royal Infirmary. Christine Newman, "Court hears case for embryo protection", *Irish Times*, 21 July 2006, p. 4; Mary Carolan, "Embryo is beginning of life, says doctor", *Irish Times*, 22 July 2006, p. 4; Mary Carolan, "Expert says inaction by lawmakers unforgivable", *Irish Times*, 22 July 2006, p. 4; Mary Carolan, "Science dictates that embryo is human being, expert tells court", *Irish Times*, 26 July 2006, p. 4; Mary Carolan, "Fertility treatment code 'unworkable'", *Irish Times*, 28 July 2006, p. 4; Mary Carolan, "IVF embryos can be adopted, expert tells court", *Irish Times*, 28 July 2006, p. 4; "British IVF laws require both parties' consent at all times", *Irish Times*, 29 July 2006, p. 4. All the expert testimony had been

heard except that of the Swiss embryologist Günter Rager. He had to return to Switzerland due to work commitments before his cross-examination was completed. Arrangements were made for the remainder of his evidence to be given by video link on 5 October. "Court adjourns embryos case", *Irish Times*, 1 August 2006, p. 4.

42   Eilis O'Hanlon, "Embryo case raises born-again question on the origins of life", *Sunday Independent*, 23 July 2006, p. 27.

43   Michael O'Regan, "Broader embryo debate urged by Dr Martin", *Irish Times*, 21 July 2006, p. 5.

44   Martin Wall, "'Informed discussion' of embryo rights urged", *Irish Times*, 21 July 2006, p. 5.

45   Martin Wall, "EU divided on stem-cell research funds", *Irish Times*, 24 July 2006, p. 7.

46   McGovern referred to Clause 24 in Section F, "Genetic Testing and Reproductive Medicine", of the *Medical Council's Guide to Ethical Conduct and Behaviour* (6th edn, 2004).

47   "Judgment of Mr. Justice McGovern delivered on the 15th day of November 2006", Neutral Citation [2006] IEHC 359 <http://www.bailii.org/ie/cases/IEHC/2006/H359.html> accessed 22 December 2009. See also articles in the *Irish Times*, 16 November 2006: Gerry Whyte, "High Court had to determine what word unborn meant" (p. 18); Mary Carolan, "Woman loses bid to have embryos implanted" (p. 4) and "Existence of embryos outside womb 'precarious'" (p. 4).

48   Catholic Communications Office, "Press Release 15 November 2006: Statement of Archbishop Diarmuid Martin" <http://www.catholiccommunications.ie/Pressrel/15-november-2006.html> accessed 21 November 2006.

49   Paul Cullen, "Mixed reactions but most agree legislation is needed", *Irish Times*, 16 November 2006, p. 4.

50   Paul Cullen, "Fertility treatment law likely to face delay" (p. 1), and Liam Reid, "Government undecided on embryo law" (p. 4); both articles in the *Irish Times*, 16 November 2006.

51   Mary Harney, "Statement by Mary Harney TD, Minister for Health and Children, on the R v R: High Court Frozen Embryos Case", 15 November 2006 <http://www.dohc.ie/press/releases/2006/20061115.html> accessed 10 March 2007. On 5 July 2006 Mary Harney had written to the Joint Committee on Health and Children to inform it that she had instructed her officials "to prepare the legislation for a specific scheme of statutory regulation of assisted human reproduction". Joint Committee on Health and Children, 29JHC 1, no. 111, 12 December 2006 (Dublin: Stationery Office), cols 3667–3668.

52   Joint Committee on Health and Children, 12 December 2006, col. 3670.

53   Ibid., col. 3672.

54 Ibid., col. 3671.
55 Ibid., cols 3666–3667.
56 Ibid., col. 3679.
57 Ibid., cols 3674, 3678.
58 Ibid., col. 3667.
59 Ibid., col. 3675.
60 Ibid., col. 3678
61 Ibid., col. 3673.
62 Ibid., cols 3669–3670.

CHAPTER FOUR

————— • —————

Embryos and the Right to Life

2006–2011

Human Embryos, Immortal Souls and the Right to Life

IN THE HIGH COURT CASE OF *MARY Roche v. Thomas Roche and Others*
(2006) the McGovern judgment seemed to be sound from a legal
perspective. It was questionable if considered in terms of moral philosophy.
Why should the status of the embryo be adversely affected if it was
located outside the womb? The Irish Catholic bishops, in their critique
of the *Report of the Commission on Assisted Human Reproduction*, asserted
that there was no scientific or philosophical basis for this.[1] Dr Berry
Kiely, spokesperson for the Pro Life Campaign, argued that the idea that
legal protection of embryos should only apply from implantation was
arbitrary.[2] Early-stage human embryos had some status – whatever that
status might be – and it seemed difficult to contend that such a status
would be affected by their location. This is not so straightforward when
potentiality is considered. An embryo in the womb has some prospect
of further development. An embryo in a laboratory environment does
not – unless it is transferred to a receptive womb.

Kiely believed that the human embryo, regardless of its location, was
"not potential human life" – it was "human life with potential". David
Quinn, a former editor of the *Irish Catholic* newspaper, placed great
emphasis on the fact that the three embryos in the Roche case were
undoubtedly human.[3] Professor William Reville, writing before the

outcome of the court case, gave the matter more extensive treatment in the *Irish Times*. He believed that there was "a strong case, consistent with science" for "the full humanity of the embryo". Human life begins at conception and every subsequent stage of development "occurs on a continuum and each is the full expression of humanity appropriate to its stage". Conception is a momentous qualitative "instant" and it is therefore logical to regard human life as beginning at this point. To choose otherwise would be arbitrary. To bolster his argument, Reville claimed that the human zygote (fertilised ovum) is not "qualitatively different" from a human adult – it is only "quantitatively different".[4]

Reville's conclusion was highly questionable. Scientific findings inform, but do not determine, conclusions in moral philosophy. Alternative interpretations of science frequently lead to entirely different conclusions. A human adult comprises billions of cells, most of which are highly specialised and highly organised. The human brain is the most complex organisation of matter known to scientists. A zygote, in stark contrast, is an unspecialised cell. It has no organs, no brain – not even the beginnings of a nervous system. No matter how special a cell it is, it is qualitatively different from a human adult, regardless of its potential. Therefore, there is a formidable argument, grounded in science, that there are a number of qualitative processes in human development, such as the formation of the "primitive streak" and the formation of synapses (connections between neurons). Both of these processes are essential for the formation of the nervous system and are momentous developments in a qualitative rather than a quantitative sense.

If by using phrases such as "the full humanity of the embryo" and "qualitatively different" Reville meant that the early-stage embryo, like the human adult, deserved full human rights, this would then have some far-reaching consequences. In this context, legal protection applied to the early-stage embryo (sometimes referred to as a "pre-embryo") would mean that IVF procedures would have to be changed so that no supernumerary embryos were generated. Restrictions against human embryonic stem cell (hESC) research would be consolidated because the harvesting of stem cells generally destroyed embryos.[5] Birth-control products which worked by preventing implantation of embryos in the womb would be illegal. The cumulative effect of all this, if legislated for, would probably have greatly weakened support for the Pro Life Campaign. If "pro-life" activists conceded on these points – i.e. if they insisted on protecting early-stage embryos only in the context of hESC research – such an inconsistency would have undermined the credibility of their position.

The logical simplicity of the pro-life argument exerted a powerful appeal. Human life begins with the union of ovum and spermatozoon. The resulting zygote is undeniably human and is definitely alive. Its genetic code is human. Yet labouring the point that human life begins when the ovum is fertilised does not settle the argument. Human zygotes and other human totipotential cells have the potential to develop into a human individual. To what extent early-stage embryos should be granted legal protection on the basis of their potentiality is highly debatable. It has been argued, for example, that terminating a pregnancy before a person exists is not morally objectionable because "the idea that a merely potential person can be harmed makes no sense."[6] Still, invoking the concept of personhood as a basis for the right to life is not without its problems – this will be examined later in this chapter and in the Appendix.

Catholic ethicists expressed different opinions about the status of early-stage embryos.[7] Ethicists who argued that early-stage embryos should not be granted full human rights tended to base their opinions on two observations. First, many early-stage embryos perish. Second, irreversible individuation is regarded as an essential precondition for personal human life.[8] The first argument is based on the idea that the importance of the early-stage embryo is greatly diminished by a very high mortality rate (estimates vary widely).[9] There is a formidable counterargument to this – the fact that nature frequently terminates human life does not give persons in positions of authority the right to do likewise. Would a high infant mortality rate, from natural causes, justify infanticide? Very few people would answer yes! Still, the high mortality rate of early-stage embryos raised a difficult question for those theologians who defended the official teaching of the Roman Catholic Church: if early-stage embryos are so highly valued, why does God, through natural/secondary causes, allow so many of them to perish?[10] Also, some cells in early-stage embryos can give rise to hydatidiform moles, some of which turn cancerous, with possibly fatal consequences for the woman.[11]

Some authors who challenged the belief that personhood begins at fertilisation emphasised the importance of individuality. They pointed out that genetic uniqueness and individuality are two different things. A unique genetic code does not inevitably give rise to an individual. An early-stage embryo can undergo fission to give identical twins.

In very rare cases two embryos, genetically different from each other, can fuse to form one individual. Twinning can occur when early-stage embryonic cells are in a totipotential state. Individuality is almost certainly established at about fourteen days post-fertilisation, when the primitive streak is formed. This is highly significant for those who advocate hESC research. Individuality, as indicated earlier, is an essential precondition for personhood.[12] Personhood is indivisible – it cannot be shared by two or more individuals. Since early-stage embryos can divide to give more than one individual there is good reason to believe that they are not entitled to full human rights. The argument from irreversible individuation is open to some disagreement, depending on how one interprets the latest data in embryology.

The Congregation for the Doctrine of the Faith asserted in *Donum Vitae* that "the human being is to be respected and treated as a person from the moment of conception and therefore from that same moment his rights as a person must be recognized." The Congregation declared itself familiar with the current debates about human individuality and "the identity of the human person". It asked rhetorically, "how could a human individual not be a human person?" But it did not attempt to elaborate. The congregation simply stated that the teaching authority had "not expressly committed itself to an affirmation of a philosophical nature".[13] Philosophers were unable to reach a consensus on personhood, and it was extremely unlikely that they would do so.[14]

It was prudent of the congregation not to attempt a definition of when personhood begins because there was so much to discover about this subject.[15] Any such definition would have been difficult to defend, and would need to be revised in the light of newly emerging data from research on neural development and psychology. And, most important of all in the context of hESC research, it would have been irrelevant. Embryonic stem cells are extracted from human early-stage embryos at about five days post-fertilisation. At this point, there is not even a primitive nervous system. Therefore, it could not have any mental faculties. How, then, could an early-stage embryo be regarded as a person? This has implications for Catholic theology concerning the spiritual soul. The immortal soul is defined as "a spiritual element" that survives death and is "endowed with consciousness and will, so that the 'human self' subsists".[16] It was argued that irreversible developmental individuation is necessary before God can infuse a soul into a physical body.[17] In other words, two or more persons cannot share a spiritual soul.

In its *Declaration on Procured Abortion* (18 November 1974), the Sacred

Congregation for the Doctrine of the Faith acknowledged that there was no consensus among Catholic scholars about when the immortal/spiritual soul is "infused".[18] Science had nothing to contribute to such a debate because the issue was deemed to be essentially philosophical and moral. Science could be marginalised because: (1) an early-stage embryo without an immortal soul "is still nothing less than a human life, preparing for and calling for a soul"; (2) the presence of an immortal soul could not be ruled out – "one can never prove the contrary" – so it was not morally permissible to risk "killing a man [*sic*] ... already in possession of his [*sic*] soul".[19] The Irish Catholic bishops were rather more optimistic about the illuminating potential of science when they declared in their pastoral letter *Human Life is Sacred* (May 1975) that the "view which is most in harmony with modern science is that the spiritual soul is present from the first moment of conception".[20] There was no rational basis for this assertion. Furthermore, there is no "moment of conception" – conception is a process of about 26 to 32 hours.[21]

That the human early-stage embryo is a person is highly implausible, but not implausible enough for the teaching authority of the Church. In his encyclical *Evangelium Vitae* (1995), Pope John Paul II stated that "the mere probability that a human person is involved would suffice to justify an absolutely clear prohibition of any intervention aimed at killing a human embryo."[22] From the text of the encyclical it is clear that the word "embryo" included the early-stage embryo. John Paul reiterated the point that the presence of a spiritual soul could not be ascertained by science. He then stated that the science of embryology provided "a valuable indication for discerning by the use of reason a personal presence at the moment of the first appearance of human life: how could a human individual not be a human person?"[23] Evidently the Pope and his advisors did not understand some of the elementary points about early-stage embryos. And what was meant by "a personal presence"? It was acknowledged by the Congregation for the Doctrine of the Faith in its *Instruction Dignitas Personae: On Certain Bioethical Questions* (8 September 2008) that – because it wished "to avoid a statement of an explicitly philosophical nature" – it had not defined the embryo as a person.[24] There was no philosophical or scientific basis for doing so.[25] Thus the congregation resorted to an arbitrary and obscure theological pronouncement to sustain its position when it declared that "there is an intrinsic connection between the ontological dimension and the specific value of every human life."[26]

The polar opposite of the official Catholic stance on the status of early-stage embryos is to view them as mere biological cells to be used without any ethical constraints. Both are extreme opinions. There is a nuanced and moderate intermediate opinion. The potential of early-stage embryos to develop into human persons is not an insignificant quality when assessing their status. The potentiality of an embryo or foetus serves as a basis for according it some value and respect.[27] It can be reasonably argued that early-stage embryos do not have an absolute right to life and that any rights that they may have should be balanced against other rights. A case in point is the judgment of the European Court of Human Rights (ECHR, not an institution of the EU)[28] concerning *Evans v. the United Kingdom*. Natalie Evans, a British national, underwent fertility treatment at Bath Assisted Conception Clinic from July 2000 to November 2001. Six embryos were created and shortly afterwards Evans had her ovaries removed because of a pre-cancerous condition. The early-stage embryos created through IVF offered her the only hope of becoming a mother of children genetically related to her. She was informed that she would have to wait for two years before the embryos could be implanted in her womb. In the meantime, her relationship with her partner, Howard Johnston, broke down. He subsequently initiated legal proceedings under the terms of the Human Fertilisation and Embryology Act 1990 to deny Evans access to the embryos and to terminate their preservation. Evans challenged this through the British courts and lost. On 26 January 2005 she was informed by the clinic that it was legally obligated to destroy the embryos and intended to do so on 23 February. Evans then took her case to the ECHR in Strasbourg to prevent this. On 10 April 2007 the ECHR ruled against her with reference to articles 2, 8, and 14 of the European Convention on Human Rights. It found that the early-stage embryos did not have a right to life in the context of Article 2. Johnston was found to have a right to withdraw consent to implantation. His assertion that he had a right not to become a father took priority.[29]

In the EU the status of the early-stage embryo seemed to be enhanced when considered in the context of hESC research. Ethics review was an important feature of the European Commission's Seventh Framework Programme (2007–2013). It was reported that research proposals which satisfied scientific criteria were subjected to rigorous ethical evaluation. There were very few research projects using human hESCs and the ethics review was especially demanding. It was essential for the grant applicant to show that hESCs were necessary for the proposed research – that is, that there were no satisfactory alternatives to achieving the same or a similar result.[30]

A philosophical and legal approach to complex issues tends to see them in terms of competing rights rather than in terms of absolute rights. The Commission on Assisted Human Reproduction did not view human early-stage embryos as persons with an absolute right to life. Otherwise it would not have recommended that supernumerary embryos from IVF procedures could be donated for research or allowed to perish. However, it also recommended that the creation of embryos specifically for research, using IVF, should not be permitted.[31]

The commission surveyed Irish public opinion in the course of its research. It noted that opinions about assisted human reproduction (AHR) ranged from opposition to all procedures relating to the treatment of infertility to the approval of every medical intervention that had been devised. Opinions about AHR and the status of embryos varied across a "continuum". At one extreme, protection of human life was obligatory from conception onwards. At the opposite extreme embryos and foetuses were seen as cellular material – undeserving of respect and sacrificed at will.[32]

The Irish Catholic bishops, in their detailed response to the *Report of the Commission on Assisted Human Reproduction*, denied the existence of a "continuum". There was no continuum because there were no intermediate positions between those who believed that early-stage embryos deserved full human rights and those who did not. The bishops were critical of the commission's survey of public opinion because they believed that important moral issues relating to respect for human life and dignity should not be decided on the basis of opinion polls.[33] This was a reasonable criticism if applied only to opinion polls. It raised the thorny question about how important moral decisions should be made. Through referendums and Acts of parliament? The bishops did not accept democracy as the final arbiter. They were aware of Pope John Paul II's teachings on the subject. In *Evangelium Vitae* John Paul condemned practices that did not respect the right to life, even when such practices were sanctioned not only by parliamentary majorities but by the majority of the people.[34] Decisions made on the basis of a democratic process are only good if consistent with Catholic moral principles. Something intrinsically evil cannot be transformed into something good simply by a majority vote. This was all very well, but who was to decide what was good or evil, moral or immoral? The Irish Catholic hierarchy claimed that the teaching authority of the Church was the infallible arbiter of morality. Many Roman Catholics, in Ireland and elsewhere, who were mindful of the Church's moral teachings did not seem to have confidence in such a claim.[35]

Senator Mullen's Bill

Breakthroughs in science seemed to diminish the importance of hESC research. In August 2006 Kazutoshi Takahashi and Shinya Yamanaka of Kyoto University in Japan announced that they had generated pluripotent cells (cells that can generate all cell types but cannot develop into an entire organism) from mouse fibroblasts. Cells were manipulated to change from a specialised condition to an embryonic-type condition. These cells were referred to as induced pluripotent stem cells (iPSCs).[36] The objective of achieving similar progress with human cells intensified and soon yielded results. In November 2007 two research teams reported success: Takahashi, Yamanaka and their fellow researchers in Japan; and James Thomson and his colleagues in the University of Wisconsin, Madison.[37] The human iPSCs were very similar to hESCs, although not identical.[38] It was anticipated that this achievement would lead to further developments which would enable scientists to generate patient- and disease-specific iPSCs. These cells were very likely to facilitate major contributions to research concerned with toxicology, diseases and drug screening.[39]

Scientists engaged in stem cell research were aware that it was easy to exaggerate the importance of what had been achieved. Viruses were used to transport four genes into adult skin cells, rather than activating the appropriate genes that were already in the cell nuclei. There was a high risk of tumour formation associated with this method. Safety issues had to be addressed before iPSCs could be used for regenerative medicine. Further research needed to be done before iPSCs could be used instead of hESCs.[40] Also, it was of major significance that both the American and Japanese research teams had relied "entirely" on data derived from embryonic stem cell research.[41]

The level of support for undertaking hESC research among Irish scientists was unclear but it was substantial. On 28 October 2008 the governing body of University College Cork issued a statement supportive of hESC research. This applied to cell lines derived from embryos, subject to strict ethical guidelines.[42] It was reported that the governing body's decision was carried by sixteen votes to fifteen with nine abstentions.[43] The narrowness of the victory for those who supported hESC research indicated just how divisive the issue was. Trinity College Dublin followed the precedent set by UCC when it put in place its own internal guidelines allowing for the use of imported hESC lines in scientific research.

The controversy about hESC research never reached centre stage in public debate, which was dominated by issues such as the government's enormous budget deficit, controversial spending cuts, rapidly growing unemployment, and the instability of the banking sector. The Irish economy was seen as particularly vulnerable in the midst of a deepening global economic crisis. All these issues distracted public attention from arguments for and against hESC research. However, those who actively opposed hESC research were not so distracted and sought allies in the Oireachtas.

On 20 November 2008 independent senator Rónán Mullen introduced his Stem-Cell Research (Protection of Human Embryos) Bill 2008 to the Seanad.[44] The purpose of the Bill was to regulate stem cell research. This required the prohibition of "embryo-destructive" research and a number of other similar kinds of research activity. These included the creation of embryos specifically for research purposes, the creation of human clones and the creation of human–animal hybrids for research. Mullen pointed to human adult stem cells (hASCs) and iPSCs as superior alternatives. He observed that sound ethics and good science were mutually supportive.[45]

The Bill received its second reading in the Seanad on 26 November. Mullen pointed to the "unilateral decision" by University College Cork as "the context for the introduction" of the Bill to the Seanad. Human adult stem cell research was presented in glowing terms. It was consistent with the highest standards of ethics and compassion in the biomedical sciences. It was "noble". It promoted social cohesion because it was not controversial. It represented an efficient use of scarce resources. Human adult stem cell research had led to "wonderful therapeutic successes" – 73 clinical treatments for diseases, including some cancers and Crohn's disease. Additionally, hundreds of clinical trials were in progress, generating confidence in future efficacy. In contrast, hESC research was unethical – the term "embryo-destructive research" was repeated a number of times for persuasive effect. It was extremely inefficient – it had not led to a single clinical trial and was nowhere near giving rise to a therapeutic treatment. The tendency for ESCs to form tumours was a major obstacle to clinical applications. The gross economic inefficiency of hESC research was more than enough to justify a denial of public funding at a time of rapidly deteriorating public finances. Ireland had to choose between investing in either hESC or hASC research. It did not have sufficient resources to achieve standards of excellence in both.[46]

Mullen anticipated that iPSCs might make hESC research obsolete "in the future" – although he prudently refrained from saying how soon that might be. Also, he claimed that the scientific advances that had led to the creation of iPSCs had not arisen from research on embryos.[47] Evidently, the intention here was to forcefully drive home the point that hESC research was not only unethical, it was also a scandalous waste of scarce resources. But this claim was simply not true. As indicated earlier, hESC research had played a central role in the creation of iPSCs.[48]

Mullen and many of his fellow senators lacked scientific expertise and had been briefed before the parliamentary session by a Professor McConnell – probably David McConnell, Professor of Genetics at Trinity College Dublin. However, Mullen disagreed with McConnell on the point that iPSC research was "inextricably tied to the continuation of embryo research."[49] This point was of great importance to Mullen and those who supported him because, if sustained, it would help to further undermine the credibility of hESC research, which now seemed to be totally without merit. Many scientists would have disagreed with Mullen's claim. The previous year, Shinya Yamanaka and his fellow scientists had observed that further research was necessary to determine whether or not iPSCs could replace hESCs in biomedical research.[50] In a "leading edge" review essay published in *Cell* (3 April 2009), Yamanaka observed that, although the potential of iPSC technology was enormous, it was still in its infancy. There were still a number of difficulties blocking the application of stem cells to clinical applications which were common to both ESCs and iPSCs – not least the tendency of both cell types to form teratomas (germ cell tumours comprising several types of cell). In a clinical application, even if a few cells in an iPSC population were undifferentiated, or were aberrantly reprogrammed, this could lead to the formation of cancer-causing cells.[51] Human ESCs were still the "gold standard" in stem cell research and would continue to be for quite some time to come.[52]

If Mullen was correct in his claims about stem cells – if hESC research was so lacking in credibility – it led to the question: why were so many scientists in favour of it? The senator's speech indicated that they were either dishonest or professionally compromised. Mullen referred to an article in the journal *Cell Proliferation* that criticised those who supported hESC research for propagating false claims and expressing unjustified optimism about its potential benefits. Generating false hope to gain government funding was condemned as unethical.[53]

Mullen had explicitly framed his arguments against hESC research on the basis of "the philosophy of human rights". He had not made any reference to either Christian or specifically Catholic ethics. In view of this, it is interesting to observe that the issue of *Cell Proliferation* (February 2008) that seems to have profoundly informed his thinking on stem cell research, was a special supplementary issue that facilitated the advocacy of opinions about stem cells consistent with the official teaching of the Roman Catholic Church.[54] The articles were based on papers presented at an international conference, *Stem Cells: What Future for Therapy? Scientific Aspects and Bioethical Problems*. Generous financial support for the conference was provided by the pro-life Jérôme Lejeune Foundation (Lejeune was a friend of Pope John Paul II and served as president of the Pontifical Academy for Life shortly before his death in 1994). The conference was jointly organised by the World Federation of Catholic Medical Associations (FIAMC) and the Pontifical Academy for Life and was held in Rome (14–16 September 2006). The guest editors for this issue of *Cell Proliferation* were Gian Luigi Gigli, professor of neurology at the University of Udine (Italy) and past president of the FIAMC; and Elio Sgreccia, former professor of bioethics, Catholic University Medical School, Rome, and president of the Pontifical Academy for Life.[55] Pope Benedict's address to the conference was published in this supplemental issue of the journal.[56] It is likely that a secular philosophy of human rights was not entirely responsible for inspiring the Bill and that orthodox Roman Catholic theology exerted a profound influence at a deeper level.

Near the conclusion of his speech Mullen referred to IVF to make the point that the Bill was not concerned with human reproduction issues. The sourcing of hESCs from supernumerary early-stage embryos indicated a strong link between hESC research and IVF – yet IVF was not to be covered by the proposed legislation. Mullen hoped to win the support of people who supported IVF as currently practised. He speculated that people who supported IVF and the use of the "morning-after" pill might support the principles upon which his Bill was based.[57] However, to do so would have been ethically inconsistent. From Mullen's perspective it seemed to be of paramount importance to save early-stage embryos from scientists willing to sacrifice them to advance biomedical science. Evidently, it was less urgent that IVF procedures be reformed so that no "supernumerary" embryos were created – a practice which, even in the absence of hESC research, frequently led to the loss of embryos. There was no sense of urgency in addressing birth control measures which, it was sometimes believed, destroyed early-stage embryos by preventing their implantation.[58] It seemed that all early-stage embryos were not of equal status after all – those that were seen as under threat from scientists were more worthy of protection than others.[59]

Senators Jim Walsh and John Hanafin jointly seconded Mullen's Bill. Walsh criticised the proactive policy of University College Cork on stem cell research and referred with approval to Professor William Reville's "Life Continuum", published in the university magazine, *UCC News* (May 2008). According to Walsh, Reville had contacted him and other politicians about hESC research.[60] It is very likely that proponents on both sides of the debate were vigorously lobbying for political support.

Jimmy Devins, Minister of State at the Department of Enterprise, Trade and Employment, addressed the Seanad to explain the government's position. The Department of Health and Children had begun the preparatory work for drafting legislation on stem cell research and a range of related issues. For guidance on such complex issues it had undertaken a detailed examination of legislation and other regulatory mechanisms in other states. A long-awaited report from the Oireachtas Joint Committee on Health and Children had still not been submitted. The High Court case of Mary Roche versus Thomas Roche had been appealed to the Supreme Court. The government did not intend to propose legislation until it had received the Joint Committee report and had the benefit of the Supreme Court judgment.[61] The decision on hESC research by the governing body of University College Cork was in stark contrast to the government's stance on the issue. As pointed out by Senator Alex White (Labour Party), the university had actually made a decision after careful consideration of the question. White rejected the claim that, in an Irish context, hESC and hASC research were mutually exclusive for economic reasons. He was also sharply critical of the tendency to demonise scientists for, supposedly, propagating false hopes to gain government funding.[62]

Senator Ivana Bacik (Labour Party) declared her opposition to the Bill. Human ESC research had greater potential than hASC research in the future treatment of diseases, especially neurodegenerative diseases such as Parkinson's and Alzheimer's. Bacik emphasised the word "potential" to avoid misrepresentation or misunderstanding of this point. She advocated that it should be permissible to use embryos up to a maximum of 14 days' development, subject to the consent of parents. To bolster her position, she argued that an early-stage human embryo stored long-term in liquid nitrogen "is not the same as a seven year old girl with leukaemia … a 32 year old woman with multiple sclerosis or a

55 year old man with Parkinson's disease."[63]

Senator David Norris (independent) did not believe that an early-stage embryo was "a full human being". Norris was trenchant in his criticism of emotive terms such as "embryo-destructive" and the invocation of human rights. The underlying influence behind the Bill, he believed, was not human rights philosophy but Roman Catholic theology. Norris pointed to an omission of central importance – Mullen had somehow omitted in his speech to the Seanad the fact that research on hESCs had enabled scientists to identify the few genes that were necessary to bring about pluripotency in adult cells.[64]

Mullen rejected Norris's contention that his Bill was inspired by theology. He asserted that his outlook was "informed by science, that human life is present in its individuality and momentum from the earliest stage".[65] This was a misunderstanding of the scientific evidence because, as already observed, individuality is not established at the "earliest stage" of human life.

Mullen's emphasis on human rights and science may have been influenced by William Reville, who was well known for his opposition to hESC research in Ireland. In his "Life Continuum" essay, Reville declared himself a Catholic, although, he informed his readers, he disagreed with the Church on some issues, including artificial contraception and IVF. His opinions were informed by "biological facts" and human rights considerations and were not based on religious doctrine. Adopting a somewhat defiant posture against ecclesiastical authority, he asserted that if the Catholic Church changed its position on hESC research, he would not do likewise.[66] To what extent Reville's outlook was shared by his co-religionists was uncertain, but his article did indicate that some Catholics were concerned to distance themselves from the official teaching of their Church on issues of sexual morality and bioethics, which has been discredited, and continued to be discredited, since the publication of *Humanae Vitae*. There seemed to be a tendency among Catholics who trenchantly opposed hESC research to deny any attribution of religious motives – as if the invocation of Catholic doctrine would damage the credibility of their views.

Roche v. Roche: Supreme Court Judgment

The economic crash, pay cuts in the public service sector, the devastating impact of flooding throughout the country, power cuts, and the ongoing revelations about paedophile priests pushed bioethical issues to the outer margins of public consciousness. On 2 December 2009 the Stem-Cell Research (Protection of Human Embryos) Bill 2008 was withdrawn from further consideration in the Seanad.[67] However, bioethical issues did not disappear from public attention. On 15 December, the Supreme Court issued its judgment on the *Roche v. Roche* case, which had been appealed from the High Court. Mr Justice Brian McGovern's ruling was upheld. It had not been established that there was any contractual agreement, express or implied, requiring the implantation of the embryos. Even if there had been an agreement it did not follow that it would have been irrevocable.

The Supreme Court found that IVF embryos were not "unborn" in the context of Article 40.3.3. A contrary judgment would have presented major difficulties for the state. Ms Justice Susan Denham observed that if the frozen embryos were "unborn" in the context of Article 40.3.3, state intervention would be necessary to facilitate their implantation. The state would be duty-bound to protect all embryos within its jurisdiction, in all hospitals, clinics, laboratories, etc. – regardless of the wishes of the parents. This in turn would clash with the rights of the family acknowledged in the Constitution (Article 41). When interpreting the Constitution, it was "appropriate to seek a harmonious construction" so that articles did not conflict with each other.[68] Furthermore, Article 40.3.3 was written on the basis of competing rights of mother and embryo (or foetus). It did not uphold the right to life of the unborn as an absolute right. This balance of rights clearly pointed to a physical connection between mother and embryo – i.e. pregnancy – which clearly did not apply in the case of frozen embryos. The balance of competing rights between the mother and father of the early-stage embryos also needed to be addressed. Denham believed that if "a party" did not already have a child and did not have any prospect of having a child, this would be "a relevant factor for consideration". All the factors needed to be considered. In this case the plaintiff already had two children. She was separated from her husband, who did not want any more children with her.[69]

Mr Justice Adrian Hardiman pointed to the problems arising from the attachment of excessive rights to early-stage human embryos. A very limited number of embryos would be produced in the course of an IVF treatment, lowering the chances of a successful outcome and exposing patients to greater stress and pain. Hardiman stated that, in normal circumstances, the "great majority" of fertilised ova perish.[70] Such events were not "generally regarded, medically, clinically, socially, legally or privately, as equivalent to a life in being". If early-stage embryos were regarded as equal in status to "a life in being", this "would lead to the outlawing of one of the most widely used methods of contraception which operates by the prevention of implantation."

Hardiman argued that human embryos deserve respect and that the state has an obligation to legislate with this in mind. This was urgent in view of the speed of scientific developments. A range of complex legal cases were bound to arise concerning AHR. Hardiman observed that experience had shown that "given a sufficient period of time, almost every conceivable set of facts will occur and may give rise to litigation." Litigation in a legislative vacuum was clearly not in the public interest. Failure to legislate could lead to circumstances where Ireland would be "an unregulated environment for practices which might prove controversial".[71]

The Supreme Court judges emphasised that there was a pressing need for the Oireachtas to address IVF and related issues. Their ruling on the *Roche v. Roche* case received widespread coverage in the national press.[72] The case was highly significant because the Supreme Court had found that constitutional protection did not extend to human embryos outside the womb. Embryos did not have any legal protection and could be used for research and/ or destroyed in the absence of regulatory controls.[73]

Arguments For and Against Human Embryonic Stem Cell Research

No legislative proposals, concerning stem cell research and AHR, had been put before parliament. It was now four years after the publication of the *Report of the Commission on Assisted Human Reproduction*. It was clear that politicians, especially those of the governing parties, had been negligent in this matter. The *Report of the Commission on Assisted Human Reproduction* had been submitted by the government to the Oireachtas Joint Committee on Health and Children to help it make decisions about recommendations requiring legislation and those that might need to be brought before the people for the purpose of amending the Constitution. It seems that there was little enthusiasm for putting forward any positive proposals based on the report of the commission. The committee did not publish a report on legislative proposals. It was against this background of political inertia that the Department of Health felt compelled to deny that it was procrastinating.[74]

Although it was now clear that hESC research was not unconstitutional, and not legally prohibited in the Republic of Ireland, this did not create conditions under which it could prosper. There was no legislation under which it could be regulated and the absence of regulation in turn created uncertainty that acted as a brake on investment. Several scientists, whose names were not disclosed, had expressed an interest in working with hESCs and a few had submitted grant applications to Science Foundation Ireland. However, as 2009 drew to a close, no public funding agency in Ireland had yet provided support for hESC research.[75]

The absence of regulation was unsatisfactory for those on both sides of the ethical divide. The Pro Life Campaign felt compelled to adopt a proactive stance. Members of the organisation expressed disappointment at the Supreme Court judgment and insisted, at a press conference in Dublin, that the ruling did not prevent the government legislating to protect early-stage human embryos. The campaign's legal adviser, Professor William Binchy of Trinity College Dublin, claimed that it was possible that constitutional and legislative protection could be put in place that did not conflict with fertility practices that were widely supported. He believed that an Oireachtas committee should examine the issue in detail.[76] Politicians, especially those of the governing parties, were not deeply committed to such an undertaking. An indication of this was the decision by the Department of Enterprise, Trade and Employment to terminate the funding of the Irish Council for Bioethics in December 2010.[77]

In ordinary circumstances the Irish Catholic bishops would have expressed strong opinions about the Supreme Court judgment – but the bishops did not find themselves in ordinary circumstances. Commissions of enquiry chaired by Justice Seán Ryan and Judge Yvonne Murphy shed new light on the horrendous sexual, psychological and physical abuse of children at the hands of religious brothers and priests over many years. The Ryan Report (May 2009) and the Murphy Report (November 2009) revealed that such abuse was pervasive. Surveys of case histories extending over the previous decades indicated a gross moral deficit in the upper echelons of the institutional Church in Ireland. It was against this backdrop that the resignation of Donal Murray, Bishop of Limerick, was announced on 17 December 2009, two days after the Supreme Court judgment. The bishop's resignation was of particular significance in the context of pro-life issues – he was chairman of the Bishops' Consultative Group for Bioethics.

Opposition to hESC research was now more frequently expressed by the Catholic laity than by the bishops, who seemed increasingly disempowered by their diminished moral authority. On 21 January 2010 William Reville, mindful of the Supreme Court judgment, reiterated, in the *Irish Times*, his opposition to hESC research. Reville speculated that the majority of scientists did not attach "full moral value" to early-stage human embryos. There was an intuitive resistance to intentionally killing human embryos, but those scientists supportive of hESC research overcame such resistance on the basis of a utilitarian ethic – "the end justifies the means." They reasoned that any ethical objection to the killing of human embryos was outweighed by the benefits of hESC research that would lead to cures for many human diseases. Reville, in contrast to the utilitarian wing of the scientific profession, embraced a "principles-based ethics" which prioritised respect for human life. Human ESC research was not only unethical – it was also impractical when compared to hASC research. Also, the use of hASCs and iPSCs was not, for the most part, burdened by ethical difficulties. Reville claimed that hASC research had led to over two hundred medical treatments, whereas hESC had not produced even one such treatment and there was no reasonable prospect of it doing so within the next ten years.[78]

If Reville's thesis was to be taken at face value, the majority of his fellow scientists were found wanting in ethical sensibilities and were additionally burdened by a persistent tendency to pursue research by inefficient means. Dr Dolores Dooley, a philosopher (formerly of University College Cork), was sharply critical of Reville's article in the *Irish Times*. In a letter to the editor she asserted that the claim of two hundred medical treatments arising from hASC research was "categorically false". She disputed Reville's claim that hASC and iPSC research were good and ethical alternatives to hESC research. Human ESCs were essential as controls in ASC and iPSC research. Dooley believed that Reville, given his professional status as a scientist, knew this but failed to include the information in his newspaper article. This omission bolstered Reville's contention that hESCs should be excluded from future stem cell research projects. False claims such as this were detrimental to the public interest.[79]

Two scientists at University College Cork, professors P.L.H. McSweeney and Tommie McCarthy, wrote to the editor of the *Irish Times* criticising Dooley.[80] Most readers may have concluded that the opinions of three science professors carried far more weight than the opinion of a philosopher on this contentious issue. Such a conclusion would not have been well founded. Dooley's credentials were strong: she had served as chairperson of the Irish Council for Bioethics and had participated in working group meetings of the Commission on Assisted Human Reproduction.[81]

McCarthy contended that hESCs were unnecessary as controls for hASC research and that iPSC research would "advance rapidly irrespective of the existence of hESCs". This claim was at odds with the opinions of the majority of scientists engaged in stem cell research.[82] Professor Patrick Cunningham, chief scientific adviser to the government, pointed out in the *Irish Times* that scientists had not yet figured out how to activate and switch off specific genes in a controlled and sequentially correct way to create cells of a specific type. His opinion was that many scientists engaged in research with hESCs would continue to do so until it could be shown that iPSCs were as effective.[83] Progress was indeed evident in iPSC research.[84] Even so, scientists generally tended not to encourage unfounded optimism. In the top-ranking scientific journal, *Nature*, it was observed that "despite much enthusiasm, it is not known whether iPS cells will be an effective treatment for human diseases." Further to this, it was stated that even embryo-derived cells had been tested in only a few settings, and their effectiveness and safety were not well established.[85]

Although there were serious problems to address in hESC research, scientists continued to place a higher value on hESCs than human iPSCs. Hence the observation, also in *Nature*, that "scientists hope that they will one day understand iPS cells well enough to substitute them for embryonic stem cells."[86] Research developments indicated that "expertise with ES cells was essential for advancing iPS-cell technology."[87] Konrad Hochedlinger, writing in *Scientific American*, stated that "Current iPSC studies rely heavily on techniques and concepts developed in work with embryonic cells over the past 30 years." He made the point that hESCs would continue to be needed as "a reference point" for iPSC research.[88] Hochedlinger was a leading stem cell researcher at Harvard University.[89]

Human iPSCs were far more difficult to culture than hESCs. Also, there was considerable evidence to indicate that various cell types generated from iPSCs were vulnerable to cellular ageing and programmed cell death after short times in culture. These problems were not experienced with cells originating from hESCs.[90] Furthermore, it was argued that iPSCs were not completely free from ethical problems because, at least theoretically, these cells could be used to create human embryos.[91] All of the above indicated that there was considerable merit in Dooley's sharp critique of Reville, despite the supportive comments of McSweeney and McCarthy. Still, Reville had the advantage in terms of influencing public opinion. His public platform – his regular column in the *Irish Times* – probably impacted significantly on the readership of that widely read national newspaper.

Developments in stem cell biology were misrepresented by those who pressed for alternatives to hESC research. Galway for Life, affiliated to the Pro Life Campaign, reported on its website that a team of scientists at Stanford University had succeeded in inducing skin cells in mice to change directly into functional nerve cells (neurons), without going through the time-consuming and inefficient process of creating iPSCs. This prompted Galway for Life to declare: "Scientists have made a major breakthrough using the process known as direct reprogramming that further renders embryonic stem cell research obsolete."[92] This claim was misleading when account was taken of the published research findings in *Nature*. Thomas Vierbuchen and his co-authors assessed the importance of their work in more modest terms when they stated that the generation of induced neurons "from non-neural lineages could have important implications for studies of neural development, neurological disease modelling and regenerative medicine".[93] It remained to be seen whether or not directly reprogrammed cells would obviate the need for stem cells sometime in the future.[94]

If a majority of biomedical scientists in Ireland approved of hESC research, they were reluctant to vigorously challenge exaggerated claims about iPSC and hASC alternatives. This did not augur well for the future of stem cell research in Ireland. Government funding and legislation for hESC research was far less likely to materialise if the pro-hESC sector of science failed to engage robustly in debate. The Irish Stem Cell Foundation (ISCF) was set up in October 2009 to promote stem cell research in Ireland and to press for appropriate legislation. Its members included scientists, medical doctors, "patient advocates", bioethicists, those with a role in policy formation, teachers and students.[95]

The ISCF received some media attention in the aftermath of the Supreme Court case of *Roche v. Roche* and the day before the publication of its policy document in April 2010.[96] Stephen Sullivan, a director and chief scientific officer for the ISCF, pointed out that Ireland was losing opportunities in cutting edge biomedical research in the absence of a legislative and regulatory framework.[97] The uncertainty created by the legislative vacuum was acting as an obstacle to investment. In its policy document the ISCF expressed support for hESC research "under certain strictly controlled conditions" and the use of supernumerary IVF embryos as sources of hESCs.[98]

There was no basis for optimism about forthcoming legislation. The Fianna Fáil–Green Party coalition collapsed in early 2011 against the backdrop of Ireland's loss of economic independence as the European Commission, the European Central Bank and the International Monetary Fund acted together to stabilise the republic's finances. Both government parties suffered heavy losses at the hands of an angry electorate on 25 February. The Green Party lost its six Dáil seats and Fianna Fáil experienced its worst defeat since its foundation in 1926. Now with only twenty Dáil seats it slipped down to third place behind the Labour Party. Fine Gael, in primary position, formed the new government with Labour.

The future for scientific research in Ireland seemed bleak. Severe reductions in public spending were seen as inevitable as part of a programme for economic recovery. Irish scientists feared that state support for science would decline in parallel with deteriorating economic conditions. Prospects for hESC research were even less promising. A report from *Nature*, which received attention in the online edition of the *Sunday Business Post*, indicated that Fine Gael was opposed to hESC research. Furthermore, the absence of legislation was a major obstacle to investment. In the absence of a legal framework, two major funding organisations, Science Foundation Ireland and the Health Research Board, did not provide funding for research that was dependent on hESCs. Although University College Cork and Trinity College Dublin had policies of permitting research on imported stem cell lines, it was reported that no scientist in either university had undertaken such research because of the uncertainty arising from the absence of relevant legislation.[99] Legislative initiatives to address this problem were far beyond the political horizon.

Endnotes

——————•——————

1   The Irish Catholic Bishops' Conference, *Towards a Creative Response to Infertility: A Detailed Response of the Irish Catholic Bishops' Conference to the Report of the Commission on Assisted Human Reproduction* (Dublin: Veritas, 2006), pp. 22–3.

2   Paul Cullen, "Mixed reactions but most agree legislation is needed", *Irish Times*, 16 November 2006, p. 4.

3   David Quinn, "'Spare' embryos are human. The courts must protect them", *Sunday Times*, 9 July 2006, p. 16.

4   William Reville, "If the embryo is fully human, we are obliged to keep it from harm", *Irish Times*, 18 May 2006, p. 15.

5   Further research may enable scientists to harvest stem cells without destroying human embryos, but restrictions may be retained because the procedure of extracting a single cell from an embryo may still entail some significant degree of risk to the embryo. See Rick Weiss, "Scientists claim advance in stem cell research", *Irish Times*, 18 October 2005 <http://www.ireland.com/newspaper/world/2005/1018/4065415237FR18STEM.html> accessed 23 May 2006; Maggie Fox, "Scientists develop stem cell harvesting without harming embryo", *Irish Examiner*, 18 October 2005 <http://archives.tcm.ie/irishexaminer/2005/10/18/story142806485.asp> accessed 23 May 2006.

6   Alberto Giubilini, "Abortion and the Argument from Potential: What we owe to the ones who might exist", *Journal of Medicine and Philosophy*, vol. 37 (January 2012), pp. 49–59; quotation from p. 59.

7   See Don O'Leary, *Roman Catholicism and Modern Science: A History* (New York and London: Continuum, 2006), pp. 224, 229–31.

8   Lisa Sowle Cahill, "The Embryo and the Fetus: New moral contexts", *Theological Studies*, vol. 54, no. 1 (March 1993), pp. 127–30.

9   Bioethicist Jeff McMahan estimates that approximately two-thirds of fertilised ova fail to result in live births. "Infanticide and Moral Consistency", *Journal of Medical Ethics*, vol. 39, no. 5 (May 2013), p. 279.

10 One estimate gives a probable spontaneous termination rate for blastocysts of up to 80%. Deirdre Madden, "*In Vitro* Fertilisation: The Embryo: The Ethical Issues", in Enda McDonagh and Vincent MacNamara (eds), *An Irish Reader in Moral Theology: The Legacy of the Last Fifty Years* (Dublin: Columba Press, 2013), p. 217. A more recent estimate is that up to 50% of pregnancies

miscarry in the first four weeks. After that there is a further significant miscarriage rate for the surviving 50%, very much influenced by the mother's age. At 30 years the miscarriage rate is about 10%; at 40 years it is at least 35%; and it increases steeply after that to reach 75% from the age of 45 years. Estimates from Institute of Obstetricians and Gynaecologists, "Repeal of the Eighth Amendment: Information for the public" <https://www.rcpi.ie/faculties/obstetricians-and-gynaecologists/repeal-the-eighth-amendment-info-for-the-public> accessed 4 April 2018.

11 Deirdre Madden, "In Vitro Fertilisation: The Moral and Legal Status of the Human Pre-Embryo", *Medico-Legal Journal of Ireland*, vol. 3 (1), 1997, pp. 12–20.

12 Thomas A. Shannon, "Delayed Hominization: A response to Mark Johnson", *Theological Studies*, vol. 57, no. 4 (December 1996), pp. 732, 734.

13 Congregation for the Doctrine of the Faith, *Instruction on Respect for Human Life in Its Origin and on the Dignity of Procreation* (Dublin: Veritas, 1987), p. 4.

14 Bertha Alvarez Manninen, "Yes, the Baby Should Live: A pro-choice response to Giubilini and Minerva", *Journal of Medical Ethics*, vol. 39, no. 5 (May 2013), p. 334.

15 John Burgess observed that, in philosophical literature, there are at least three – and very probably more than three – categories of ideas of what a person is. "Could a Zygote be a Human Being?", *Bioethics*, vol. 24, issue 2 (February 2010), p. 62. See also C.A.J. Coady, "The Common Premise for Uncommon Conclusions", *Journal of Medical Ethics*, vol. 39, no. 5 (May 2013), p. 286.

16 Sacred Congregation for the Doctrine of the Faith, "The Reality of Life after Death" (11 May 1979), in Austin Flannery (general ed.), *Vatican Council II: More Postconciliar Documents* (Collegeville, Minn.: Liturgical Press, 1982 (1st edn)), p. 502. See also *Catechism of the Catholic Church* (Dublin: Veritas, 1995), paragraph 366.

17 Mark Johnson, "Delayed Hominization: Reflections on some recent Catholic claims for delayed hominization", *Theological Studies*, vol. 56, no. 4 (December 1995), p. 745. See also Jean Porter, "Individuality, Personal Identity, and the Moral Status of the Preembryo: A response to Mark Johnson", *Theological Studies*, vol. 56, no. 4 (December 1995), p. 764.

18 Sacred Congregation for the Doctrine of the Faith, *Declaration on Procured Abortion (Quaestio de abortu)*, 18 November 1974, note 19, in Flannery, *Vatican Council II*, p. 452. For a discussion of a major change in church teaching on the status of embryos arising from a decree by Pope Pius IX in 1969, see Stephen T. Asma, "Abortion and the Embarrassing Saint", *The Humanist*, vol. 54, no. 3 (May–June 1994), pp. 30–3.

19 Sacred Congregation for the Doctrine of the Faith, *Declaration on Procured Abortion* paragraph 13 and note 19, in Flannery, *Vatican Council II*, pp. 445–6, 452.

20 Archbishops and Bishops of Ireland, *Human Life is Sacred: Pastoral Letter of*

the Archbishops and Bishops of Ireland to the Clergy, Religious and Faithful (n.p.: Archbishops and Bishops of Ireland, May 1975), paragraph 19.

21 Madden, "*In Vitro* Fertilisation", p. 217.

22 Pope John Paul II, *Evangelium Vitae* (London: Catholic Truth Society, 1995), paragraph 60.

23 Ibid.

24 Congregation for the Doctrine of the Faith, *Instruction Dignitas Personae: On Certain Bioethical Questions*, 8 September 2008, paragraph 5 <http://www.vatican.va/roman_curia/congregations/cfaith/documents/rc_con_cfaith_doc_20081208_dignitas-personae_en.html> accessed 2 December 2011.

25 For philosophical arguments in relation to this point see Michael Tooley, "Philosophy, Critical Thinking and 'After-birth Abortion: Why should the baby live?'", *Journal of Medical Ethics*, vol. 39, no. 5 (May 2013), pp. 266–72.

26 *Instruction Dignitas Personae*, paragraph 5.

27 See Coady, "The Common Premise for Uncommon Conclusions", p. 285.

28 The ECHR adjudicates on issues of human rights for member states of the Council of Europe, of which Ireland is one. Ireland is a signatory to the council's European Convention on Human Rights.

29 ECHR, "Grand Chamber Judgment: *Evans v. The United Kingdom*", press release issued by the Registrar, 10 April 2007 <http://cmiskp.echr.coe.int/tkp197/view.asp?item=3&portal=hbkm&action=html&highlight=&sessionid=12215313&skin=hudoc-pr-en> accessed 12 April 2007.

30 See Mary Fitzgerald, "The EU gets Tough on Ethics", *Technology Ireland*, vol. 38, issue 1 (March–April 2007), pp. 27–30.

31 *Report of the Commission on Assisted Human Reproduction* (Dublin: Stationery Office, 2005), pp. xv, xvii (recommendations 10 and 34).

32 Ibid., pp. xii, 29–31.

33 Irish Catholic Bishops' Conference, *Towards a Creative Response to Infertility*, pp. 34–6.

34 Pope John Paul II, *Evangelium Vitae*, paragraph 20.

35 For an indication of this in Ireland see Carl O'Brien, "Majority of women want abortion legalised", *Irish Times*, 29 September 2007, p. 1 <http://www.ireland.com/newspaper/frontpage/2007/0929/1191014902496.html> accessed 8 October 2007; and Patsy McGarry, "Bishops warn of crisis over sanctity of life", *Irish Times*, 8 October 2007, p. 1 <http://www.ireland.com/newspaper/frontpage/2007/1008/1191668714883.html> accessed 8 October 2007.

36 Kazutoshi Takahashi and Shinya Yamanaka, "Induction of Pluripotent Stem Cells from Mouse Embryonic and Adult Fibroblast Cultures by Defined Factors", *Cell*, vol. 126 (25 August 2006), pp. 663–76.

37 The Japanese team had used a similar technique, and the same four factors, to generate human iPSCs from human dermal fibroblasts (a type of skin cell). Thomson and his colleagues had also used four genes, although two of these

were different from those used by Takahashi and Yamanaka.

38 Gretchen Vogel and Constance Holden, "Field Leaps Forward With New Stem Cell Advances", *Science*, vol. 318, no. 5854 (23 November 2007), pp. 1224–5 <http://www.sciencemag.org/cgi/content/full/318/5854/1224> accessed 23 November 2007.

39 When Ian Wilmut (who had played a supervisory role in the team of scientists who cloned Dolly the sheep in 1996) heard about the research breakthrough with mice he declared that his research team made plans to cease work on human somatic cell nuclear transfer (SCNT) so that resources could be reallocated to exploit the new methods of generating iPSCs. The subsequent research breakthrough with human iPSCs dispelled any reluctance to proceed with such a decision. Vogel and Holden, "Field Leaps Forward".

40 Ibid.; Kazutoshi Takahashi, Shinya Yamanaka *et al.*, "Induction of Pluripotent Stem Cells from Adult Human Fibroblasts by Defined Factors", *Cell*, vol. 131 (30 November 2007), pp. 8–9; and "Simple Recipe Turns Human Skin Cells into Embryonic Stem Cell-Like Cells", press release, *Cell Press*, 20 November 2007 <http://www.cellpress.com/misc/page?page=misc20> accessed 23 November 2007.

41 Alan I. Leshner and James A. Thomson, "Standing in the way of stem cell research", *Washington Post*, 3 December 2007; sourced from the website of the American Association for the Advancement of Science (AAAS) on 18 February 2010. Alan I. Leshner, at the time of writing, was chief executive of the AAAS and executive publisher of the AAAS journal *Science*. Thomson was professor of anatomy at the University of Wisconsin and was the first scientist to culture human embryonic stem cells. He was the senior scientist in the American team (mentioned earlier) that, in parallel with Takahashi *et al.* (see previous note), reprogrammed human skin cells to iPSCs.

42 "UCC Statement following Governing Body Meeting of 28/10/2008 at which consideration was given to embryonic stem cell research recommendations" <http://www.ucc.ie/en/mandc/news/fullstory,63377,en.html> accessed 28 October 2008.

43 Michelle McDonagh, "UCC approves use of embryonic stem cells by single vote", *Irish Independent*, 29 October 2008 <http://www.independent.ie/health/latest-news/ucc-approves-use-of-embryonic-stem-cells-by-single-vote-1511912.html> accessed 1 November 2008.

44 Seanad Debates, vol. 192 (20 November 2008), p. 335.

45 Rónán Mullen, Jim Walsh and John Hanafin, *Stem-Cell Research (Protection of Human Embryos) Bill 2008: Explanatory Memorandum* (Dublin: Stationery Office, 20 November 2008).

46 Seanad Debates, vol. 192 (26 November 2008), pp. 462–4.

47 Ibid., p. 463.

48 To substantiate this point it is appropriate to refer to an article by Shinya

Yamanaka, one of the leading scientists in iPSC research. Although at the time mainly concerned with generating iPSCs from mouse fibroblasts, Yamanaka observed that reprogramming cells by fusion with human ESCs had been reported in 2005. ESCs, human and otherwise, contain factors that induce pluripotency in somatic cells. S. Yamanaka, "Induction of Pluripotent Stem Cells from Mouse Fibroblasts by Four Transcription Factors", *Cell Proliferation*, vol. 41, no. s1 (February 2008), 51–6. Furthermore, as pointed out earlier, the creation of iPSCs by the Japanese and American research teams had relied entirely on the use of hESCs. See Leshner and Thomson, "Standing in the Way of Stem Cell Research".

49 Seanad Debates, vol. 192, p. 463

50 Takahashi, Yamanaka *et al.*, "Induction of Pluripotent Stem Cells from Adult Human Fibroblasts", p. 9.

51 Shinya Yamanaka, "A Fresh Look at iPS Cells", *Cell*, vol. 137 (3 April 2009), pp. 13–17. See also Yamanaka, "Elite and Stochastic Models for Induced Pluripotent Stem Cell Regeneration", *Nature*, vol. 460, issue no. 7251 (2 July 2009), pp. 49–52.

52 Editorial, "Still the Gold Standard: Halting Embryonic Stem Cell Research Now would be Nothing Short of Rash", *New Scientist*, vol. 198, no. 2654 (3 May 2008), p. 3; and Alice McCarthy, "Will Human Embryonic Stem Cell Therapies Finally Grow Up?" *Chemistry & Biology*, vol. 16, issue 5 (29 May 2009), pp. 471–2.

53 Seanad Debates, vol. 192, p. 463.

54 Mullen stated that the issue was published "earlier" in 2008 but gave no further details. An examination of the volumes for that year indicates that it was volume 41, no. s1 (February 2008), published online on 20 December 2007.

55 Gian Luigi Gigli and Elio Sgreccia, Editorial, *Cell Proliferation*, vol. 41, no. s1 (February 2008), pp. 1–3.

56 "Address of His Holiness Pope Benedict XVI to Participants of the Symposium on the Theme: 'Stem Cells: What Future for Therapy? Scientific Aspects and Bioethical Problems'", *Cell Proliferation*, vol. 41, no. s1 (February 2008), pp. 4–6. The author, Richard M. Doerflinger, who alleged that there were frequent exaggerations and misrepresentations by some scientists working with hESCs, was associated with the National Catholic Bioethics Center (Philadelphia, USA). R.M. Doerflinger, "The Problem of Deception in Embryonic Stem Cell Research", *Cell Proliferation*, vol. 41, no. s1 (February 2008), 65–70. See also J.L. Sherley, "The Importance of Valid Disclosures in the Human Embryonic Stem Cell Research Debate" in the same issue of *Cell Proliferation*, pp. 57–64.

57 Seanad Debates, vol. 192, p. 464.

58 The Congregation for the Doctrine of the Faith acknowledged that there was "not always complete knowledge" of the way contraceptive

pharmaceutical products worked in the human body. Despite this, it condemned the use of "interceptive" contraceptive methods. It stated that: "anyone who seeks to prevent the implantation of an embryo which may possibly have been conceived and who therefore either requests or prescribes such a pharmaceutical, generally intends abortion". Congregation for the Doctrine of the Faith, *Dignitas Personae*, paragraph 23.

59   It can be argued that not all early-stage embryos are equal. The moral status of the embryo can be judged with reference to the probability of it developing to become a person. If this "gradualist approach" is accepted, an implanted embryo should have a higher status, and greater legal protection, than an embryo which is not implanted. An embryo in the womb (*in vivo*) should have a higher status than an embryo in a laboratory petri dish (*in vitro*). See Ciara Staunton, "A Moral Gap? Examining Ireland's Failure to Regulate Embryonic Stem Cell Research" in Mary Donnelly and Claire Murray (eds), *Ethical and Legal Debates in Irish Healthcare: Confronting Complexities* (Manchester: Manchester University Press, 2016), p. 154.

60   Seanad Debates, vol. 192, pp. 465–6.

61   Ibid., pp. 471–2.

62   Ibid., pp. 481–2.

63   Ibid., pp. 475–6.

64   Norris spoke about the induction of pluripotency in "adult stem cells" (ibid., p. 476). These cells are already multi-potent or pluripotent. Presumably Norris meant "adult cells".

65   Seanad Debates, vol. 192, p. 486.

66   William Reville, "Life Continuum", *UCC News*, issue 40 (May 2008), p. 1.

67   Seanad Debates, vol. 199 (2 December 2009), p. 12.

68   Susan Denham, "Judgment delivered the 15th day of December, 2009 by Denham J.", Neutral Citation [2009] IESC 82, Supreme Court Record No. 469/06 & 59/07, accessed from the Supreme Court of Ireland website 19 December 2009.

69   Ibid.

70   Hardiman's words were "fertilised embryos". The correct term is fertilised ova or zygotes.

71   Adrian Hardiman, "Judgment delivered the 15th day of December, 2009, by Mr. Justice Hardiman", Neutral Citation [2009] IESC 82, Supreme Court Record No. 469/06 & 59/07, accessed from the Supreme Court of Ireland website, 19 December 2009. See also Deirdre Madden, *Medicine, Ethics and the Law* (Haywards Heath, UK: Bloomsbury Professional, 2016 (3rd edn)), pp. 269–71.

72   *Irish Examiner* (16 December 2009) coverage included: Claire O'Sullivan, "Supreme Court ruling: meaning of life", p. 1; Vivion Kilfeather, "'Unborn' refers to child within the womb, rules court" and "'Science will not wait for us to update our laws'", both p. 6; Editorial: "Supreme Court Ruling:

Decisions put off for too long", p. 16. The *Irish Times* coverage (16 December 2009) included: Mary Minihan and Carol Coulter, "Harney to propose law on assisted human reproduction: Supreme Court finds failure to legislate 'disturbing'", p. 1; Mary Carolan, "Embryos are not the 'unborn', court rules" and "'Disturbing' failure to enact laws on fertility treatment criticised", both p. 4; Mary Minihan, "Lack of legislation puts judiciary in 'unenviable' position, says FG", p. 4; Jimmy Walsh, "'Cowardice' being shown on reproduction issue: Seanad Report", p. 8; Carol Coulter, "Court again calls for law on assisted human reproduction", p. 15; Editorial: "Political failings and embryo case", p. 17.

73 Deirdre Madden, "Assisted Reproduction in Ireland – Time to Legislate" (guest editorial), *Medico-Legal Journal of Ireland*, vol. 17, no. 1 (2011), pp. 3–5.

74 See Claire O'Sullivan, "Lack of enthusiasm blocked report on law", *Irish Examiner*, 16 December 2009, p. 6.

75 Gretchen Vogel, "Ireland: Embryo Ruling Keeps Stem Cell Research Legal", *Science*, vol. 327, issue 5961 (1 January 2010), p. 25.

76 Evelyn Ring, "Calls for legislation to protect embryos", *Irish Examiner*, 16 December 2009, p. 6.

77 Dick Ahlstrom, "'Retrograde' closure of bioethics body criticised", *Irish Times*, 17 December 2009 <http://www.irishtimes.com/newspaper/ireland/2009/1217/1224260838471_pf.html> accessed 11 January 2010.

78 William Reville, "Killing of embryos in human stem-cell research is wrong", *Irish Times*, 21 January 2010 <http://www.irishtimes.com/newspaper/sciencetoday/2010/0121/1224262767052_pf.html> accessed 21 January 2010.

79 Dolores Dooley, letter to the editor, *Irish Times*, 28 January 2010 <http://www.irishtimes.com/newspaper/letters/2010/0128/1224263288324_pf.html> accessed 28 January 2010.

80 P.L.H. McSweeney, letter to the editor, *Irish Times*, 29 January 2010 <http://www.irishtimes.com/newspaper/letters/2010/0129/1224263355254_pf.html> accessed 29 January 2010; and Tommie McCarthy, letter to the editor, *Irish Times*, 3 February 2010 <http://www.irishtimes.com/newspaper/letters/2010/0203/1224263647755_pf.html> accessed 3 February 2010.

81 Irish Council for Bioethics, *Ethical, Scientific and Legal Issues Concerning Stem Cell Research: Opinion* (Dublin: Irish Council for Bioethics, 2008), preface, p. 116; and *Report of the Commission on Assisted Human Reproduction*, p. iii.

82 Scientists in a number of states pressed for a loosening of very tight restrictions on hESC research and for greater funding. See Alan I. Leshner, AAAS Response to the "National Institutes of Health (NIH) Guidelines for Human Stem Cell Research, published in the *Federal Register* on April 23", 20 May 2009 (accessed from the AAAS website, 20 February 2010).

The American Association for the Advancement of Science (AAAS) claimed to be the largest multidisciplinary science society, representing ten million scientists worldwide. For additional examples of support for hESC research in international science see Alison Abbott, "Italians Sue over Stem Cells", *Nature*, vol. 460, issue no. 7251 (2 July 2009), p. 19; and David Cyranoski, "Japan Relaxes Human Stem-Cell Rules", *Nature*, vol. 460, issue no. 7259 (27 August 2009), p. 1068.

83 Patrick Cunningham, "Advances in stem-cell research may resolve ethical issues", *Irish Times*, 22 April 2009 <http://www.irishtimes.com/newspaper/opinion/2009/0422/1224245127531_pf.html> accessed 28 April 2009.

84 In March 2009 a team of scientists reported that they had sourced fibroblasts from five patients with idiopathic Parkinson's disease. These cells were manipulated to generate iPSCs and later induced to differentiate into dopaminergic neurons – which die in large numbers as the disease develops. These cells were patient-specific; therefore no complications would arise from immune rejection. Reprogramming was achieved using viruses which could later be extracted from the cells. The research team acknowledged that iPSC and ESC therapies were "at an early stage of development". Patient-specific iPSCs were seen as extremely valuable for research, especially concerning central nervous system diseases such as Parkinson's. Frank Soldner, Dirk Hockemeyer *et al.*, "Parkinson's Disease Patient-Derived Induced Pluripotent Stem Cells Free of Viral Reprogramming Factors", *Cell*, vol. 136 (6 March 2009), pp. 964–77.

85 Valery Krizhanovsky and Scott W. Lowe, "The Promises and Perils of p53", *Nature*, vol. 460, issue no. 7259 (27 August 2009), pp. 1085–6.

86 Alison Abbott, "Faster Route to Stem-like Cells", *Nature*, 10 November 2009 <http://0-www.nature.com.library.ucc.ie/news/2009/091108/full/news.2009.1070.html> accessed 16 February 2010. See also Lisa Fullam and William R. O'Neill, "Bioethics and Public Policy", *Theological Studies*, vol. 71 (March 2010), pp. 173–4.

87 Cyranoski, "Japan relaxes human stem-cell rules", p. 1068.

88 There was also the possibility that iPSCs would retain a "memory" of their previous specialised status which in turn would limit their ability to be converted into another type of cell. Konrad Hochedlinger, "Your Inner Healers", *Scientific American*, vol. 302, no. 5 (May 2010), pp. 30, 35.

89 Konrad Hochedlinger was associate professor of stem cell and regenerative biology at Harvard University and a faculty member of the Harvard Stem Cell Institute and the Howard Hughes Medical Institute.

90 Gretchen Vogel, "Reprogrammed Cells Come Up Short, for Now", *Science*, vol. 327 (5 March 2010), p. 119.

91 Hochedlinger, "Your Inner Healers", pp. 34, 35. See also Sally Lehrman, "Undifferentiated Ethics: Stem cells from adult skin are as morally fraught

as the embryonic kind", *Scientific American*, vol. 303, no. 3 (September 2010), pp. 11–12.

92 Galway for Life, "Scientists' Advance Further Renders Embryonic Stem Cell Research Obsolete", 10 February 2010 <http://galwayforlife.blogspot.com/2010/02/scientists-advance-further-renders.html> accessed 23 August 2010.

93 Thomas Vierbuchen, Austin Ostermeier *et al.*, "Direct Conversion of Fibroblasts to Functional Neurons by Defined Factors", *Nature*, vol. 463, no. 7284 (25 February 2010), p. 1035.

94 Vierbuchen and his colleagues stated: "Future studies will be necessary to determine whether iN [induced neuronal] cells could represent an alternative method to generate patient-specific neurons" (p. 1040). See also Cory R. Nicholas and Arnold R. Kriegstein, "Cell Reprogramming gets Direct", *Nature*, vol. 463, no. 7284 (25 February 2010), pp. 1031–2.

95 Irish Stem Cell Foundation, "About Us" <http://www.irishstemcellfoundation.org/aboutus.htm> accessed 24 May 2010; and ISCF home page <http://www.irishstemcellfoundation.org/index.html> accessed 24 May 2010. The ISCF's main spokespersons were Dr Orla Hardiman (Chief Medical Officer) and Dr Stephen Sullivan (Chief Scientific Officer).

96 Stephen Sullivan and Fionnuala Gough, "Crux of the unborn", *Irish Examiner*, 15 December 2009; Stephen Sullivan and Martin Codyre, "A legal limbo", *Irish Examiner*, 17 December 2009; Catherine Shanahan, "Warning over lack of laws on stem cell research", *Irish Examiner*, 27 April 2010 <http://www.examiner.ie/ireland/warning-over-lack-of-laws-on-stem-cell-research-118297.html> accessed 24 May 2010.

97 Shanahan, "Warning over lack of laws".

98 Irish Stem Cell Foundation, "Irish public policy and human embryonic stem cell research: A policy document by the Irish Stem Cell Foundation, April 2010" <http://www.irishstemcellfoundation.org/docs/policy.pdf> accessed 24 May 2010.

99 Alison Abbott, "Irish Election Raises Questions for Stem Cell Research", *Nature*, 28 February 2011 <http://blogs.nature.com/news/2011/02/irish_election_raises_question.html> accessed 20 November 2011; and Susan Mitchell, "Warning over stem cell research in Ireland", ThePost.ie (the *Sunday Business Post* online), 6 March 2011 <http://www.thepost.ie/story/text/ojeysnojmh/> accessed 31 March 2011.

CHAPTER FIVE

·

Assisted Suicide

Catholic Doctrine

It is frequently claimed that human life is sacred and that only God has the right to end a human life. This belief is forcefully expressed in Roman Catholic doctrine. In its *Pastoral on the Church in the Modern World* (*Gaudium et spes*, 7 December 1965) the Second Vatican Council included "wilful suicide" and euthanasia alongside genocide, murder and abortion as offences against life, offences against God, and incompatible with a civilised way of life.[1] Those who oppose assisted suicide and euthanasia for religious reasons are not without recourse to non-religious arguments. These may be described as (1) the "slippery slope" argument, (2) the medical ethics argument, and (3) the "alternative" argument.

The "slippery slope" perspective anticipates unintended consequences where a dangerous precedent is set. Assisted suicide might lead to voluntary euthanasia and, with changing social attitudes, to non-voluntary euthanasia, and perhaps even to involuntary euthanasia. People with severe disabilities, in very poor health, and in constant care, may be subjected to pressure to request assisted suicide or euthanasia, so that they are not a burden on their families. Some patients might choose assisted suicide or euthanasia on the basis of a wrong diagnosis.

The legalisation of assisted suicide and euthanasia is widely seen as contrary to a fundamental principle of medical practice – the importance of preserving human life. Any departure from this principle, it is argued, could have an adverse impact on the attitude of doctors to their patients, and on the patient–doctor relationship. Doctors might become so at ease with the termination of human life that they might lack compassion when treating severely disabled, terminally ill or elderly patients. Patients, in turn, might distrust their doctors, suspecting that the professional preference was for termination as a simpler option, rather than the more challenging course of medical treatment in a complex case.

The "alternative" argument is based on both advances in palliative care and mental health treatment. Effective end-of-life treatments are available, so assisted suicide and euthanasia are not seen as valid treatment options. Palliative sedation is frequently given to terminally ill people to make them unconscious and unaware of pain. Needless suffering is avoided.[2] It has been argued that major improvements should be made to healthcare services before legal reforms are contemplated. These include a high standard system of equitable and accessible palliative care services and major improvements to services necessary to support those with chronic physical conditions, disability or mental illness. The optimisation of services would reduce, to a minimum, requests for assistance in dying.[3]

It may be that arguments about slippery slopes, heartless doctors and manipulative relatives of terminally ill people are pressed too far, notwithstanding the need for vigilance. In some medical cases it is already legally permissible for a doctor to bring about death sooner than would otherwise occur. Physicians may prescribe medical treatment to relieve pain and suffering even when such treatments shorten life. This is referred to as the "double effect principle". The intention is to reduce or eliminate suffering, not to hasten death – although this inevitably occurs. Doctors are permitted to place a "do not attempt resuscitation" order on a patient's chart when they anticipate such resuscitation would be futile. Life-sustaining treatments, such as dialysis, ventilation or intravenous nutrition, may be withdrawn when there are no prospects of the patient's recovery and the life-support system is only prolonging the dying process. Under Irish law, all adult patients of sufficient mental capacity are entitled to refuse medical treatment – even when that treatment is necessary to save their lives. Patients suffering from cancer, for example, may decline chemotherapy to avoid its distressing side-effects when such treatment would only slightly prolong their lives. Patients who refuse nutrition and fluids are still entitled to medical care to alleviate consequential pain and discomfort. This, as observed by Deirdre Madden (professor of law at University College Cork) could be viewed as "tantamount to a right to assisted dying".[4] Mr Justice P. Kearns argued in the High Court (*Fleming v Ireland*) that, in cases of mentally competent patients declining life-saving medical treatment, there was "a real and defining difference" between such decisions and the act of one person terminating the life of another, even when such an act was done in response to an expressed wish to hasten death. However, Kearns acknowledged that, in some cases, the difference between "the two types of decisions may sometimes be nuanced and blurred".[5]

Medical science and technology can in many cases extend life, but it does not always, in such cases, improve or maintain health to the point where life is valued, not simply endured. In view of this it is not surprising that consideration was given in some jurisdictions to changing the law on assisted suicide and euthanasia. It was against this background that the Sacred Congregation for the Doctrine of the Faith issued its *Declaration on Euthanasia* (5 May 1980).[6]

The congregation defined euthanasia as "an act or omission which of itself or by intention causes death, in order that all suffering may in this way be eliminated. Euthanasia's terms of reference, therefore, are to be found in the intention of the will and in the methods used."[7] The moral issues associated with assisted suicide and euthanasia were not new, but they were now much more complex because of developments in the medical sciences. Should every means necessary be availed of to sustain human life in all circumstances? The traditional response was that there is no moral obligation to resort to "extraordinary" means to sustain life. The word "extraordinary" was later deemed too imprecise in the light of modern medicine.[8] Words such as "proportionate" and "disproportionate" now seemed more precise.[9] But there was also a persistent lack of precision about all these terms.[10] There was no easily identifiable line of demarcation between such terms as "proportionate" or "disproportionate". Every case required careful judgement, with due consideration given to the costs, risks, and benefits of treatment, and any additional suffering that might be imposed on the patient. It was morally permissible for a patient to decline medical treatment that was excessively "burdensome" and to "make do" with "normal" medical care. Such a decision was considered "an acceptance of the human condition" – not suicide.[11] In its *Catechism of the Catholic Church* (1992) the teaching authority declared that the use of painkillers to alleviate suffering was morally permissible, even when this shortened life, provided that this secondary effect was not intended as a means or an objective.[12]

The Marie Fleming Case, 2012–2013

Assisted suicide, in a legal context, is an act of intentionally giving assistance or encouragement to a person who commits suicide or attempts to commit suicide. Euthanasia may be defined as a deliberate act of terminating a person's life to prevent intractable suffering, and not for personal gain.[13] In most cases the person is given an overdose of sedatives or muscle relaxants, initially inducing coma and then death. In this chapter the main focus will be on assisted suicide, which was the subject of High Court and Supreme Court proceedings in Ireland in 2012–2013.

Assisted suicide is illegal in most jurisdictions, including Ireland. The few jurisdictions where it is legal include the Netherlands, Luxembourg, Switzerland, a few states in the USA, and Canada. In Ireland, Section 2 of the Criminal Law (Suicide) Act 1993 states that a "person who aids, abets, counsels or procures the suicide of another, or an attempt by another to commit suicide, shall be guilty of an offence and shall be liable on conviction on indictment to imprisonment for a term not exceeding fourteen years".[14] It also stated that suicide would no longer be a crime. Therefore, it was illegal to assist someone to commit an act which was not in itself a criminal act.

Some people, suffering debilitating incurable illnesses and in constant pain, express a wish to die and seek help in doing so, sometimes because physical impairment prevents them acting without assistance. Proponents of assisted suicide argue on the basis of personal autonomy. People have a right to choose. They have a right to make decisions about their own lives if they do not violate the rights of others. Legal arguments for the right to assisted suicide have been made in Ireland and other jurisdictions with reference to Article 8 of the European Convention on Human Rights. But Article 8 is a qualified right, subject to interference by the state to uphold the rights of others. The European Court of Human Rights acknowledges the right of contracting parties to impose a ban on assisted suicide when it is considered necessary to protect vulnerable citizens who might feel under pressure to end their own lives if assisted suicide became legally permissible.[15]

Ireland's blanket prohibition on assisted suicide was challenged in the High Court case of *Marie Fleming v Ireland and Others* (2012). The plaintiff, Marie Fleming, was 59 years of age and had suffered her first episode of multiple sclerosis at the age of 32. Multiple sclerosis is an incurable immune system-mediated disease that causes progressive neurological deterioration, eventually causing death. By 2010 Marie Fleming had lost the use of her hands, was almost completely physically helpless, and was suffering constant pain which was frequently intense.

Her mental faculties were unimpaired. She was losing the power of speech and was suffering choking episodes even when not attempting to swallow. The disease, she felt, had robbed her of her dignity. What lay ahead was months of pain, helplessness and isolation due to her impending loss of speech.

Marie Fleming was not afraid of death – it was the process of death that distressed her. She regretted not ending her life before she lost the use of her arms. What she wished for was a peaceful death with her family in attendance. She anticipated that, with help, she could self-administer lethal gas through a face mask; or, with medical assistance, she could apply a lethal injection. She did not wish her partner, daughter or son to assist her if such assistance exposed them to the risk of prosecution. There were alternatives. A patient could legally decline nutrition and hydration. She did not wish to die this way. Palliative care was not acceptable either. Heavy doses of analgesics would dull the pain but would induce a comatose state, which she wished to avoid.[16]

The High Court judges were not indifferent to the suffering of Marie Fleming. Even so they felt compelled to issue a reserved judgment against her on 10 January 2013. To issue a judgment in her favour would put other lives at risk – which they acknowledged was contrary to her wishes. Unintended consequences would arise. Vulnerable groups in society, such as the elderly, the disabled, and those who were suffering from mental illness, would be exposed to risk. Any safeguards in the new system would be "vulnerable to laxity and complacency and might well prove difficult or even impossible to police adequately".[17] It was "impossible to craft a solution specific to the needs of a plaintiff such as Ms. Fleming without jeopardising an essential fabric of the legal system … respect for human life". Protections for other citizens would be compromised.[18]

The case was appealed to the Supreme Court. It was argued on behalf of Marie Fleming that disabled people who were suffering severe pain from a terminally degenerative disease, and who were mentally competent in expressing their wishes, should not be prohibited in law from receiving assistance to end their lives. It was not beyond the competence of the Oireachtas to legislate for safeguards that addressed issues of consent, and verification of medical evidence. A blanket prohibition was disproportionate.[19] Furthermore, Section 2 (2) of the Criminal Law (Suicide) Act 1993, although apparently neutral, discriminated against disabled persons "in practice".[20] Article 40 of the Constitution grants all citizens equality before the law and imposes a duty on the state to protect their personal rights.

On 29 April 2013 the Supreme Court found that none of Marie Fleming's constitutional rights had been violated. Although suicide was no longer a crime, there was no explicit right in the Constitution to commit this act.[21] If there were such a right to suicide, it would have "to be found as part of another expressed right or in an unenumerated right". The issue of proportionality did not arise in the absence of a constitutional right.[22] Article 40.3.2 imposed a duty on the state to protect life. However, the "precise extent of the State's obligation in any given circumstances" was not entirely clear and in some cases might "require a careful balancing of other constitutional considerations". It was open to the Oireachtas to legislate for cases similar to that of Marie Fleming. The constitutionality of such legislation, and the practicability of its provisions, was likely to be tested in the courts.[23]

Marie Fleming died on 20 December 2013. The controversial issue of assisted suicide did not die with her. An advocacy group, Right to Die Ireland, was set up with three objectives in mind: (1) protecting the right to live; (2) respecting the right to die; and (3) the legalisation of assisted peaceful dying for rational people who were either seriously or terminally ill. Its founding members included Tom Curran, the partner of the late Marie Fleming.[24]

It was inevitable that further cases would arise similar to that of Marie Fleming. There seemed to be some basis for believing that prosecutions would not always be taken against those suspected of assisting suicide. Section 2 of the Criminal Law (Suicide) Act stated that no prosecution would be taken against a suspected offender without the consent of the Director of Public Prosecutions (DPP). The High Court anticipated that the DPP would be guided by "humane and sensitive" considerations in deciding whether or not to prosecute.[25] This soon proved to be at least unreliable, if not unfounded, when Gail O'Rorke was prosecuted for allegedly assisting her friend, Bernadette Forde, to commit suicide in 2011. Ms O'Rorke was acquitted in April 2015 after a three-week trial.[26] But the legal implications were clear enough for anyone who might find themselves in similar circumstances. It was very likely that such a person, motivated by compassion and acting on the wishes of a rational, well-informed and terminally ill adult, would be prosecuted, notwithstanding speculative comments expressed by the High Court. Tom Curran argued that the law prohibiting assisted suicide was not in harmony with public opinion. He referred to an *Irish Times* Ipsos MRBI poll that found that 54 per cent of respondents would be prepared to help another person to die, despite the possibility of a prison sentence of up to fourteen years. Over 80 per cent believed that the law needed to be changed. It seemed anomalous that it was a criminal act to help someone do something which was "perfectly legal". It also seemed contrary to the constitutionally supported principle that all citizens are equal before the law. A disabled person could not do something that was legally permissible in the case of an able-bodied person. Curran was mindful that vulnerable people needed to be protected if legislation was passed.[27]

Drafting legislation on such a sensitive and complex issue would prove to be a very challenging task with a considerable risk of political fallout. The main political parties left it to independent TD John Halligan to take the initiative. On 15 December 2015 he submitted his Dying with Dignity Bill (2015) for consideration by the Dáil. His proposal was to give "clearly consenting adults" who were experiencing extreme physical pain legal entitlement to seek medical assistance to die. He claimed that a number of opinion polls indicated that about 70 per cent of the electorate approved of assisted suicide in cases of terminal illness. Safeguards would have to be put in place to ensure that a decision by a terminally ill person was informed and had not been made under duress. Doctors who conscientiously objected would not be obligated to participate in an assisted suicide. Halligan pointed to increasing life expectancy and an ageing population, and how these were giving rise to greater frequencies of debilitating illnesses.[28]

International case law indicated that it would be extremely difficult to lift the blanket prohibition on assisted suicide in Ireland. The High Court judgment pointed to "a preponderance of judicial opinion" against assisted suicide in Canada, the USA, the UK, and at the European Court of Human Rights.[29] International law concerning human rights did not – in contrast to the issue of abortion – offer much support to the cause of assisted suicide. This, together with lack of political support, indicated very poor prospects for change within a few years. However, demographic trends have indicated quite the opposite – not just for Ireland but for the EU generally. Ageing populations, greater frequencies of age-related illnesses such as dementia, and escalating healthcare costs, indicate that attitudes are likely to change towards assisted suicide and euthanasia.[30]

There are unavoidable economic costs associated with enhancing the quality of life and extending longevity. All healthcare systems are restricted to varying degrees by finite resources. A case in point is the recommendation of the National Centre for Pharmacoeconomics (NCPE Ireland) in June 2016 that the drug Orkambi not be reimbursed because it was found to be not cost-effective for the treatment of cystic fibrosis in about 505 patients at the submitted price by Vertex Pharmaceuticals. The cost per patient per annum was about €159,000. The impact of this cost on the national health budget was so high that it imposed "an associated opportunity cost".[31] It provoked the question: "How do you put a price on a life?"[32] It can be argued that the state, in the context of providing healthcare services, has to make decisions about competing needs, and in some circumstances will have to put a price on human life due to limited resources.[33] Although quite separate issues, there is an inconsistency in public policy when there is a legal prohibition against assisted suicide for rational, well-informed and terminally ill persons who wish to avoid needless suffering in parallel with the state denying life-saving medical treatment to dangerously ill patients to prolong and enhance the quality of life.

The economic dimension to healthcare is inescapable, but it should not be permitted to feature prominently in lifting the total legal ban on assisted suicide. The central issue is one of balancing the right of self-determination with the need to protect those who are vulnerable. It is essentially a question of human rights. In Ireland, Catholic moral principles are likely to exert a considerable influence for many years to come in shaping public opinion on this highly sensitive ethical issue.

Endnotes

———————•———————

1   *Pastoral Constitution on the Church in the Modern World* (*Gaudium et spes*, 7 December 1965), paragraph 27, in Austin Flannery (general ed.), *Vatican Council II: The Conciliar and Post Conciliar Documents* (Dublin: Dominican Publications, new revised edn, 1992), p. 928.

2   Health Service Executive, "Euthanasia and assisted suicide" <http://hse.ie/eng/health/az/E/Euthanasia-and-assisted-suicide/Alternatives-to-euthanasia-and-assisted-suicide.html> accessed 29 March 2016.

3   Louise Campbell, "Current Debates about Legislating for Assisted Dying: Ethical Concerns", *Medico-Legal Journal of Ireland*, vol. 24, no.1 (2018), pp. 20–7 <https://login-westlaw-ie.ucc.idm.oclc.org/maf/wlie/app/document?src=toce&docguid=ID47A32FC7D524948A7F3527560CE1085&crumb-action=append&context=13> accessed 2 December 2018.

4   Deirdre Madden, "Is there a Right to a 'Good Death'?", *Medico-Legal Journal of Ireland*, vol. 19(2), 2013, pp. 60–7.

5   P. Kearns, *Fleming v Ireland and Ors*, High Court Judgment, [2013] IEHC 2, 10 January 2013 <http://www.courts.ie/Judgments.nsf/597645521f07a-c9a80256ef30048ca52/911cb02a6531c7a380257aef0037c379?OpenDocument> accessed 16 April 2016, paragraphs 53–5.

6   Pádraig Corkery, *Bioethics and the Catholic Moral Tradition* (Dublin: Veritas, 2010), p. 84.

7   Sacred Congregation for the Doctrine of the Faith, *Declaration on Euthanasia* (5 May 1980), in Austin Flannery (general ed.), *Vatican Council II: More Post Conciliar Documents* (Collegeville, Minn.: Liturgical Press, 1982), p. 512.

8   Domingo Bañez (1528–1604) introduced the terms "ordinary" and "extraordinary" to distinguish between what is morally obligatory and morally optional in treatments intended to prolong human life. His terminology, shortly afterwards, became part of Catholic moral philosophy and informed secular medical practice for centuries. See Joan McCarthy, Mary Donnelly, Dolores Dooley, Louise Campbell and David Smith, *End-of-Life Care: Ethics and Law* (Cork: Cork University Press, 2011), p. 278.

9   Sacred Congregation for the Doctrine of the Faith, *Declaration on Euthanasia*, p. 515.

10 See Corkery, *Bioethics and the Catholic Moral Tradition*, pp. 86–7.

11 *Declaration on Euthanasia*, pp. 515–16.

12 *Catechism of the Catholic Church* (Dublin: Veritas, 1995), paragraph 2279, p. 491.

13 There are different types of euthanasia. Active euthanasia occurs when a person intentionally intervenes to terminate another person's life. Passive euthanasia is withdrawing or withholding treatment necessary to sustain life, such as not giving antibiotics to treat pneumonia. Voluntary euthanasia is the termination of a person's life in response to their request for termination. Involuntary euthanasia occurs when a person is killed contrary to their expressed wishes and is almost always regarded as murder. Non-voluntary euthanasia occurs when the issue of consent does not arise, as in, for example, a severely brain damaged person. Health Service Executive, "Euthanasia and assisted suicide".

14 Criminal Law (Suicide) Act (1993) <http://www.irishstatutebook.ie/ eli/1993/act/11/enacted/en/print> accessed 15 April 2016.

15 McCarthy *et al.*, *End-of-Life Care*, p. 176; and Madden, "Is there a Right to a 'Good Death'?".

16 Kearns, *Fleming v Ireland and Ors*, paragraphs 10–24.

17 Ibid., paragraph 76.

18 Ibid., paragraph 120.

19 Louise Campbell (clinical ethicist and lecturer in medical ethics at National University of Ireland, Galway) observed that the actions of Ms Fleming were those of a "competent, rational individual with a clear and settled desire to end a life which she found incompatible with her sense of what life should be. It is difficult to see how the interests of the vulnerable can be served by condemning someone in Ms Fleming's situation to live a life so entirely at odds with her own purposes." Louise Campbell, "The Limits of Autonomy: An Exploration of the Role of Autonomy in the Debate about Assisted Suicide" in Mary Donnelly and Claire Murray (eds), *Ethical and Legal Debates in Irish Healthcare: Confronting Complexities* (Manchester: Manchester University Press, 2016), p. 66.

20 C.J. Denham, *Fleming v Ireland & Ors*, paragraph 24; Neutral Citation [2013] IESC 19, Supreme Court Record Number 019/2013 <http:// www.supremecourt.ie/Judgments.nsf/60f9f366f10958d1802572ba003d-3f45/94ff4efe25ba9b4280257b5c003eea73?OpenDocument&Highlight=0,-Fleming> accessed 9 June 2015.

21 Deirdre Madden, *Medicine, Ethics and Law* (Haywards Heath, UK: Bloomsbury Professional, 2016 (3rd edn)), pp. 628–33, 639–41.

22 Denham, *Fleming v Ireland*, paragraphs 99–100.

23 Ibid., paragraphs 106–8.

24 Right to Die Ireland website <http://rtdireland.com/about/> accessed 23 April 2016.

25 Madden, "Is there a Right to a 'Good Death'?".

26 Dearbhail McDonald, "'Justice done' as jury acquits carer Gail O'Rorke of

assisting sick woman's suicide", Independent.ie, 29 April 2015 <http://www.
independent.ie/irish-news/courts/justice-done-as-jury-acquits-carer-gail-
ororke-of-assisting-sick-womans-suicide-31180940.html> accessed 30 July
2016.

27 Tom Curran, "Helping a person to die – why new compassionate laws are
needed", *Irish Times*, 29 April 2015, <http://www.irishtimes.com/opinion/
helping-a-person-to-die-why-new-compassionate-laws-are-needed-
1.2192306?mode=print&ot=example.AjaxPageLayout.ot> accessed 29 April
2015.

28 Dying with Dignity Bill 2015: First Stage, Dáil Debates, vol.
901, no.1 (15 December 2015) <http://oireachtasdebates.
oireachtas.ie/debates%20authoring/debateswebpack.nsf/takes/
dail2015121500035?opendocument#NN01200> accessed 21 April 2016.

29 Kearns, *Fleming v Ireland*, paragraph 119.

30 See David Smith, "Euthanasia: Conflicting Positions" in Enda MacDonagh
and Vincent MacNamara (eds), *An Irish Reader in Moral Theology: The Legacy
of the Last Fifty Years* (Dublin: Columba Press, 2013), p. 344; Ciarán D'Arcy,
"Issue of assisted suicide 'coming down the tracks' for Ireland", *Irish Times*,
16 October 2015, report on Emily O'Reilly's address to the Conference on
Strengthening the Voice of Older People (Dublin) <http://www.irishtimes.
com/news/social-affairs/issue-of-assisted-suicide-coming-down-the-tracks-
for-ireland-1.2394640?mode=print&ot=example.AjaxPageLayout.ot>
accessed 17 October 2015.

31 "Cost-effectiveness of Lumacaftor/Ivacaftor (Orkambi) for cystic fibrosis
in patients aged 12 years and older who are homozygous for the F508del
mutation in the CFTR gene", National Centre for Pharmacoeconomics
(NCPE Ireland) (June 2016) <http://www.ncpe.ie/wp-content/
uploads/2015/12/Website-summary-orkambi.pdf> accessed 8 August
2016. The NCPE is a team of clinicians, pharmacologists, pharmacists and
statisticians who advise the Health Services Executive about the costs and
benefits of medical technologies.

32 Muiris Houston, "A doctor writes: Cost of high-tech drugs a bitter pill
to swallow", *Irish Times*, 3 June 2016 <http://www.irishtimes.com/
news/health/a-doctor-writes-cost-of-high-tech-drugs-a-bitter-pill-to-
swallow-1.2670565> accessed 3 June 2016.

33 For example, funding the cost of Pembrolizumab ("Pembro") for melanoma
cancer treatment at a cost of €70,000 per annum per patient, and declining to
fund the cost of Orkambi for cystic fibrosis treatment at about €159,000 per
patient per annum. Houston, "A doctor writes".

CHAPTER SIX

———•———

Assisted Human Reproduction

2013–2019

Surrogacy

INCREASED RATES OF INFERTILITY ARE OFTEN ATTRIBUTED to social and lifestyle factors such as delayed parenthood (frequently for career purposes and financial security), sexually transmitted diseases, and obesity. Many couples affected by infertility or impaired fertility have opted for treatments arising from developments in assisted human reproduction (AHR) technologies, such as IVF, gamete (ova and spermatozoa) donation from third parties, and surrogacy. In a surrogacy agreement the surrogate mother consents to artificial insemination or to the transfer of an embryo to her womb. She agrees to hand over the child shortly after birth to the commissioning couple (or sometimes commissioning person). There are – potentially – up to five participants in surrogacy procedures: the commissioning mother, the commissioning father, the surrogate mother, the egg donor, and the sperm donor.[1]

Thousands of children were born in Ireland due to IVF and other AHR procedures, but fertility clinics in Ireland operated in a legislative vacuum.[2] Legitimate expectations of a comprehensive regulatory framework – by couples availing of AHR services, staff in fertility clinics, and the general public – were not being met. Couples contemplating AHR services were confronted by legal uncertainties. Before access to IVF and surrogacy, there was no rational basis for challenging the legal maxim *mater semper certa est* – "motherhood is always certain". The mother was always the birth mother and the identity of the father could be challenged. Science changed all this: DNA tests could confirm the identity of the father of a child; in surrogacy agreements science split motherhood into its genetic and gestational elements. Who then was the real mother?

It was inevitable that surrogacy cases would come before the courts. In the absence of an adequate legislative framework such cases would be difficult to resolve – even those that were relatively straightforward. A landmark High Court case (*M.R. & Anor v An tArd Chlaraitheoir & Ors*) in early March 2013 drew public attention to the urgent need for legislation. It concerned a married couple, genetic parents of twins, whose application to be registered as the children's parents on their birth certificates had been denied in 2011.[3] The surrogate mother was the sister of the genetic mother and was in full agreement that her sister should be registered as the infants' mother. The state authorities disagreed, asserting that "as a matter of law" the gestational mother was the mother of the twins.[4] Their case was heard in the High Court and on 5 March 2013 Mr Justice Henry Abbott delivered his judgment. He found that the Latin maxim *mater semper certa est* could no longer be sustained because of access to IVF. Surrogacy was not illegal because "positive legislation" on the issue was "totally absent".[5] Mindful of the need to issue a judgment consistent with "constitutional and natural justice" for both genetic parents, the judge stated that the genetic mother should be registered as the mother under the Civil Registration Act 2004.[6] Expert evidence had been submitted concerning how the gestational mother influenced foetal growth and development.[7] Even so, DNA was acknowledged as the dominant determining factor. Mr Justice Abbott believed that the main consideration was the blood relationship as determined through chromosomal DNA.[8]

This landmark case had the potential to raise legal difficulties for some couples who had children by means of assisted human reproduction. For example: what would be the status of a child whose mother had become pregnant through the use of donor gametes? Previously, legal difficulties did not arise because birth/gestational mothers were "lawful mothers".[9] In the absence of adequate legislation, parents would feel compelled to undertake time-consuming, costly and stressful legal actions to address a range of problems concerning their children relating to inheritance, taxation, passports and medical procedures. Passport issues arose when couples resorted to surrogacy services abroad.[10]

Catholics who wished to stay loyal to the teachings of their Church were confronted by an additional challenge. It was clear from the Vatican's *Donum Vitae*, and from the Catechism, that the Roman Catholic Church opposed all forms of surrogacy. The Church declared that:

> Techniques that entail the dissociation of husband and wife, by the intrusion of a person other than the couple (donation of sperm or ovum, surrogate uterus), are gravely immoral. These techniques … infringe the child's right to be born of a father and mother known to him and bound to each other by marriage. They betray the spouses' "right to become a father and a mother only through each other." Techniques involving only the married couple … are perhaps less reprehensible, yet remain morally unacceptable. They dissociate the sexual act from the procreative act.[11]

Abbott's judgment received coverage in the national press, but there was little criticism that was explicitly Catholic. The Iona Institute, set up to promote "the place of marriage and religion in society", and Roman Catholic in its outlook, observed that surrogacy imposed on society the question: who was the "true" mother of the child – the birth mother, the genetic mother, or the "social"/ "intentional"/ "commissioning" mother? The institute urged the government to bring forward legislation to prohibit surrogacy. This would, it claimed, be consistent with the laws of most European states.[12] The institute also published a detailed paper arguing that surrogacy was unethical. Surrogacy violated the dignity of both the mother and child and was against their best interests. There was a danger that surrogate mothers and children would be treated as commodities. Even when surrogacy arrangements were motivated by altruism they were "a violation of the human dignity of mother and child".[13] The institute constructed its argument on the basis of legal considerations and the welfare of children and women rather than invoking religious or theological opinions.

The Iona Institute pointed to ethical problems and legal difficulties. Commercial surrogacy was thriving in some countries where vulnerable women were subjected to exploitation.[14] If an Irish couple resorted to surrogacy services abroad (in India, for example), problems were likely to arise in relation to the child concerning nationality and entitlement to an Irish passport. Surrogacy was a legal minefield. What would the law dictate if the surrogate mother changed her mind and wished to keep the child? The commissioning couple might also decide not to take the child in the event of their relationship breaking down or if the child was born with a disability. If disability was diagnosed during pregnancy, would the surrogate mother be legally required to terminate the pregnancy? Sharp differences of opinion might also emerge about the appropriate course of action if there was a serious risk to the mother's health or life during pregnancy.[15]

On 6 June 2013 the Department of Social Protection issued a press release stating that the Fine Gael–Labour coalition government intended to legislate for surrogacy and other issues concerning assisted human reproduction. The department acknowledged that these were matters of "exceptional public importance". Legislation was being drafted for consideration by the government later in the year. The High Court judgment presented difficulties on two main fronts. By "linking motherhood exclusively to genetic connection" it would potentially have adverse consequences for many families. It was anticipated that the judgment would also limit the freedom of the Oireachtas to legislate for surrogacy and related issues. The government therefore intended to appeal the landmark judgment to the Supreme Court.[16]

On 5 November 2013 the Department of Justice and Equality expressed concern about the increasing frequency of commercial surrogacy arrangements by Irish citizens, both at home and abroad. The Children and Family Relationships Bill 2013 was intended to provide a legislative framework for parental duties and responsibilities "in diverse family forms", including those created through assisted human reproduction. Commercial surrogacy was to be prohibited.[17] There was some speculation that the Minister for Justice, Alan Shatter, a barrister who had practised family law, had himself drafted most of the legislation over the summer.[18]

Shatter published a draft General Scheme of Children and Family Relationships Bill on 30 January 2014 to facilitate a consultative process that would include the Oireachtas Committee on Justice, Equality and Defence, the Oireachtas Committee on Health and Children, "relevant interest groups" and the general public. The "diverse family forms" referred to earlier included single parent families, families where children were cared for by a parent and a step-parent, by extended family members, by cohabiting couples, and by couples in civil partnerships. It was to be a comprehensive scheme with the best interests of children as its most important principle. Parental rights and responsibilities were to be clarified in legal terms for all families. Irish legislation would "set out how parentage is to be assigned in cases of assisted reproduction and non-commercial surrogacy".[19]

The ideal family from an orthodox Catholic perspective was "a man and a woman united in marriage, together with their children".[20] The Church declared that there was a moral imperative for public authorities to acknowledge this and to implement policies supportive of family life.[21] However, both law and society in Ireland had strayed far from the norms of Catholic moral teaching and there were no indications that this trend would be reversed or halted. For example, single gay and lesbian individuals could adopt children.[22] This was far beyond the bounds of what was legally permissible, or deemed morally acceptable by mainstream public opinion, before the decriminalisation of homosexuality in 1993. Shatter had little reason to fear pronouncements from the Catholic hierarchy; but traditionalist Catholic opinion in general was a different matter.

Shatter's draft scheme was published only a few days before the state's challenge to the Abbott judgment was heard in the Supreme Court. The case title was *M.R. and D.R. (suing by their father and next friend O.R.) & Ors v An t-Ard-Chláraitheoir & Ors.* Michael McDowell SC, acting on behalf of the state, pointed out that there would be "massive" and "radical" consequences if the High Court judgment was upheld.[23]

McDowell argued that the birth mother was legally the mother of the child and that the High Court was not empowered to amend public law in this way by changing the meaning of motherhood. McDowell was questioned thoroughly by the Supreme Court judges. What had the Constitution to say about motherhood? McDowell replied that motherhood was not defined by the Constitution, but Article 40.3.3 (asserting the equal right to life of the mother and unborn child) implied that the woman who gives birth is the mother. Even so, the Constitution permitted motherhood to "shift in certain circumstances", as in cases of adoption.[24]

The judges "wanted to talk about science." *Mater semper certa est* was no longer sustainable. Reality and the law were in conflict here and would remain so until the Oireachtas brought about reconciliation. McDowell distributed copies of the government's draft General Scheme of Children and Family Relationships Bill to the seven Supreme Court judges, to impress upon them that the law concerning surrogacy would be decided by the Oireachtas.[25]

It was clear that the definition of motherhood needed to be broadened – otherwise some women who had used donor eggs to have children were at risk of becoming "demothered".[26] The Supreme Court judges, mindful that the state was busy drafting legislation on the issue, reserved their judgment.[27] David Quinn, a former editor of the *Irish Catholic*, evidently felt that he had seen enough of what was in the legislative programme to deliver a caustic commentary. Shatter's legislative proposals were "riddled ... with the ideology of choice" – as if there was something inherently objectionable or unethical about the element of choice in becoming a parent. In Quinn's ideal world, nature rather than "intention" was the true determinant of parenthood. There was of course the complication presented by adoption, which Quinn felt some obligation to acknowledge, but his dismissive attitude was evident in the comment: "we know from adoption that no matter how well children are loved by their adoptive parents, they will frequently go looking for their natural parents anyway."[28] There was, then, it seemed, something very deficient about love in the absence of genetic parentage.

Quinn's point that issues of personal identity arose in the absence of information about genetic origins was a source of genuine concern, yet there was a lack of balance in his analysis. After all, many children not conceived through AHR were unintended, frequently unwanted, and sometimes unloved. There was also the welfare of women to be addressed. Quinn simply assumed the worst, pointing to the gross exploitation of women in India while ignoring the Abbott judgment, which presented an entirely different case in an Irish context. Shatter's declared objective was to introduce legal reforms so that different types of family would have legal clarity concerning parental responsibilities and rights based on the best interests of children.

In May 2014 Alan Shatter was replaced by Fine Gael TD Frances Fitzgerald as Minister for Justice and Equality. Surrogacy was removed from the General Scheme of the Children and Family Relationships Bill on which Shatter had worked so extensively. The reasons given were that, first, a Supreme Court decision was pending on the state's appeal against the Abbott judgment. Second, "critical issues needed to be resolved" concerning commercial surrogacy and the rights of children born through surrogacy arrangements.[29]

The Supreme Court delivered its judgment on 7 November 2014.[30] The interpretative process was narrowly focused, addressing the question: who was to be registered as the mother of the children? What was the meaning of the word "mother" in the text of the 2004 Act?[31] Science had undermined or altered underlying assumptions, but this did not alter the interpretation of the Act.[32] It was not for the courts to lay down principles regulating the legal status of genetic and gestational mothers in the wide range of circumstances that would inevitably arise in surrogacy arrangements. Value judgements needed to be applied to the legislative process, especially in relation to the welfare of children. This was the function of the Oireachtas, not the courts. The courts could only interpret and apply the law as they found it, or, in the case of the Supreme Court, deliver final judgment on its constitutionality. It was clear from the provisions of the Civil Registration Act that such terms as "particulars of the birth" and "when a child is born in the state" dictated that the birth mother was to be legally registered as the mother.[33] If the Abbott judgment was upheld, it was possible that women who had become pregnant through the use of donor genetic material would lose their status as mothers in a legal sense.[34]

The Constitution did not define motherhood. There was no constitutional impediment to legislation on surrogacy. Therefore, the Oireachtas was free to legislate on this issue. In the meantime, children were being born into a "legal limbo". This created problems for parents and children alike.[35] In the above case, for example, the genetic mother was not legally permitted to sign for her children's participation in a school excursion or to give consent for a medical procedure. Passports had to be signed for by the surrogate mother, which could be especially difficult in cases of commercial surrogacy where the surrogate mother was living abroad.

The Supreme Court judgment upheld the rights of birth mothers whose children had been donor conceived. But the state failed to address the rights of genetic mothers, leaving them and their children in a legal limbo. Author Jill Allison observed that "Their social, emotional and financial commitment to parenting a child is eclipsed by the fact of birth and another woman, who may have no social investment in that child [and] will be designated as the mother."[36] There was a clear need for a new approach to the onerous task of framing legislation for surrogacy – legislation which was long overdue to remedy the ongoing injustice to many families in Ireland.

Same-sex Marriage

The Convention on the Constitution was established by the Oireachtas in 2012 to put forward recommendations on several issues concerning constitutional reform, one of which was same-sex marriage. The government committed to responding to each recommendation of the Convention in the Oireachtas but not necessarily to hold a referendum on any proposed constitutional amendment. On 17 December 2013, Alan Shatter, then Minister for Justice and Equality, informed the Dáil that a referendum facilitating same-sex marriage would, in response to a recommendation of the Convention, be held on or before mid-2015.[37] The Fine Gael–Labour coalition government had hoped to have had the Children and Family Relationships Bill passed by both the Dáil and Seanad well in advance of the onset of public debates about the referendum, probably because of the complexity of the issues in the Bill. Even if this had been achieved, it was probably inevitable that same-sex marriage would still have become entangled in controversies about the adoption of children and assisted human reproduction.[38] It was in the interests of those who opposed same-sex marriage to interlink these issues.

The impending legislation was described by Taoiseach Enda Kenny as the most important reform of family law since the foundation of the state.[39] The Children and Family Relationships Bill provided a legal framework for parentage, custody, guardianship and access to children across a range of family situations not satisfactorily addressed in existing legislation. Single-parent families and cohabiting couples with children totalled over 275,000 citizens.[40] The Bill provided for the adoption of children by same-sex couples and it created a legal standing for children born through donor-assisted reproduction. The Bill was drafted to prioritise the welfare of children in diverse family circumstances. It elicited broad cross-party support and it was signed into law by President Michael D. Higgins on 6 April 2015 after approval by both Houses of the Oireachtas.

The Children and Family Relationships Act 2015 is complex and long, extending to 117 pages. The Act addressed legal issues arising from donor-assisted human reproduction (DAHR). Surrogacy was excluded! The Department of Health was given responsibility for drafting legislation on this complex issue. But, as Taoiseach Enda Kenny made clear in May 2015, there would be no legislation on surrogacy before the next election.[41]

The Act was consistent with the Supreme Court judgment in the surrogacy case – the birth mother was still the legal mother of the child. Provisions of the Act enabled civil partners and cohabiting couples to jointly adopt children, although this would not have immediate effect.[42] The parents of a donor-conceived child would be the birth mother and her husband, civil partner or cohabitant (intending parent) when the mother and the intending parent had given consent in advance. If such consent had not been given, then the birth mother alone would be the parent of the child. Donors of spermatozoa, ova or embryos had no parental rights or duties towards the child.[43] The Act also provided for the use of DNA testing to determine parentage in some circumstances.

When the Children and Family Relationships Act 2015 was signed into law the referendum on marriage equality was only a few weeks away (set for 22 May). Concerns were expressed that it might be defeated, especially if it became entangled with the issue of adoption of children. *Irish Times* columnist Stephen Collins observed that the outcomes of referendums in Ireland and elsewhere were frequently influenced by extraneous issues.[44] This observation proved accurate in the case of same-sex marriage. The Thirty-Fourth Amendment to the Constitution (Marriage Equality) Bill 2015 proposed to add the following words to Article 41: "Marriage may be contracted in accordance with law by two persons without distinction as to their sex." And who could argue against the principle of equality? Opponents of same-sex marriage would have to find some other issue as a basis for their arguments if they were to secure rejection – and they did so.

The Irish Catholic Bishops' Conference published a booklet, *The Meaning of Marriage*, in December 2014, to inform the electorate of its stance on the issue. It reaffirmed its opposition to same-sex marriage, arguing that the "rational basis" of marriage was that it should be "reserved for the unique and complementary relationship between a man and a woman from which the generation and upbringing of children is uniquely possible". Children had "a natural right to a mother and a father" and this was "the best environment for them where possible". Heterosexual marriage was "therefore deserving of special recognition and promotion by the State". Marriage was "the single most important institution" in all societies and if it was redefined it would be undermined as "the fundamental building block" of society.[45] The bishops were adamant that same-sex marriage was not about equality or about a civil versus a religious view of marriage. It was not about civil rights or a denial of dignity. It was about the fundamental nature of marriage, its importance to society, and the welfare of children.[46]

Same-sex relationships were, by their very nature, different from marriage. A same-sex couple, unlike a heterosexual couple, could not procreate without recourse to a third party. The "biological bond" between children and their natural parents was important. The bishops of course acknowledged that sometimes it was not possible for children to be raised by their biological parents. In these circumstances adoption and fostering by heterosexual married couples would provide the next best type of environment for children. If the state failed to protect marriage

– as understood by the Church – it would "in effect, deprive children of the right to a mother and a father".[47] The bishops' *Meaning of Marriage* was launched at St Patrick's College, Maynooth on 3 December 2014 and distributed to about 1,300 parishes.[48]

The bishops were not alone in their opposition to the proposed constitutional amendment. A few organisations, including the Iona Institute and Mothers and Fathers Matter, campaigned for a No vote. Professor Ray Kinsella of University College Dublin, fathers' rights campaigner John Waters, disability rights campaigner Kathy Sinnott, and senators Jim Walsh and Rónán Mullen, campaigned against the amendment.

Senator Mullen argued that same-sex marriage could not simply be restricted to the issue of equality. The government was manipulating the electorate. If people expressed opposition, it might seem that they were against equality – that they were "homophobes". The proposed constitutional amendment was essentially dishonest. It would "create a situation where a child had no right to a mother". It would impose restrictions on government when legislating on surrogacy. It was dishonest to claim that matters of marriage and children could be isolated from each other.[49] David Quinn, writing in the *Irish Catholic*, observed that Article 41 was entitled "The Family", not "Marriage". The article made it clear that the family was founded on marriage. Marriage had "always been understood" as a union of a man and a woman. Quinn believed that the Constitution bestowed the right to have children. Therefore, same-sex couples would have the right to have children underpinned by the Constitution. This had profound implications for future legislation on assisted human reproduction. Quinn attached high importance to "biological ties", which could not be severed without adverse consequences – even if a child was reared in a loving environment.[50]

Opponents of same-sex marriage observed, with reference to the European Court of Human Rights (ECHR), that "marriage equality" was not a human right. Access to civil partnership had been available since 2011 and an estimated 1,500 couples had availed of it. The rights bestowed by civil partnership were "almost identical" to the rights given by marriage. Same-sex marriage was a redefinition of marriage and the family that violated the rights of children. The morally appropriate alternative was to extend the rights associated with civil partnership to grant better social and legal support to same-sex couples.[51] This argument failed to acknowledge the key point that married couples enjoyed the benefit of constitutional as well as legal protection. Civil partnerships granted only legal protection, which could be overturned, diminished or amended by parliament, whereas constitutional protection could only be removed by the people through a referendum.

Those for and those against same-sex marriage agreed that marriage was of central importance for any healthy society. Activists on both sides expressed support for the role of families in Irish social life and for enhancing the rights of children. Beyond that there was little common ground. Advocates for a Yes vote argued that the constitutional status of marriage would remain unchanged and that extending the right to marry to same-sex couples would not damage or diminish the status of those who already had that right. The right of same-sex couples to marry was essentially about inclusivity, justice and equality. It was about civil marriage – not religious marriage. No Church would be legally obligated to conduct a marriage ceremony inconsistent with its own doctrines[52] – therefore religious liberty was not an issue.

Concern was expressed that the welfare of children would be somehow at risk if same-sex marriage was legally permitted. This was potentially the Achilles heel of the Yes campaign. Proponents of a Yes vote therefore endeavoured to assuage public concern by pointing out that they enjoyed the support of all the major children's charities, including Barnardos, the Irish Society for the Prevention of Cruelty to Children, Foróige and Children's Rights Alliance.[53] The clear implication was that such support was hardly likely if there were credible doubts on this point.

Diametrically opposing claims by the Yes and No campaigns created confusion in the minds of many voters. There was a pressing need for clarification. In mid-May, Kevin Cross, a High Court judge and chairperson of the Referendum Commission, issued public statements providing legal clarification on key issues that undermined claims made by the No campaign. The Constitution did not define marriage. The constitutional status of marriage would not change if the Thirty-Fourth Amendment was carried.[54]

Opponents of the proposed amendment claimed that "Marriage comes with the Constitutional right to start a family. For same-sex couples this would require AHR and / or surrogacy."[55] This was misleading. There was some basis for the claim that a couple had the right to procreate naturally, although such a right was not unlimited.[56] There was no constitutional right to access AHR. Access to AHR would be regulated by law. The specific issue of surrogacy was unregulated – there were neither legal rights or prohibitions – nor was there any constitutional provisions on surrogacy. There was no link between surrogacy and same-sex marriage, or between adoption and same-sex marriage.[57]

The issue of adopting children was raised by No campaigners. But nobody had a right to adopt a child – this would not change if the Thirty-Fourth Amendment was passed. There was a right to apply for adoption, which was very different. Same-sex couples were already eligible to apply. Adoption, unlike surrogacy, was regulated by law and would only occur where it was deemed to be in the best interests of the child. There was no right to a mother and a father – contrary to claims by those against the amendment.[58]

Same-sex married couples would have the same constitutional status as opposite-sex married couples. But could legislation be passed that treated same-sex married couples differently from opposite-sex couples? The answer was not straightforward. If, for example, evidence was presented that children fared better with opposite-sex parents than with same-sex parents, it was possible that legislation could introduce differential measures in response to this. The evidence would have to be subjected to rigorous review and would be tested by the judiciary. Parenting capacity rather than marital status would be the central issue. Legislation could not be arbitrary.[59]

Was homosexuality psychologically abnormal or pathological? Was there something about it that was harmful to children whose parents were of the same gender? The interpretation of scripture by the Roman Catholic Church presented homosexual acts as "acts of grave depravity".[60] The Church toned down the intemperate language of scripture but declared that homosexual acts were "intrinsically disordered". The Church teaches that such acts "are contrary to natural law" and "close the sexual act to the gift of life ... Under no circumstances can they be approved."[61] Homosexuals were "called to chastity". The Church acknowledged that homosexuals did not choose their "condition" – for the majority of them it was "a trial". They were not to suffer "unjust discrimination".[62]

As early as December 1975 the Church had indicated its awareness that research in psychology was influencing people to "judge homosexual relationships indulgently and even to excuse them completely" – contrary to the teachings of the Church.[63] Catholic doctrine and science had reached different conclusions on this issue. Forty years later, in Catholic Ireland, nothing had changed to suggest that agreement had been reached. A group of thirteen psychiatrists practising in Ireland wrote to the *Irish Times* with a strong argument in favour of a Yes vote:

> A fundamental tenet of medical care is the acceptance of patients

as they are and for who they are. From a psychiatric point of view, there is no medical or psychiatric pathology related to same-sex preferences. Nor is there any abnormality related to same-sex relationships. Discrimination, however, is harmful to mental health. Therefore, in the interests of promoting happiness and better mental health, we intend to vote Yes for the marriage referendum.[64]

A group of eight psychologists, writing "on behalf of 316 independent Irish Psychologists", presented further scientific evidence:

We are an independent group of psychologists in Ireland. From a psychological point of view same-sex preference is part of the spectrum of human sexuality and is in no way abnormal or pathological. Same-sex couples are similar to heterosexual couples in many regards. All the available research shows that children of same-sex couples are similar to children of heterosexual couples. Inequality and discrimination, however, are damaging to mental health. It is for these reasons that we intend to vote Yes in the marriage referendum.[65]

Scientific evidence and expert legal opinion weighed heavily in favour of same-sex marriage. There was broad support for it in the main political parties, the press, voluntary and professional organisations, and the youth sector of the electorate. The Thirty-Fourth Amendment was carried by a large majority of approximately 62 per cent. All constituencies except Roscommon–South Leitrim voted Yes.[66] Opponents of same-sex marriage had observed that most countries in Europe had not "redefined" marriage. In countries where same-sex marriage had been introduced it was "imposed" either by politicians or the court system. No country had introduced it by means of a referendum.[67] Ireland was now the first country in the world to have done so. Its reputation as a conservative Catholic country was shattered, both at home and abroad.[68]

Yes voters celebrated in the streets, many of them evidently enjoying the attention of journalists and press photographers. Extensive international coverage followed, including commentary from the BBC's World Service, the *Daily Telegraph* (Britain), the TV news channel CNN (USA), the *New York Times*, the Qatari TV news channel Al Jazeera, the *Hindustan Times* (India), the *South China Morning Post* (Hong Kong), *El Pais* (Spain) and the *Sydney Morning Herald*.[69] Most significant, for the Catholic Church in Ireland, was the comment by Cardinal Pietro Parolin, the Vatican's Secretary of State, an experienced diplomat who was well known for his tact and discretion. Observers of Vatican current affairs were surprised at his intemperate comment that the referendum result was a "disaster for humanity". The margin of the Yes victory in Ireland provoked those in the higher echelons of the international Church to think about the poor outcomes of the Church's dialogue with western culture. Something had gone very badly wrong, because western society was experiencing "an accelerated process of secularisation".[70] To simply attribute the Yes victory in Ireland to the emergence of a highly secularised society was an oversimplification. Many conscientious Catholics voted Yes – including Mary McAleese, former President of Ireland and highly educated in theology; and Sister Stanislaus Kennedy ("Sister Stan"), well known for her work among the poor. It was not simply about the weakening of Catholicism in western society; it was very much about internal transformations within Catholicism – including regular church-going Catholics.

The bishops were clearly shocked at the outcome of the referendum. Catholic Primate of Ireland, Archbishop Eamon Martin, mindful of Cardinal Parolin's reaction, expressed a sense of "bereavement ... something very unique and precious had been lost."[71] It seemed as if that something was not just about the meaning of marriage. It was very much about the bishops' loss of power and growing sense of isolation in a Church that had experienced radical change. Archbishop Diarmuid Martin believed that the Church needed to do "a reality check right across the board". He was cautious in that he did not explicitly criticise the abysmally poor leadership in the top echelons of the Church. A "social revolution" had been under way for quite some time and this had been poorly understood. Of particular significance was the drifting away of young people from the Church. Twelve years of indoctrination in Catholic schools was not working well. The Church needed to find "a new language" – one that was expressed in terms of love and was not condemnatory. It had to consider the complexities of how people lived their lives![72]

Martin's speech led to the question of what kind of "reality check" the Church needed. Fr Gerry O'Hanlon, a former provincial of the Jesuits in Ireland, believed that Martin had not addressed the essence of the problem when he spoke about the need of the Church to find "a new language" to communicate its teachings. The problem was not so much with the communication as the message itself. The Church had lost credibility – especially with the young – on gender and sexual issues. Church teaching could not be "simply" changed to harmonise with contemporary culture. It was essential for the Catholic hierarchy to promote a "culture of dialogue" within the Church to ascertain "the sense of the faithful," and to empower the laity.[73] Yet the bishops were likely to resist to the utmost any demands for such empowerment. If conceded, it was most likely to overturn some of their cherished doctrines on sexual morality and the status of women in the Church. But such resistance was likely to further damage the Church and might prove futile. As journalist Patsy McGarry observed in the *Irish Times*, the average age of Irish Catholic priests was 64, and the retirement age was 75. Some of those priests decided not to read out their bishops' pastoral letters to the faithful during the marriage equality referendum campaign, while others publicly expressed support for the proposed amendment to the Constitution.[74]

About 734,000 people had voted No. Weekly Mass-going adults in the Republic numbered about one million. David Quinn, writing in the *Irish Catholic*, deduced from these figures that many of these Catholics had voted Yes, effectively handing victory to the Yes side. Opponents of same-sex marriage found little if any support from "famous celebrities", "the major institutions of society", the print and broadcast media, or the political parties. The major cause of the widespread dissent from the Church's teaching was, in Quinn's opinion, the failure of the Church to teach catechesis on marriage for many years.[75] Quinn's fellow columnist Michael Kelly was more perceptive when addressing the reasons why Catholics did not conform to their Church's teachings on sexual morality. He observed:

> Of course, it's no surprise that it is the teachings that people find personally difficult that are largely rejected. I've never heard a Catholic say they struggle to understand the Hypostatic union or the procession of the Holy Spirit from the Father and the Son. Instead, it is areas that touch very directly on sexuality and relationships.[76]

Robust catechesis and nurturing a culture of dialogue was not likely to make much of an impact on this problem. Vast numbers of Catholics were quite willing to accept obscure theological concepts that they did not understand. But religious faith had its limits – for many it would not dictate decisions on life-and-death issues. Catholics were independently exercising their own judgement on abortion, AHR, sexual relationships and contraception. Many Catholics, including some regular Mass-going Catholics, had "walked away from the teaching without walking away from the practice of the Faith".[77]

The General Scheme of the Assisted Human Reproduction Bill 2017

After the general election on 26 February 2016 a new minority coalition of Fine Gael and independent TDs formed the new government after more than two months of negotiations. Enda Kenny was re-elected Taoiseach on 6 May and was succeeded by Leo Varadkar on 14 June 2017. On 3 October the Minister for Health, Simon Harris, announced the government's approval of the General Scheme of the Assisted Human Reproduction Bill 2017 (GSAHR).[78] It was a broad-ranging scheme, extending to 190 pages. The main guiding principle was that due consideration would be given to the wellbeing and health of children born as a result of AHR. Appropriate measures were to be taken to protect the health of intending parents, donors and surrogates.[79]

Part 3 outlined the conditions and restrictions relating to the donation of gametes and embryos for use in AHR treatments for other people and for research. Further provisions of the Bill allowed for posthumous assisted reproduction (Part 4); pre-implantation genetic diagnosis (PGD), gender selection for medical reasons, and human leucocyte antigen (HLA) matching (Part 5); and the establishment of an Assisted Human Reproduction Regulatory Authority (Part 8).[80] Part 7 of the GSAHR stipulated the conditions under which research could be undertaken using hESCs, iPSCs and embryos, subject to obtaining a licence from the regulatory authority.[81]

Part 6 outlined the conditions under which surrogacy would be permitted. Commercial surrogacy agreements were to be prohibited. Surrogacy agreements were to be pre-authorised by the regulatory authority. At least one intending parent had to be "ordinarily resident" in Ireland. The surrogate had to be "habitually resident" in Ireland and the embryo transfer had to occur within the state.[82] Surrogacy was permissible for married couples, civil partners, cohabiting couples, and single intending parents.[83] It was not permissible to use the surrogate's egg to create the embryo. At least one intending parent had to be genetically related to the child. The GSAHR outlined a court-based process through which the parentage of the child could be transferred from the surrogate (and her husband, if applicable) to the intending parent or parents.

The Joint Committee on Health (JCH) began pre-legislative

scrutiny of the GSAHR on 17 January 2018. This series of deliberations was an important part of the legislative process, facilitating a detailed examination of the draft legislation in the light of written submissions and oral evidence by advocacy groups, stakeholders and experts. The committee was to issue a report to the government before the final version of the Bill was drafted.[84]

IVF, using gametes from both parents, was the most common form of AHR in Ireland. There were relatively few cases of surrogacy because fertility clinics did not provide the service.[85] Dr Tony Holohan, Chief Medical Officer at the Department of Health, informed the committee that one in six couples worldwide experience infertility at some point. The rate of infertility was increasing, including in Ireland.[86] It was estimated, on the basis of information received from the Health Products Regulatory Authority, that AHR procedures carried out in fertility clinics in Ireland increased from 7,589 cycles in 2009 to nearly 9,000 in 2016.[87] Demand for AHR services was clearly rising. The categories of people seeking treatment had increased to include not only heterosexual couples, but also same-sex couples, single people, and those who wished to avoid passing on serious hereditary diseases to their offspring. Advances in AHR technologies had increased the number of treatment options available. Furthermore, AHR was one of the most innovative and rapidly developing specialist areas of medicine. Therefore, all the indicators pointed towards increasing demand in the years ahead. The need to legislate could only increase. Representations were being made to the Minister for Health on behalf of citizens who were experiencing infertility problems.[88]

Progress was evidently very difficult, given the complexity of the issues. The GSAHR and the Children and Family Relationships Act 2015 were interconnected. The 2015 Act had reformed family law to address the needs of children in diverse types of family. Parts 2 and 3 of the Act regulated: (1) aspects of parentage rules for children born through DAHR procedures; (2) obligations of clinics providing such procedures; and (3) the establishment of a donor-conceived person national register. The Department of Health was endeavouring to solve "some technical issues" so that the procedures relating to Parts 2 and 3 of the 2015 Act could be "commenced".[89]

Officials in the Department of Health were mindful of the critically important principle of safeguarding the welfare of children when working out details of the GSAHR. Reference was made to Article 42A of the Constitution and to the UN Convention on the Rights of the

Child.[90] Despite this, the rights of the child were to become the main focus of criticism of the GSAHR.

Traditionalist Catholic advocacy organisations objected strongly to the legislative proposals in the GSAHR. Human Life International (Ireland) criticised the scheme outright with reference to the *Catechism of the Catholic Church, Evangelium Vitae* and *Donum Vitae*.[91] However, explicit reference to Catholic doctrine was not usual when expressing opposition to AHR. The Iona Institute adopted a secular approach when it submitted its critical observations on the GSAHR to the JCH. The six-page document was jointly authored by Dr Joanna Rose, who was herself donor-conceived and had won a landmark court case in Britain that ruled against anonymous donation of gametes.[92] The Iona Institute and Rose were implicitly critical of the use of supernumerary embryos for research, surrogacy, posthumous conception and the creation of "saviour siblings" for donation of stem cells and bone marrow to severely ill siblings. But they chose to limit their criticisms and recommendations to the use of donor gametes. They believed that DAHR was "a massive experiment with the lives of children." They acknowledged that the GSAHR prohibited anonymity in DAHR but still concluded that the scheme devalued the connection between the child and its genetic parents. Children would not have a right to access information about their genetic origins until they were 18 years old.

The authors pointed to the experiences of adopted people to emphasise the importance of genetic kinship. There were many instances where people who had been adopted had searched extensively for their biological parents and siblings – "no matter how well loved they were by their adoptive parents". A critically important distinction between adoption and DAHR was that the natural connection in adoption was mostly broken by "circumstance". In the case of DAHR, the severing of the genetic connection was done by "deliberate design". The authors acknowledged that many adopted and donor-conceived people never search for their genetic kin, but many do. The experiences of this latter group of people needed to be "seriously considered".

Dr Rose and her fellow authors were critical of the GSAHR because it granted greater status to the intending parents than the biological parents. It was "extremely adult-centred".[93] The identity issues created by the severing of natural ties was further exacerbated by the "underlying philosophy" of the GSAHR – based on the assumption that the number of parents, their gender, and whether or not they were married, did not impact on the welfare of the child. The authors acknowledged that there would be no reversal on the DAHR elements of the GSAHR or a return to the traditional concept of family structure. Their main purpose was to submit eleven recommendations to mitigate the harm that would be done to children if the GSAHR was enacted. One such recommendation was that the Assisted Human Reproduction Regulatory Authority should, as far as possible, assist donor-conceived children to trace their genetic kin both in Ireland and overseas.[94]

Dr John Waterstone, President of the Irish Fertility Society, gave evidence to the JCH on 28 February 2018. His outlook contrasted sharply with that of the Iona Institute and Dr Rose. He told the JCH that IVF clinics were already strictly regulated, licensed and inspected by the Health Products Regulatory Authority in compliance with directives of the EU on tissues and cells. Control was already strict. Legislation in northern and western Europe was very restrictive. Restrictions drove European citizens to seek AHR outside Europe, giving rise to "reproductive tourism". It was important not to "slavishly" imitate regulatory systems in other jurisdictions that were evidently failing their citizens. Waterstone emphasised the importance of protecting patients against financial exploitation and the need to enhance the probability of successful outcomes. He found that the proposed legislation was mainly "progressive", but excessively restrictive concerning gamete donation and surrogacy. He expressed concerns that Parts 2 and 3 of the Children and Family Relationships Act 2015 would infringe on the reproductive rights of patients. He objected to the state having the right to inform an 18-year-old who requested a birth certificate that they had been conceived using a donor gamete. Dr Waterstone believed, in common with many of his colleagues, that both identifiable and anonymous gamete donation were ethical.[95]

It was intended that Part 9 of the Children and Family Relationships Act 2015 would amend the Civil Registration Act 2004, which provided the legal framework for the registration of birth. In this scheme the registrar of births would retain "additional information" on donor-conceived children which could be requested when the person reached 18 years. Mary Hallissey, a journalist writing for the *Law Society Gazette*, observed that anonymous gamete donation was to be prohibited, but parents were not legally obliged to inform their children about their biological origins. Hallissey believed that Ireland was "sleepwalking into the possibility of large-scale human tragedy and emotional devastation" as the government was preparing legislation in relation to birth certificates that would be "legal fictions" in cases of AHR. She saw striking similarities between the proposed legislation and the bitter legacy of past abuses in the adoption system, when birth certificates containing false information had been issued.[96] A few months earlier, the Minister for Children, Katherine Zappone, disclosed that there were at least 126 illegally registered adoptions in the state that were based on "fictitious" birth certificates.[97] But drawing parallels between these cases and the GSAHR was highly questionable considering that, in the proposed legislation, children would have a right to obtain information about their biological parents from the National Surrogacy Register and the National Donor-Conceived Person Register when they reached 18 years of age.[98]

Hallissey referred to the Convention on the Rights of the Child that had been ratified by the General Assembly of the UN on 20 November 1989. She quoted Article 7 to make the point that "it could not be clearer on the right of every child to its genetic identity, and to know and be cared for by its natural parents." Contrary to Hallissey's interpretation, no such right was clearly stated. Article 7 makes no reference to "genetic identity". It declares that "The child shall be registered immediately after birth and shall have the right from birth to a name, the right to acquire a nationality and, as far as possible, the right to know and be cared for by his or her parents."[99] The word "parents" was not defined to exclude intending parents who were not genetically related to the child. Hallissey also quoted Article 8 of the UN document, which placed a human rights obligation on states to "respect the rights of the child to preserve his or her identity, including nationality, name and family relations as recognised by law". In this context, identity was not necessarily synonymous with genetic identity. Therefore, the rights of the child in the context of DAHR were very much in question.

Hallissey quoted at length psychologist Emma O'Friel, who saw DAHR as contrary to the best interests of the child. Fertility clinics were "running a business" and "had a profit motive". This criticism of fertility clinics was not reasonable, especially considering the lack of public funding and facilities for AHR. It was not reasonable to expect investors, scientists and other personnel to provide a service without profit or remuneration. Scientists were permitted to undertake DAHR procedures, but, according to O'Friel, they had refused to engage with its consequences. This characterisation of scientists was unduly harsh. Scientists in Ireland had been actively engaged in addressing ethical issues arising from scientific and technological developments, both generally, and specifically in the area of AHR. They (especially medical scientists) had been well represented on the Commission on Assisted Human Reproduction (2000–2005) and the Irish Council for Bioethics (2002–2010). They served on ethical committees in hospitals and universities. Leading clinical scientists who were providing fertility services had not been reluctant to give evidence to the JCH on 28 February 2019.[100]

On 19 December 2018 the JCH heard evidence from Emma O'Friel, Dr Joanna Rose, Professor Deirdre Madden (School of Law, University College Cork), and Professor Nóirín Hayes (School of Education, Trinity College Dublin). Marian Barnard and Gillian Keegan gave evidence on behalf of the National Infertility Support and Information Group. Madden and Hayes had served as members of the Commission on Assisted Human Reproduction and welcomed the GSAHR, despite concerns about some aspects of the scheme, especially in relation to the best interests of children. They proposed revisions to remedy flaws in the proposed legislation.[101] O'Friel and Rose were resolutely opposed to the scheme on the basis that DAHR, no matter how well regulated, was detrimental to the best interests of children born through such procedures. Rose described DAHR as "about child production, not child protection". Disruption of identity and kinship created grief in adulthood. DAHR was a "social experiment" and the "adverse impacts and consequences" were "unravelling over time around the world". Rose pointed to illegal adoptions and misleading birth certificates. She saw surrogacy as "a fragmentation and sacrifice of children's maternal integrity". Members of the JCH were urged to remember "the pain that has come to light in the likes of Philomena".[102]

Rose's reference to the case of Philomena Lee pointed to cases of illegal and forced adoptions in mid-twentieth-century Ireland – where children who were born out of wedlock and their mothers were harshly treated by the Catholic Church.[103] Mothers and their grown-up children who subsequently tried to trace each other encountered deception and obstruction. The comparison of the Philomena Lee case with the anticipated adverse consequences of DAHR and surrogacy failed to take a broad view of both adoption and the newly emergent AHR technologies. Adoption was widely regarded as beneficial to society when it was regulated in a manner consistent with optimising the care of children and with due consideration of the rights of parents. An argument against adoption in principle would not have been rationally tenable if it was based only on cases similar to the experiences of Philomena Lee and her son, Michael Hess. Similar points are applicable to cases of DAHR and surrogacy.

Emma O'Friel's submission to the JCH emphasised, at length, the importance of genetics, associating it with "a sense of self" which was essential for psychological well-being. She concluded her submission by identifying two main driving forces behind the provision of AHR services. Fertility services were (1) "adult-centric, run by adults for adults, and not in a child's best interest"; and (2) motivated by a desire for financial gain.[104] The second point, addressed earlier, requires no further comment. The first point was based on assumptions that were highly questionable. It was true that the DAHR "industry" was "run by adults for adults", but it did not follow that this was contrary to the best interests of children, if properly regulated. The word "adult-centric" in this context was without substance, considering that human reproduction without medical intervention could also be seen as "adult-centric" – especially when it is unplanned.

The submissions of Rose and O'Friel raised the question: was there evidence that DAHR and surrogacy harmed mothers and children even if well regulated? The evidence of Hayes and Madden referred to scientific research. Longitudinal studies of children up to the age of fourteen, born through surrogacy and donor-conceived, found no evidence of harm. No evidence of psychopathology was found in cases of surrogate mothers. Madden had thirty years of research experience on issues concerned with AHR. She informed the JCH that there was no evidence of harm to surrogate mothers, intended parents or children. Research indicated that surrogate mothers did not regard the children they carried as theirs and did not wish to be the legal mothers of these children.[105]

There was no extensive scientific research on the contentious issue of whether or not DAHR and surrogacy caused harm to mothers and children. Further longitudinal studies needed to be done for adolescents older than fourteen years of age. O'Friel and Rose's contentions of harm to children and mothers were not scientifically based (i.e. with reference to peer-reviewed studies). When pressed in the course of debate to point to such evidence they were unable to do so.[106]

Madden informed the JCH that, in her opinion, it was possible to create a scheme for AHR, including surrogacy, consistent with human rights. She expressed concerns about some aspects of the GSAHR, especially in relation to surrogacy. The Bill did not assume that the parents of the child, to be born through surrogacy, were the commissioning/intended parents, contrary to what had been recommended in the *Report of the Commission on Assisted Human Reproduction*.[107] The regulation of surrogacy in Ireland, as proposed in the GSAHR, would not work. The exploitation of women in surrogacy agreements was of major concern, but the Bill imposed such excessively stringent measures to prevent this in Ireland that it was counterproductive. Intending parents would continue to travel abroad as before. The Bill did not provide legally for couples who would try to bring their children home from another jurisdiction. This would leave children potentially stateless and legally parentless pending the outcome of legal proceedings.[108]

Approval of surrogacy and DAHR did not necessarily lead to a denial that genetic and gestational elements of a child's personal history were important features of a sense of self and a sense of belonging. Madden advised that donor anonymity should not be permitted. Children had the right to know about their biological parents if they requested it. Hayes pointed out that early disclosure about biological origins favoured the best psychological outcomes. And, of course, as pointed out by Rose, access to the medical history of the donor was important – sometimes critically important for timely and appropriate medical treatment for patients who were donor-conceived.

Dr Angelo Bottone, research officer at the Iona Institute, responded on 21 December, on the institute's website, to the proceedings of the JCH. He complained that the "well-reasoned objections" of O'Friel and Rose had been "dismissed as mere opinions". This was inaccurate; Bottone failed to acknowledge that they were unable to refer to scientifically validated research to support their claims. His criticisms of Madden's testimony were especially misleading on the issue of surrogacy. Madden informed the JCH that the GSAHR provisions for surrogacy would not work and would not prevent the exploitation of women – it would instead ensure that such exploitation occurred outside the jurisdiction. Bottone commented that this assessment was "totally defeatist. It says that if a law can be circumvented then law must be changed but all laws can be circumvented, does this means [*sic*] we should haven [*sic*] laws?"[109] Bottone missed a point of central importance in Madden's argument. She did not simply criticise the provisions on surrogacy without putting forward constructive proposals. She recommended that legislators follow the examples of New Hampshire and California – not Britain, where the legislation was unfit for purpose.[110] Also, her contention that prohibiting surrogacy would drive it abroad was difficult to refute. For example, when India introduced prohibitions and restrictions, agencies redirected their services abroad to countries such as Laos, Ukraine, and several African countries. Indian women who applied to be surrogates travelled to countries where they were even more vulnerable to exploitation and abuse.[111] Internationally, demand for surrogacy was rising due to the proliferation of liberal ideas about diverse types of family, and declining numbers of children available for adoption.[112] This did not dissuade many countries from banning surrogacy. These included France, Germany, Italy and Switzerland. Religious conservatives and left-wing feminists in Europe frequently found common cause in opposing the loosening of restrictions.[113] The widespread prohibition of surrogacy, especially in liberal democracies, seemed to offer a *prima facie* case against the legalisation of surrogacy. The stance of the Roman Catholic Church on surrogacy seemed to be far less at variance with public policies in Western Europe relative to the issues of contraception, abortion and divorce.

Senator Rónán Mullen made the point in the course of JCH deliberations on 19 December 2018 that Sweden, frequently regarded as "enlightened", was giving serious consideration to the prohibition of surrogacy – including altruistic surrogacy. The clear implication was that if a liberal democratic state was moving in a conservative direction, there must be a very strong case against the legalisation of surrogacy. Bottone also referred to Sweden, informing his readers that Swedish feminist organisations expressed approval of the Swedish government's announcement that surrogacy would not be legalised. The Swedish Women's Lobby took a strong position against all forms of surrogacy, seeing it as "trade with women's bodies and children" and a threat to women's basic human rights.[114] The Swedish government's announcement was influenced by the recommendations of a government commission on the issue.[115]

Since the 1980s, traditionalist Catholic opposition to AHR in Ireland was very much eclipsed by its ongoing opposition to abortion. Its main focus, in relation to AHR, was concerned with the integrity of marriage, the inseparability of sexual intercourse from reproduction, the wellbeing of children, and genetics. Inadequate attention was given to the rights and wellbeing of women. The excessive emphasis on genetics in DAHR seemed inconsistent with a spiritual and social outlook and more consistent with a reductionist and areligious view of parenthood. The psychological and social aspects of parenthood were diminished with reference to sexual intercourse, genetics and the circumstances of birth. "Choice" and "intention" in the context of "the wanted child" were not ranked high in the vocabulary of Catholic moral teaching! In *Donum Vitae* the Congregation for the Doctrine of the Faith stated that married couples who experienced infertility could not resort to IVF without contravening the Church's moral teaching – even when there was no third-party gamete donor. The "good intention" of having a child was "not sufficient for making a positive moral evaluation".[116] The congregation urged politicians to legislate for the prohibition of surrogacy, embryo banks and post-mortem insemination.[117]

Surrogacy is probably the most ethically and legally challenging aspect of AHR. It is multidimensional – genetic, gestational, psychological, social, legal and ethical. From a conservative Catholic perspective, all the complexity is swept aside by a dogmatic moral prohibition. Conservative Catholics emphasised the importance of procreation exclusively through sexual intercourse within marriage, thus ruling out surrogacy. Although they frequently presented their arguments in secular terms, their foundational beliefs were unwaveringly religious. But they were unlikely to exert enough influence to obstruct the passing of legislation providing for the regulation of AHR services in Ireland. Opinion polls indicated that public opinion in Ireland was supportive of AHR. An extensive survey of public opinion in March 2013 found that majorities favoured IVF, gamete donation, embryo donation, surrogacy and preimplantation genetic diagnosis.[118] The proceedings of the JCH indicated that Catholic moral philosophy exerted little influence.[119] Defeats on the issues of same-sex marriage (2015) and abortion (2018) signalled that conservative Catholicism in Ireland was no longer powerful enough to obstruct constitutional and legislative reforms.

Endnotes

———————•———————

1   Fiona Gartland, "Calls made for surrogacy legislation", *Irish Times*, 6 March 2013, p. 2. Surrogacy can proceed using any of the following: (1) the commissioning mother's ova and the commissioning father's sperm; (2) the commissioning mother's ova and donor sperm; (3) the commissioning father's sperm and the surrogate mother's ova; (4) the commissioning father's sperm and donor ova; (5) the surrogate mother's ova and donor sperm; (6) donor ova and sperm, or donor embryo. Citizens Information Board, "Surrogacy" <http://www.citizensinformation.ie/en/birth_family_relationships/adoption_and_fostering/surrogacy.html> accessed 9 November 2013.

2   Carl O'Brien, "The reproduction revolution", *Irish Times*, 19 November 2011 <https://search-proquest-com.ucc.idm.oclc.org/docview/904689669/fulltext/238C39D788CB4D01PQ/6?accountid=14504> accessed 28 March 2018. The estimate of the number of children born through AHR was between 2,500 and 3,000 per annum.

3   "Genetic parents win surrogate twins case", *Irish Times*, 6 March 2013, p. 2.

4   Judgment by Mr Justice Henry Abbott, *M.R. & Anor v An tArd Chlaraitheoir & Ors*, paragraph 5, Neutral Citation [2013] IEHC 91, High Court Record Number 2011 46 M, 5 March 2013 <http://www.courts.ie/Judgments.nsf/597645521f07ac9a80256ef30048ca52/e3f0dc917872554c80257b250052dab3?OpenDocument> accessed from the Court Services website on 9 November 2013 and 8 February 2014.

5   Ibid., paragraph 105.

6   Ibid., paragraph 104.

7   Poor diet, alcohol consumption and high blood pressure impact adversely on foetal growth and development. Short-term immunity against some infections is acquired by the foetus after maternal antibodies cross the placental barrier. Small numbers of cells from the gestational mother pass through the placenta into the foetus (microchimerism) and were considered a risk factor for autoimmune diseases. Epigenetics revealed that a number of biochemical substances turned some genes on and others off. Most epigenetic effects were reversed postnatally, but there was some uncertainty as to whether all such effects are reversed. Ibid., paragraphs 8–15, 23–6.

8   He observed that this prioritisation of genetics was consistent with current legislative practice arising from the Adoption Act 2010. Ibid., paragraphs 102–5. The High Court directed that the identities of the genetic parents, surrogate mother and children were not to be disclosed by the newspapers or through social media. Ibid., paragraph 122.

9   Ibid., paragraph 90.

10 Fiona Whyte and Seán Malone, *Without a Doubt: An Irish Couple's Journey through IVF, Adoption and Surrogacy* (Dublin: Merrion Press, 2017), pp. 81–7. Mary Carolan, "Irish father wins surrogacy case over child born in India", *Irish Times*, 6 March 2013, p. 2.

11 *Catechism of the Catholic Church* (Dublin, Veritas, 1995), paragraphs 2375 and 2376; in reference to the Congregation for the Doctrine of the Faith, *Donum Vitae*, II, 1 and 5.

12 Iona Institute, "Government must move to prohibit surrogacy in the interests of children: Surrogacy splits motherhood between up to three women: Surrogacy illegal in most European countries", press release, 5 March 2013 <http://www.ionainstitute.ie/index.php?id=2810> accessed 1 January 2014. The Iona Institute issued a similar press release on 26 September 2013: "State must consider why most European countries ban surrogate motherhood" <http://www.ionainstitute.ie/index.php?id=3200> accessed 1 January 2014.

13 Iona Institute, "The Ethical Case Against Surrogate Motherhood: What we can learn from the law of other European Countries" (n.d.), Conclusion <http://ionainstitute.org/assets/files/Surrogacy%20final%20PDF.pdf> accessed 1 January 2014.

14 Commercial surrogacy thrives in India, driven by relatively low cost and a lack of regulation. The case of an Irish couple, broadcast on RTÉ 1 television on Monday 13 January 2014, under the title *Her Body, Our Babies*, was followed by a *Prime Time* discussion that examined the ethical issues. Of particular concern was the vulnerability of Indian women who volunteered as surrogate mothers to help their families escape poverty. Other countries facilitating commercial surrogacy included the USA, Mexico, Russia, Ukraine, Poland, Georgia, Nepal and Thailand.

15 Iona Institute, "The Ethical Case Against Surrogate Motherhood", p. 4.

16 Department of Social Protection, "Statement in Relation to High Court judgment in the case of MR, DR, OR and CR v An tÁrd Chlaraitheoir [Registrar General], Ireland and the Attorney General", 6 June 2013 <https://www.welfare.ie/en/pressoffice/pdf/pr060613a.pdf> accessed 8 January 2014.

17 Department of Justice and Equality, "Children and Family Relationships Bill 2013: Briefing Note", 5 November 2013 <http://www.justice.ie/en/ JELR/Children%20and%20Family%20Relationships%20Bill%202013%20 141113.pdf/Files/Children%20and%20Family%20Relationships%20 Bill%202013%20141113.pdf> accessed 11 January 2014.

18 Carl O'Brien, "Updating family law for the needs of the 21st century", *Irish Times*, 18 November 2013 <http://www.irishtimes.com/news/social-affairs/ updating-family-law-for-the-needs-of-the-21st-century-1.1598175> accessed 19 November 2013.

19 "Minister Shatter publishes General Scheme of Children and Family
    Relationships Bill for consultation", press release, 30 January 2014
    <http://www.merrionstreet.ie/index.php/2014/01/minister-shatter-
    publishes-general-scheme-of-children-and-family-relationships-bill-for-
    consultation/?cat=12> accessed 2 February 2014.
20 *Catechism of the Catholic Church* (Dublin: Veritas, 1995), paragraph 2202.
21 Ibid., paragraphs 2210–11.
22 "Minister Shatter publishes General Scheme", 2 February 2014.
23 "Surrogacy appeal to Supreme Court underway", 3 February 2014 <http://
    www.independent.ie/irish-news/courts/surrogacy-appeal-to-supreme-court-
    underway-29974763.html> accessed 7 February 2014.
24 Ruadhán Mac Cormaic, "State's message on surrogacy: 'Leave it to the
    Oireachtas'", *Irish Times*, 4 February 2014 <http://www.irishtimes.com/
    news/crime-and-law/courts/state-s-message-on-surrogacy-leave-it-to-the-
    oireachtas-1.1678316> accessed 7 February 2014.
25 Ibid.
26 Mary Carolan, "Agencies urge broad definition of motherhood in Supreme
    Court surrogacy case", *Irish Times*, 6 February 2014 <http://www.irishtimes.
    com/news/crime-and-law/courts/agencies-urge-broad-definition-of-
    motherhood-in-supreme-court-surrogacy-case-1.1681015> accessed 7
    February 2014.
27 Ibid., p. 6.
28 David Quinn, "Shatter's Brave New World attacks children's rights: The
    Government is trying to set aside nature and replace it with choice",
    Irish Catholic, 6 February 2014 <http://www.irishcatholic.ie/article/
    shatter%E2%80%99s-brave-new-world-attacks-children%E2%80%99s-
    rights> accessed 9 February 2014.
29 Department of Justice and Equality, "Minister Fitzgerald publishes General
    Scheme of the Children and Family Relationships Bill", press release, 25
    September 2014 <http://www.justice.ie/en/JELR/Pages/PR14000257>
    accessed 27 September 2014.
30 The central issue was one of statutory interpretation concerning some
    provisions of the Civil Registration Act 2004. The Status of Children Act
    1987 also required examination. J. Murray, Supreme Court judgment,
    *M.R. and D.R. (suing by their father and next friend O.R.) & Ors v An
    t-Ard-Chláraitheoir & Ors*, 7 November 2014, Neutral Citation [2014]
    IESC 60, Appeal No. 263/2013, paragraphs 1, 5, 54–6 <http://www.
    supremecourt.ie/Judgments.nsf/1b0757edc371032e802572ea0061450e/
    b8659a33e49cda9f80257e90003f5e6f?OpenDocument> accessed 1 October
    2015.
31 Ibid., paragraph 1; C.J. Denham; Supreme Court judgment, *M.R.
    and D.R. (suing by their father and next friend O.R.) & Ors v An
    t-Ard-Chláraitheoir & Ors*, 7 November 2014, Neutral Citation

[2014] IESC 60, Appeal No. 263/2013, paragraph 60 <http://www. supremecourt.ie/Judgments.nsf/1b0757edc371032e802572ea0061450e/ e238e39a6e756ab480257d890054dcb6?OpenDocument> accessed 12 December 2014; Donal J. O'Donnell; Supreme Court judgment, *M.R. and D.R. (suing by their father and next friend O.R.) & Ors v An t-Ard-Chláraitheoir & Ors*, 7 November 2014, Neutral Citation [2014] IESC 60, Appeal No. 263/2013, paragraph 27 <http:// www.supremecourt.ie/Judgments.nsf/1b0757edc371032e802572 ea0061450e/516ac26fc227e31780257d890055587a?OpenDocument> accessed 12 December 2014.

32 O'Donnell judgment, paragraph 32; and J. MacMenamin; Supreme Court judgment, *M.R. and D.R. (suing by their father and next friend O.R.) & Ors v An t-Ard-Chláraitheoir & Ors*, 7 November 2014, Neutral Citation [2014] IESC 60, Appeal No. 263/2013, paragraph 19<http://www.supremecourt.ie/ Judgments. nsf/1b0757edc371032e802572ea0061450e/6a0d5025c1ba0a3a8 3a80257d890055e902?OpenDocument> accessed 12 December 2014.

33 Denham judgment, paragraph 60; O'Donnell judgment, paragraphs 30–4, 38.

34 J. Hardiman, Supreme Court judgment, *M.R. and D.R. (suing by their father and next friend O.R.) & Ors v An t-Ard-Chláraitheoir & Ors*, 7 November 2014, Neutral Citation [2014] IESC 60, Appeal No. 263/2013, paragraph 18 <http://www.supremecourt.ie/Judgments.nsf/1b0757edc371032e802572e- a0061450e/1ef9e77e549c328a80257d8c0050ebbd?OpenDocument> accessed 12 December 2014. Mr Justice Frank Clarke, mindful of this problem, proposed that in this case "the genetic mother is the mother of the twins without prejudice to the status of the birth mother." The "least bad solution" was to register both the birth mother and the genetic mother "in some way". However, he was in a minority of one and the Supreme Court overturned the Abbott judgment. J. Clarke, Supreme Court judgment, *M.R. and D.R. (suing by their father and next friend O.R.) & Ors v An t-Ard-Chláraitheoir & Ors*, 7 November 2014, Neutral Citation [2014] IESC 60, Appeal No. 263/2013, paragraph 10.5 <http://www.supremecourt.ie/Judgments.nsf/1b0757edc371032e802572e- a0061450e/928bd82eb3b32ece80257d890055b1f6?OpenDocument> accessed 12 December 2014.

35 Deirdre Madden, "Assisted Reproduction in Ireland – Time to Legislate" (guest editorial), *Medico-Legal Journal of Ireland*, vol. 17, no. 1 (2011), pp. 3–5.

36 Jill Allison, "Enduring Politics: The Culture of Obstacles in Legislating for Assisted Reproduction Technologies in Ireland", *Reproductive Biomedicine and Society Online*, vol. 3 (December 2016), pp. 134–41 <https://www. sciencedirect.com/science/article/pii/S2405661816300399> accessed 18 February 2019.

37 Dáil Debates, vol. 825, no. 1 (17 December 2013), p. 35 <http:// oireachtasdebates.oireachtas.ie/debates%20authoring/DebatesWebPack.nsf/ takes/dail2013121700035?opendocument> accessed 10 October 2015.

38 Stephen Collins, "Bill will recognise and protect diverse family units", *Irish Times*, 18 February 2015, p. 14.

39 Stephen Collins, "Family law legislation hailed as 'major step'", *Irish Times*, 18 February 2015, p. 1.

40 David Stanton, "Child-centred Bill will improve lives of many families", *Irish Times*, 18 February 2015, p. 14, in reference to the 2011 census.

41 Sarah Bardon, "No surrogacy legislation before election, says Kenny", *Irish Times*, 20 May 2015 <http://www.irishtimes.com/news/politics/oireachtas/no-surrogacy-legislation-before-election-says-kenny-1.2219658?mode=print&ot=example.AjaxPageLayout.ot> accessed 20 May 2015.

42 Provisions concerning assisted human reproduction would not come into effect for at least a year. This was to protect couples undergoing fertility treatment at the time.

43 Citizens Information Board, "Children and Family Relationships Act 2015", *Relate*, vol. 42, issue 5 (May 2015) <http://www.citizensinformationboard.ie/publications/relate/relate_2015_05.pdf> accessed 8 September 2015. The meaning of donor-assisted human reproduction, in a legal sense, is given in the Children and Family Relationships Act 2015, Part Two: Parentage in Cases of Donor-Assisted Human Reproduction, p. 11. Office of the Attorney General, Children and Family Relationships Act 2015 <http://www.irishstatutebook.ie/eli/2015/act/9/enacted/en/pdf> accessed 28 August 2015.

44 Collins, "Bill will recognise and protect diverse family units". See also Noel Whelan, "No side posters may prove counterproductive", *Irish Times*, 24 April 2015 <http://www.irishtimes.com/opinion/noel-whelan-no-side-posters-may-prove-counterproductive-1.2186624?mode=print&ot=example.AjaxPageLayout.ot> accessed 24 April 2015.

45 Irish Catholic Bishops' Conference, *The Meaning of Marriage* (n.d.), p. 2 <http://www.accord.ie/images/uploads/docs/The_Meaning_of_Marriage.pdf> accessed 17 October 2015.

46 Ibid., pp. 3, 9.

47 Ibid., pp. 8–11.

48 Rónán Duffy, "'God's Plan for Marriage' is being distributed to 1,300 parishes ahead of referendum", TheJournal.ie, 3 December 2014 <http://www.thejournal.ie/same-sex-marriage-bishops-1813682-Dec2014/> accessed 17 October 2015.

49 Sarah Bardon, "Mullen calls on Kenny to debate in same-sex marriage campaign", *Irish Times*, 28 April 2015 <http://www.irishtimes.com/news/politics/mullen-calls-on-kenny-to-debate-in-same-sex-marriage-campaign-1.2191262?mode=print&ot=example.AjaxPageLayout.ot> accessed 28 April 2015.

50 David Quinn, "'Yes Equality' family values leaflet is deeply hypocritical", *Irish Catholic*, 14 May 2015 <http://irishcatholic.ie/article/%E2%80%98yes-

equality%E2%80%99-family-values-leaflet-deeply-hypocritical> accessed 20 May 2015.

51 Iona Institute, *A Mother's Love is Irreplaceable: Vote No* (2015); Mothers and Fathers Matter, *Don't Deny a Child the Right to a Mother and a Father: Vote No on 22 May* (2015).

52 Yes Equality, *Marriage and Family Matter: Vote Yes on May 22nd* (2015).

53 Yes EqualityCork, *Vote Yes for Equality on May 22nd* (2015).

54 Referendum Commission, *Marriage Referendum and Age of Presidential Candidates Referendum* <http://refcom2015.ie/marriage/> accessed 16 May 2015.

55 Iona Institute, *A Mother's Love is Irreplaceable.*

56 Case law indicated that the state had a right to impose "reasonable and proportionate restrictions ... in the pursuit of legitimate aims", as in the case of prisoners, for example. Clearly, the state had similar rights in relation to AHR. Conor O'Mahony, "The Constitution, the Right to Procreate and the Marriage Referendum", Constitution Project @UCC <http://constitutionproject.ie/?p=503> accessed 24 April 2015.

57 Carol Coulter, "Why surrogacy has nothing to do with same-sex marriage", *Irish Times*, 27 April 2015 <http://www.irishtimes.com/opinion/why-surrogacy-has-nothing-to-do-with-same-sex-marriage-1.2189717?mode=print&ot=example.AjaxPageLayout.ot> accessed 28 April 2015; Ruadhán Mac Cormaic, "State to introduce parts of Children and Family Relationships Act", *Irish Times*, 20 May 2015 <https://www.irishtimes.com/news/politics/state-to-introduce-parts-of-children-and-family-relationships-act-1.2218743?mode=print&ot=example.AjaxPageLayout.ot> accessed 20 May 2015; Sarah Bardon, "Referendum body to clarify position on surrogacy and adoption", *Irish Times*, 13 May 2015 <http://www.irishtimes.com/news/politics/referendum-body-to-clarify-position-on-surrogacy-and-adoption-1.2210110?mode=print&ot=example.AjaxPageLayout.ot> accessed 13 May 2015.

58 Ruadhán Mac Cormaic, "Marriage referendum Q&A: What you need to know", *Irish Times*, 14 May 2015 <http://www.irishtimes.com/news/politics/marriage-referendum-q-a-what-you-need-to-know-1.2212840?mode=print&ot=example.AjaxPageLayout.ot> accessed 15 May 2015.

59 Ibid. See also O'Mahony, "The Constitution", Constitution Project @UCC.

60 Reference was made to Genesis 19:1–29, Romans 1:24–27, I Corinthians 6:10 and I Timothy 1:10.

61 *Catechism of the Catholic Church* (Dublin, Veritas, 1995), paragraph 2357, pp. 504–5.

62 Ibid., paragraphs 2358–9, p. 505.

63 Sacred Congregation for the Doctrine of the Faith, Declaration on Certain Problems of Sexual Ethics (*Personae Humanae*, 29 December 1975),

paragraph 8, in Austin Flannery (general ed.), *Vatican Council II: More Postconciliar Documents* (Collegeville, Minn.: Liturgical Press, 1982 (1st edn)), pp. 490–1.

64 Brendan McCormack *et al.*, *Irish Times*, 21 May 2015 <http://www.irishtimes.com/opinion/letters/marriage-referendum-countdown-to-polling-day-1.2220003?mode=print&ot=example.AjaxPageLayout.ot> accessed 25 May 2015.

65 Alan Carr *et al.*, *Irish Times*, 21 May 2015 <http://www.irishtimes.com/opinion/letters/marriage-referendum-countdown-to-polling-day-1.2220003?mode=print&ot=example.AjaxPageLayout.ot> accessed 25 May 2015.

66 Jody Corcoran and Daniel McConnell, "A new beginning: Historic Yes for gay marriage after surge in youth vote", *Sunday Independent*, 24 May 2015, pp. 1, 5.

67 Iona Institute, *A Mother's Love is Irreplaceable*.

68 See Johan A. Elkink, David M. Farrell, Theresa Reidy and Jane Suiter, "Understanding the 2015 Marriage Referendum in Ireland: Context, Campaign, and Conservative Ireland", *Irish Political Studies*, vol. 32, issue 3 (2017), pp. 361–81.

69 Shane Doran, "The world looks on as Irish voters make history", *Sunday Independent*, 24 May 2015, p. 5.

70 Paddy Agnew, "Vatican stands by Cardinal's remarks on referendum", *Irish Times*, 27 May, 2015 <http://www.irishtimes.com/news/social-affairs/religion-and-beliefs/vatican-stands-by-cardinal-s-remarks-on-referendum-1.2227805?mode=print&ot=example.AjaxPageLayout.ot> accessed 28 May 2015.

71 Aine McMahon, "Catholic Church 'bereavement' after same-sex marriage vote", *Irish Times*, 2 June 2015 <http://www.irishtimes.com/news/social-affairs/religion-and-beliefs/catholic-church-bereavement-after-same-sex-marriage-vote-1.2234500?mode=print&ot=example.AjaxPageLayout.ot> accessed 29 October 2015.

72 Alison Healy, "Diarmuid Martin: Catholic Church needs reality check", *Irish Times*, 23 May 2015 <http://www.irishtimes.com/news/ireland/irish-news/diarmuid-martin-catholic-church-needs-reality-check-1.2223872?mode=print&ot=example.AjaxPageLayout.ot> accessed 29 October 2015.

73 Gerry O'Hanlon, "Catholic Church needs to empower the laity", *Irish Times*, 1 June 2015.

74 Patsy McGarry, "All churches in Ireland in need of 'reality check'", *Irish Times*, 24 May 2015 <http://www.irishtimes.com/news/social-affairs/religion-and-beliefs/all-churches-in-ireland-in-need-of-reality-check-1.2224081?mode=print&ot=example.AjaxPageLayout.ot> accessed 25 May 2015; and "Same-sex marriage vote an 'unmitigated disaster' for Church",

Irish Times, 25 May 2015 <http://www.irishtimes.com/news/social-affairs/religion-and-beliefs/same-sex-marriage-vote-an-unmitigated-disaster-for-church-1.2225680?mode=print&ot=example.AjaxPageLayout.ot> accessed 25 May 2015.

75 David Quinn, "A 'reality check', but which kind?", *Irish Catholic*, 28 May 2015 <http://irishcatholic.ie/article/%E2%80%98reality-check%E2%80%99-which-kind> accessed 28 May 2015.

76 Michael Kelly, "Church does need a 'reality check' after the referendum", *The Irish Catholic*, 27 May 2015 <http://irishcatholic.ie/article/church-does-need-%E2%80%98reality-check%E2%80%99-after-referendum> accessed 28 May 2015. For a similar point see Louise Fuller, *Irish Catholicism Since 1950* (Dublin: Gill and Macmillan, 2002), p. 250.

77 Kelly, "Church does need a 'reality check'".

78 Department of Health: "Government approves the drafting of the Assisted Human Reproduction Bill", 3 October 2017 <https://health.gov.ie/blog/press-release/government-approves-the-drafting-of-the-assisted-human-reproduction-bill/ accessed 24 January 2019); and "General Scheme of the Assisted Human Reproduction Bill 2017", 6 October 2018 <https://health.gov.ie/blog/publications/general-scheme-of-the-assisted-human-reproduction-bill-2017/> accessed 4 January 2019.

79 Department of Health, General Scheme of the Assisted Human Reproduction Bill 2017 <https://health.gov.ie/wp-content/uploads/2017/10/AHR-general-scheme-with-cover.pdf> accessed 4 January 2019.

80 HLA matching would be used when an existing child of the intending parents suffered from a severe disease. The objective of the parents resorting to AHR was (1) to prevent a future sibling suffering the same inheritable disease and (2) to provide a tissue match between the existing child and its future sibling, provided that tissue donation would not be detrimental to the welfare of the intended sibling.

81 It was not permissible to create embryos specifically for research purposes. Cloning human embryos was prohibited; neither was it permissible to transfer a human embryo clone into the body of an animal or a human. Other prohibited procedures included mitochondrial donation and replacement involving human gametes or embryos, and the creation of human–animal hybrid embryos.

82 Department of Health, General Scheme of the Assisted Human Reproduction Bill 2017.

83 This was consistent with the Equal Status Acts 2000–2004, which prohibit direct or indirect discrimination on grounds that include sexual orientation, marital status and gender. Deirdre Madden, *Medicine, Ethics and the Law* (Haywards Heath, UK: Bloomsbury Professional, 2016 (3rd edn)), p. 177.

84 "Health Committee to commence PLS on General Scheme of the Assisted Human Reproduction Bill 2017", press release, 16 January 2018 <https://

www.oireachtas.ie/en/press-centre/press-releases/20180116-health-committee-to-commence-pls-on-general-scheme-of-the-assisted-human-reproduction-bill-2017/> accessed 24 January 2019.

85 Deirdre Madden, evidence to the Joint Committee on Health, 19 December 2018 <https://www.oireachtas.ie/en/debates/debate/joint_committee_on_health/2018-12-19/2/> accessed 21 January 2019.

86 In 1999 it was reported that 1 in 10 couples in Ireland experienced infertility. About 1,000 Irish couples were receiving IVF treatment. Richard Oakley, "Options for treating infertility", *Sunday Tribune*, 11 July 1999, p. 5.

87 Joint Committee on Health, 17 January 2018, General Scheme of the Assisted Human Reproduction Bill 2017 <https://www.oireachtas.ie/en/debates/debate/joint_committee_on_health/2018-01-17/3/> accessed 21 January 2019; evidence of Dr Tony Holohan.

88 There was very little regulation in relation to the use of gametes and embryos. In 2006 the Health Products Regulatory Authority was designated as the competent authority to monitor and regulate fertility clinics in relation to standards of safety and quality concerning gametes and embryos. Evidence of Dr Tony Holohan.

89 Ibid., evidence of Dr Tony Holohan.

90 Ibid.

91 Human Life International (Ireland), "Submission to the Oireachtas Joint Committee on Health, on the General Scheme of the Assisted Human Reproduction Bill 2017" <https://humanlife.ie/latest-news/ivf-submission/> accessed 18 February 2019.

92 Ingrid Torjesen, "Five Minutes with ... Joanna Rose", *British Medical Journal*, vol. 351 (4 November 2015) <https://www-bmj-com.ucc.idm.oclc.org/content/351/bmj.h5864> accessed 13 February 2019.

93 Objections to the GSAHR, similar to those expressed by the Iona Institute and Dr Joanna Rose, were expressed by the institute's director, David Quinn, in the *Irish Catholic*. David Quinn, "The more things change ...", *Irish Catholic*, 22 February 2018 <https://www.irishcatholic.com/the-more-things-change/> accessed 18 February 2019.

94 Iona Institute and Dr Joanna Rose, "General Scheme of the 2017/18 Assisted Human Reproduction Bill: Comments and recommendations concerning donor-conceived children", 2018 <https://ionainstitute.ie/submission-to-health-committee-on-assisted-human-reproduction-bill/> accessed 21 January 2019.

95 Joint Committee on Health, 28 February 2018, General Scheme of the Assisted Human Reproduction Bill 2017 <https://www.oireachtas.ie/en/debates/debate/joint_committee_on_health/2018-02-28/3/> accessed 21 January 2019.

96 Mary Hallissey, "Who do You Think You Are?", *Law Society Gazette*, August–

September 2018 <https://www.lawsociety.ie/globalassets/documents/gazette/gazette-pdfs/gazette-2018/sept-2018-gazette.pdf> accessed 23 January 2019. Hallissey's article was the basis of Dr Angelo Bottone's criticisms of the GSAHR: "'Mother', 'father' to be replaced by 'parent 1', 'parent 2'", Iona Institute, 12 September 2018 <https://ionainstitute.ie/mother-and-father-to-be-replaced-by-parent-1-and-parent-2/> accessed 23 January 2019.

97 The organisation responsible was the former adoption society, St Patrick's Guild (set up by the Sisters of Charity in 1910). At the peak of its activities it was one of the largest adoption societies. The illegal registrations, which gave false information about the parents, occurred in the years from 1946 to 1969. It was probable that many more cases would be brought to light with a further examination of adoption records. "126 had births incorrectly registered by former adoption society St Patrick's Guild", RTÉ News, 30 May 2018 <https://www.rte.ie/news/ireland/2018/0529/966890-st-patricks-guild-adoptions-tusla/> accessed 16 February 2019.

98 General Scheme of the Assisted Human Reproduction Bill 2017, Head 53.

99 UN General Assembly, Convention on the Rights of the Child (ratified on 20 November 1989) <https://www.ohchr.org/en/professionalinterest/pages/crc.aspx> accessed 10 February 2019.

100 These clinicians were Dr John Waterstone, Prof. Mary Wingfield (clinical director of Merrion Fertility Clinic, affiliated to Holles Street Hospital), and Dr John Kennedy (National Fertility Centre, Rotunda Hospital and medical director of Sims IVF in Clonskeagh and Cork).

101 Deirdre Madden, Opening Statement to the Joint Committee on Health on the General Scheme of the Assisted Human Reproduction Bill 2017, 17 December 2018 <https://data.oireachtas.ie/ie/oireachtas/committee/dail/32/joint_committee_on_health/submissions/2018/2018-12-19_opening-statement-professor-deirdre-madden-school-of-law-ucc_en.pdf> accessed 5 February 2019; and Nóirín Hayes, Opening Statement to the Joint Committee on Health, 19 December 2018 <https://data.oireachtas.ie/ie/oireachtas/committee/dail/32/joint_committee_on_health/submissions/2018/2018-12-19_opening-statement-professor-noirin-hayes-school-of-education-tcd_en.pdf> accessed 5 February 2019.

102 Dr Joanna Rose, Opening Statement to the Joint Committee on Health, 19 December 2018 <https://data.oireachtas.ie/ie/oireachtas/committee/dail/32/joint_committee_on_health/submissions/2018/2018-12-19_opening-statement-dr-joanna-rose_en.pdf> accessed 5 February 2019.

103 Philomena Lee's son Anthony (later Michael Hess) was born on 5 July 1952. He was taken from her, against her wishes, in December 1955. Martin Sixsmith, "The Catholic church sold my child", *Guardian*, 19 September 2009 <https://www.theguardian.com/lifeandstyle/2009/sep/19/catholic-church-sold-child> accessed 20 February 2019.

104 Emma O'Friel, Opening Statement to the Joint Committee on Health, 19

December 2018 <https://data.oireachtas.ie/ie/oireachtas/committee/dail/32/joint_committee_on_health/submissions/2018/2018-12-19_opening-statement-emma-o-friel_en.pdf> accessed 5 February 2019.

105 Joint Committee on Health, 19 December 2018.

106 Ibid. Rose pointed to the longitudinal studies of adoption as a source of evidence for the JCH to consider, referring to the work of Pauline Ley (awarded the Order of Australia) and Alexina McWhinnie MBE. Her opinions about parallels between adoption and donor-conceived children were not accepted as valid comparisons by members of the committee. This was especially evident in the responses of Kate O'Connell TD (Fine Gael) and Louise O'Reilly TD (Sinn Féin). O'Friel pointed to "people's lived experience" expressed through Donor Offspring Europe, Tangled Webs, Anonymous Us (USA) "and many other organisations around the world". It was in this context that Kate O'Connell referred to the testimonies of O'Friel and Rose as "opinions". What the JCH sought was scientific evidence from longitudinal studies of surrogacy and donor-conceived children with which they could engage critically.

107 See Commission on Assisted Human Reproduction, *Report of the Commission on Assisted Human Reproduction* (Dublin: Stationery Office, 2005), p. 52.

108 Joint Committee on Health, 19 December 2018.

109 Angelo Bottone, "Refusing to engage with the ethical harms of surrogacy and donor-conception", Iona Institute, 21 December 2018 <https://ionainstitute.ie/refusing-to-engage-with-the-ethical-harms-of-surrogacy-and-donor-conception/> accessed 23 January 2019.

110 Deirdre Madden, Joint Committee on Health, 19 December 2018.

111 "Help wanted; surrogacy", *Economist*, vol. 423, no. 9040 (13 May 2017) <https://search-proquest-com.ucc.idm.oclc.org/docview/1898476635/12A62D38D6F1454APQ/47?accountid=14504> accessed 23 January 2019.

112 "The gift of life; surrogacy", *Economist*, vol. 423, no. 9040 (13 May 2017) <https://search-proquest-com.ucc.idm.oclc.org/docview/1898478309/12A62D38D6F1454APQ/6?accountid=14504> accessed 23 January 2019.

113 For details see Anna Momigliano, "When Left-Wing Feminists and Conservative Catholics Unite", *The Atlantic*, 28 March 2017 <https://www.theatlantic.com/international/archive/2017/03/left-wing-feminists-conservative-catholics-unite/520968/> accessed 8 March 2019.

114 Swedish Women's Lobby, "Feminist No to Surrogacy Motherhood" <http://sverigeskvinnolobby.se/en/project/feminist-no-to-surrogacy-motherhood/> accessed 23 January 2019.

115 Kajsa Ekis Ekman, "All surrogacy is exploitation – the world should follow Sweden's ban", *Guardian*, 26 February 2016 <https://www.theguardian.com/commentisfree/2016/feb/25/surrogacy-sweden-ban> accessed 6 March 2019.

The conclusions of this government commission provide some insights into evaluating traditionalist Catholic criticisms of the JCH and the broader issues of surrogacy and DAHR. See *Olika vägar till föräldraskap*, Stockholm 2016 <http://www.sou.gov.se/wp-content/uploads/2016/02/SOU-2016_11_webb. pdf> accessed 23 January 2019, pp. 51–8.

116 Congregation for the Doctrine of the Faith, *Instruction on Respect for Human Life in Its Origin and on the Dignity of Procreation* [*Donum Vitae*], "Homologous Artificial Fertilization", paragraph 5.

117 Ibid., "Moral and Civil Law".

118 David J. Walsh, E. Scott Sills, Gary S. Collins, Christine A. Hawrylyshyn, Piotr Sokol and Anthony P.H. Walsh, "Irish Public Opinion on Assisted Human Reproduction Services: Contemporary Assessments from a National Sample", *Clinical and Experimental Reproductive Medicine*, vol. 40, no. 4 (December 2013), pp. 169–73 <https://www.ncbi.nlm.nih.gov/pmc/articles/ PMC3913896/> accessed 17 March 2019.

119 The Joint Committee on Health published submission documents from 33 organisations and individual authors on 10 July 2019. Explicit reference to Catholic moral teaching is made in only one submission: Patrick McCrystal, Human Life International (Ireland), pp. 89–91. Joint Committee on Health, *Report on Pre-Legislative Scrutiny of the General Scheme of the Assisted Human Reproduction Bill*, 10 July 2019 <https://data. oireachtas.ie/ie/oireachtas/committee/dail/32/joint_committee_on_health/ submissions/2019/2019-07-10_submissions-report-on-pre-legislative- scrutiny-of-the-general-scheme-of-the-assisted-human-reproduction-bill_ en.pdf> accessed 30 July 2019.

CHAPTER SEVEN

———•———

Abortion

1992–2016

Morality and Law

MANY CATHOLICS DISAGREE WITH THE DOCTRINAL TEACHINGS of their Church that human life is sacred from conception, but others defend the hierarchy's stance on the basis of the "slippery slope" or "domino effect" argument. For example, "pro-lifers" may argue that if experimentation is permitted on *in vitro* embryos up to fourteen days it will lead inevitably to experimentation on embryos at more advanced stages of development. Simon Lee, professor of jurisprudence at Queen's University Belfast, writing in the aftermath of the Supreme Court judgment on the X Case (1992), criticised this approach to bioethics on the basis that it was "extraordinarily difficult" to change the law on abortion and related issues. Besides, "we are always already on the slope, holding a position. Most legal systems already allow abortion in some circumstances and prohibit it in others."[1] Legal and philosophical arguments generally focus on balancing rights rather than clinging to the idea that human life is an absolute right.[2]

Many voters disagreed with a liberal abortion regime but approved of abortion in a limited range of circumstances, such as in cases of rape or severe to fatal foetal abnormalities. In doing so they defied neat categorisations such as "pro-life" and "pro-choice". Biomedical issues were rarely, if ever, adequately addressed by simple choices between right and wrong, or between one extreme and another. For example, a legal prohibition of abortion in all circumstances would violate the human rights of pregnant women. The other extreme of abortion without any legal restrictions fails to address any rights pertaining to the human foetus. Neither extreme was likely to find majority support in Ireland.

When viewed in the context of the EU, Ireland's abortion law was very restrictive – as was legislation in Poland and Malta. The UK (excluding Northern Ireland), the Netherlands, Belgium and Sweden were at the liberal end of the spectrum. If it was moral or immoral to terminate the life of a human foetus in Ireland, then it was equally moral or immoral to terminate such a life in Britain. It was hard to refute such an argument in terms of moral philosophy alone. Still, there is another way of addressing this issue and that is by considering the political dimension. At what political level should policy formation and reform occur? Should Ireland reform its laws in response to the findings of the UN Human Rights Committee (UN HRC)? Pro-life activists argued that Ireland should be free to decide its own laws on abortion without dictation from any outside body. There was merit to this argument – but only up to a point. When Ireland was judged to have violated human rights by the UN HRC, on the basis of an international treaty it had freely signed, its moral credibility on the issue was difficult to sustain. The politics of the EU, relating especially to the principle of subsidiarity, also needed to be considered. Member states of the EU compromised their sovereignty to some extent, but not on biomedical ethics. The principle of subsidiarity applied so that public policy was worked out at national parliamentary level. Even so, member states were obliged to take account of judgments issued by the European Court of Human Rights (ECHR).

Pro-choice activists frequently referred to the thousands of Irish women who were travelling to Britain for abortions. Advocates of pro-choice contended that the Republic of Ireland was "exporting" its abortion problem to Britain. There was some validity to this view, but it was somewhat flawed in that it seemed to overlook the right of Ireland to exercise independent judgement or simply assumed that British legislation placed that jurisdiction in a morally superior position on the matter. Pro-choice advocates frequently failed to address the question of what rights, if any, attach to unborn human life.

The principle of subsidiarity, in the context of Ireland's membership of the EU, served the interests of the pro-life lobby in Ireland quite well. If decisions were made at European level it was likely that Irish law concerning the termination of pregnancy would have been less restrictive – considering that most EU states were governed by laws more liberal than Ireland's. Any attempt to impose a liberal abortion regime on Ireland would most likely have provoked strong opposition from the majority of the electorate – hence the protocol for Ireland in the Treaty on European Union (Maastricht, 1992) giving assurances about the application of Article 40.3.3 "in Ireland".[3] The Irish electorate, asserting the right to make its own decision, could not credibly have sought to impose its will on any other member state. Neither would it have been sustainable or morally justified to have imposed travel restrictions on Irish women seeking abortions in a jurisdiction where it was legal to do so. This was affirmed by the Irish electorate in the Thirteenth Amendment (1992) to the Constitution.

The X Case and the European Court of Human Rights

In August 2005 three women (referred to as A, B and C) resident in Ireland lodged a complaint to the ECHR claiming that the state's restrictions on abortion breached their human rights. The ECHR observed that the Irish state had failed to legislate or put in place any procedures relating to how the risk to a woman's life was to be determined or quantified. Sections 58 and 59 of the Offences Against the Person Act 1861 had not been amended, creating great legal uncertainty for those women who sought lawful abortions in Ireland. The ECHR found that the criminal provisions of the Act imposed "a significant chilling factor" on both doctors and their patients because a decision taken about entitlement to abortion might subsequently be judged unlawful.

On 16 December 2010, the Grand Chamber of the ECHR turned down the applications of A and B but found that human rights had been breached in the case of C. The Republic of Ireland was legally obligated to implement a legislative or regulatory scheme to provide effective and accessible procedures so that pregnant women could ascertain whether or not they had a right to a lawful termination of pregnancy under the terms of Article 40.3.3 of the Constitution as interpreted by the Supreme Court in the X Case. In cases where entitlement was established, access to abortion services in the state would have to be put in place. Ireland was a signatory to the European Convention for the Protection of Human Rights and Fundamental Freedoms and was under a legal obligation to comply with the judgments of the ECHR.[4] The Irish government responded by setting up an advisory committee with expertise in medicine, law and administration to advise it on how best to implement the ECHR judgment. The *Report of the Expert Group on the Judgment in A, B and C v Ireland* was published in November 2012. The committee submitted a number of options that were "practical and consistent with the Constitution and the law of the State".[5]

The bishops were quick to react. They observed that the terms of reference of the expert group did not include ethical considerations for determining public policy. After their general meeting at Maynooth on 5 December 2012 they held a press conference, at which they expressed criticism of the absence of ethical analysis in the expert group's report. They did not oppose medical treatment for any gravely ill pregnant woman that put her unborn child at risk, provided that every effort was made to save both mother and child. This was fundamentally different from a medical intervention undertaken to deliberately terminate the life of the unborn. The bishops believed that the options put forward by the expert group could end the practice in Irish hospitals of making this ethical distinction. The judgment of the ECHR did not mean that it was necessary for the state to legislate for abortion. It was open to the government to hold another referendum on abortion to amend the Constitution for the purpose of overturning the Supreme Court X Case judgment. Guidelines, consistent with sound ethics, were also seen as potentially beneficial for those in the healthcare professions who needed legal clarity about medical treatment for pregnant women. The bishops argued that there was evidence from other jurisdictions that "the floodgates for abortion" opened when abortions were performed on the basis of mental health issues.[6]

The Catholic hierarchy's press release was issued against the background of controversy arising from the death of Savita Halappanavar at University Hospital Galway on 28 October 2012. This tragedy intensified pressure for legislative reforms in relation to abortion. Halappanavar was 17 weeks pregnant and was denied a termination, despite being dangerously ill from complications associated with the pregnancy. She died shortly afterwards. Savita Halappanavar's death received coverage in the national press and in social media, and also received attention abroad. It was widely reported that the termination she sought was not granted because Ireland was a "Catholic country".[7]

Dr Ciarán McLoughlin, coroner for the West Galway district, asked Dr Peter Boylan to assist the inquest as an expert witness. Boylan's report pointed to deficiencies in the clinical care of Halappanavar, but he "effectively" attributed her death to the Eighth Amendment. In so doing, he anticipated that this would provoke a response, which he was willing to engage with.[8] The inquest returned a verdict of medical misadventure, but there was also another key finding. McLoughlin, evidently mindful of Boylan's evidence, found a lack of clarity in law and in Medical Council guidelines. He pointed out that doctors who work to professional standards and in good faith should not have to contend with the threat of such extremely punitive measures as imprisonment or removal from the medical register.[9]

Boylan did not have to wait long for a response to his findings about the impact of the Eighth Amendment on women's healthcare. On 1 May 2013 eight obstetricians and three other medical consultants wrote to the *Irish Times*, challenging Boylan's opinion that "Irish law prevented necessary treatment to save Ms Halappanavar's life." The signatories, well-known defenders of the Eighth Amendment, included Dr John Monaghan, Dr Trevor Hayes and Professor John Bonnar. They suggested that Boylan's conclusion was "a personal view, not an expert one".[10] The signatories to the *Irish Times* letter argued that:

> [I]t is impossible for Dr Boylan, or for any doctor, to predict with certainty the clinical course and outcome in the case of Savita Halappanavar where sepsis arose from the virulent and multi drug-resistant organism, E.coli ESBL. What we can say with certainty is that where ruptured membranes are accompanied by any clinical or bio-chemical marker of infection, Irish obstetricians understand they can intervene with early delivery of the baby if necessary. Unfortunately, the inquest shows that in Galway University Hospital the diagnosis of chorioamnionitis was delayed and relevant information was not noted and acted upon.[11]

Boylan believed that his professional reputation had been impugned by the suggestion that his professional competence was compromised by personal bias and lost no time in vigorously defending the medical report he had submitted to the coroner. He had not predicted with certainty any clinical outcome in the Halappanavar case. His prediction was made "on the balance of probabilities". (Medical judgements are generally based on probabilities, not on certainties.) The signatories had unwisely used the term "any clinical or bio-chemical marker of infection". Boylan found this "truly astonishing".[12] Years later, in *In the Shadow of the Eighth* (2019) he was not so polite, dismissing the point about non-specific markers as "nonsense" and "rubbish".[13] Why such a caustic response? Boylan pointed out that a non-specific marker of infection/inflammation implied that "an elevated white blood cell count … on its own would justify a termination of pregnancy."[14] If true, this would indeed have opened "the floodgates" to abortion in Ireland, considering that the common cold could cause an increase in the white blood cell count. There was, of course, no prospect that such a radical shift of opinion towards abortion was imminent in Ireland.

Conservative Catholicism, although much weakened since the 1990s, was still powerful enough to act as a brake on constitutional reform. It pressed for a referendum to reverse the X Case judgment. The Fine Gael–Labour coalition was determined to resist its demands. On 18 December, after examining the expert group's report, it decided that the best way forward was a combination of legislation and regulations consistent with Article 40.3.3 of the Constitution as interpreted by the Supreme Court in the X Case. The legislation was to provide "clarity and certainty" about the termination of pregnancy when there was a substantial risk to the life of the mother and when such a risk could only be eliminated by a termination of pregnancy.[15]

The government decided not to draft heads of a Bill until after the Joint Committee on Health and Children had concluded hearings from medical and legal experts, and advocacy organisations, in early January 2013. Psychiatric evidence submitted to the committee indicated that suicide was extremely rare in pregnancy; but it was a risk that always had to be considered. If legislation was implemented, psychiatrists would be asked to consider if there was "a real and substantial risk" to the mother's life arising from suicidal ideation or intent, and whether termination of pregnancy was the only way of eliminating that risk. The Joint Committee was informed that no psychiatric evidence had been submitted to the Supreme Court in the X Case. Patricia Casey, professor of psychiatry at University College Dublin and clinical psychiatrist at the Mater Misericordiae University Hospital, argued that suicide risk should not be included in the legislation. She referred to an extensive review of research papers by the Royal College of Psychiatrists to make the point that abortion made no difference generally to risks of mental illness. The outcome was the same whether women gave birth to unwanted children or had an abortion. But risk of mental illness increased for those women who previously had mental health problems or had been coerced. Adolescents were also at higher risk of mental illness in cases of unwanted pregnancies.[16] The report Professor Casey referred to was probably *Induced Abortion and Mental Health* (London, 2011). Its authors – mainly psychiatrists – did find, as Casey had pointed out, that "the rates of mental health problems for women with an unwanted pregnancy were the same whether they had an abortion or gave birth." However, the authors found that many research papers were of low quality and with a significant risk of bias. There was a need for good-quality longitudinal research. Significantly, the authors did not recommend restricting access to abortion.[17]

Casey argued that a provision for suicide risk in legislation for the X Case would not be supported by scientific evidence. She told the Joint Committee that "the two tests envisaged in the X case – that suicide will occur, on the balance of probability, and can only be averted by abortion – cannot be met." Risk assessment was not an exact science and psychiatrists would err on the side of caution to avoid the risk of a woman committing suicide. This would lead to a higher number of abortions.

Casey believed that legislation on abortion in relation to suicide risk would be "bad law" because it was not evidence-based. She spoke of a "floodgates phenomenon". She believed that increasing demands to extend the law to include mental health as well as suicidality would lead to "widespread abortion in a short period". She anticipated that the law would initially be found "cumbersome" and would eventually be dismantled, opening the way for a liberal abortion regime similar to those in many other jurisdictions.[18] Her prediction that the law would be cumbersome was to prove correct, but her concerns about widespread abortion were groundless considering the restrictions imposed by Article 40.3.3. of the Constitution as interpreted by the Supreme Court.

In psychiatric terms, Professor Casey had presented a plausible argument against legislating for suicide as grounds for termination of pregnancy. Still, the issue of scientific evidence in psychiatry was far from straightforward. Veronica O'Keane, professor of psychiatry at Trinity College Dublin and clinical psychiatrist at Tallaght Hospital (Dublin), pointed to a "discrepancy" between the evidence as adduced by experts and what was happening in "real life". Women who were suicidal due to an unwanted pregnancy did not go to an obstetric unit and did not consult a perinatal psychiatrist. They went to their GP. Most people in Ireland who committed suicide did not go to a psychiatrist. About 5,000 Irish women per annum had travelled abroad for abortions since 1983. O'Keane argued that if the option to travel, especially to Britain, for abortion services was blocked, the result would be injury and death to women, and death to babies – as had happened in countries where women had no access to abortion. There was no information about how many of the thousands of women who had travelled abroad for abortion were suicidal or suffered from mental illness. Only inferences could be made from examining the reasons why women undergo terminations of pregnancy in other jurisdictions.[19]

Obstetricians Dr Rhona Mahony (master of the National Maternity Hospital), Dr Sam Coulter-Smith (master of the Rotunda Hospital) and Dr Mary McCaffrey (Kerry General Hospital) were asked if any avoidable maternal deaths had occurred because of a lack of legal clarity. Had any doctors felt unable to perform a life-saving procedure because they believed that it might have been illegal to do so? At this point official enquiries into the death of Savita Halappanavar had not been concluded. Coulter-Smith did not know of any such case. Mahony gave a more nuanced answer. She questioned the accuracy of available data. In relation to suicide, she argued that it was very difficult to ascertain its frequency because open verdicts were frequently delivered by the Coroner's Court. Also, since many women travelled abroad for terminations of pregnancy, there was considerable uncertainty about the frequency of suicide ideation, suicide intent and suicide. She made similar points in relation to physical health issues. Some women with cancer or with some other serious medical problem travelled discreetly to other jurisdictions, where they terminated their pregnancies.[20]

Several advocacy organisations – religious and non-religious – were represented at the proceedings of the Joint Committee on Health and Children. Bishop Christopher Jones of the diocese of Elphin and Fr Timothy Bartlett attended on behalf of the Irish Catholic Bishops' Conference. From the bishops' perspective, there was nothing in Irish law, in medical guidelines or in Catholic ethics that prevented mothers and their unborn babies from receiving medical care and life-saving treatment when necessary. The Supreme Court judgment on the X Case was unsound because it had "overturned the pro-life intention" of the Irish electorate as expressed in the 1983 referendum and it had heard no psychiatric evidence. The Catholic hierarchy's position was that a referendum should be held so that the people would have the opportunity to reverse the X Case judgment. It was not necessary to legislate for the X Case to satisfy the ECHR. Concerns expressed by doctors that they were vulnerable to prosecution could be addressed by issuing professional guidelines reviewable by the courts.

Bishop Jones believed "totally in the equal right of mother and child".[21] However, the principle of equality was not without complications. Fr Pádraig McCarthy, writing in *The Furrow*, argued that if legislation permitted a termination of pregnancy to save the life of the mother, it would give rise to a disturbing and unintended corollary. Considering the equal right to life imposed by the Constitution, this could be interpreted to "mean that it would also be legally permitted to take the life of the mother in order to save the life of the child". Not satisfied with this finding, Fr McCarthy concluded that it "would be difficult to accept".[22] Fr McCarthy seems to have had in mind the delaying of chemotherapy or some other life-saving medical procedure for the mother that would extend gestation long enough for the foetus to be safely delivered but would greatly diminish the mother's prospects of survival. In an earlier article in *The Furrow* he had proposed guiding principles for discussion. A life-saving treatment for the mother, which was considered to endanger the life of the unborn, should be made accessible to the mother and applied only with her permission. This treatment was not to be delayed if it endangered the life of the mother.[23] Fr McCarthy had, apparently without intending to do so, added considerable weight to the opinion that the rights of mother and unborn child should not be seen as equal.

Catholics who resolutely opposed abortion as a response to the threat of suicide saw the Supreme Court judgment in the X Case as deeply flawed. They believed, in common with the Catholic bishops, that it had overturned the pro-life intentions of the Irish electorate as expressed in Article 40.3.3 – but this claim was no longer sustainable because the electorate had rejected proposals in the referendums of 1992 and 2002 to exclude the risk of suicide as a basis for lawful abortion. Despite this, opponents of abortion argued that legislation based on the X Case judgment would have dire consequences for human rights – the right to life being the most fundamental.[24] Public representatives were urged to vote in accordance with their conscience – conscience was "the only whip that matters".[25] The risk of suicide was extremely difficult to assess – this added considerable clout to the anti-abortion case. If abortion was permitted on the basis of a perceived risk of suicide, this, it was argued, would lead to relatively easy access to abortion. The Catholic bishops insisted that abortion had no constructive role to play in the treatment of depression or suicidal tendencies in pregnant women.[26]

Protection of Life During Pregnancy Act 2013

Government ministers were not unduly influenced by the bishops on abortion and this was very much in evidence on 1 May 2013 when the publication of the General Scheme of the Protection of Life during Pregnancy Bill 2013 was announced.[27] No referendum was to be held concerning the Supreme Court judgment in the X Case. The definition of unborn human life was based on the Supreme Court judgment in *Roche v Roche and Others*. Legal protection of the unborn was from implantation to birth (including the birth process). It was incompatible with Catholic doctrine, which maintained that there was a moral imperative to protect human life from the point of conception. The reason why implantation was chosen was to avoid legally prohibiting emergency contraception and the treatment of ectopic pregnancies (implantation outside the womb) under the terms of the Bill.[28]

The Irish Catholic bishops condemned the Bill as morally unacceptable, asserting that intentionally terminating the life of an unborn child was never a "remedy" for suicide ideation. They understood that hospitals under Catholic management would be duty bound to offer abortion services, which would in turn be a violation of the autonomy and ethos of religious institutions. Citizens of a similar outlook were urged to make their views known to members of the Oireachtas.[29] There was now conflict between the intentions of the legislators and Catholic moral teaching! News media reports indicated that Catholic members of the Dáil who voted for the proposed legislation might be "automatically" excommunicated. When pressed on the matter, Cardinal Seán Brady declined to give a definitive answer. However, he was very clear on the intentions of the hierarchy to frustrate the intentions of the government. He did not see this as unwarranted Church interference in the political domain. Brady argued that abortion was contrary to the public interest. He acknowledged that politicians derived their power from the people but neither people nor politicians had the right to terminate human life.[30] The Taoiseach, Enda Kenny, responded forcefully. Although Kenny is Roman Catholic he was, in this instance, taking instructions from "the people's book" – the Constitution – as interpreted by the Supreme Court.[31] Kenny didn't elaborate on the interaction between his religious beliefs and his sense of political duty. His political philosophy took precedence over his Catholic beliefs in this context.

Kenny's riposte was calculated to steady the nerves of his party colleagues – and with good reason. Cardinal Raymond Burke, prefect of the Supreme Tribunal of the Apostolic Signatura at the Vatican, asserted that bishops and priests were duty-bound to refuse Roman Catholic parliamentarians Holy Communion if they voted in favour of legislation for abortion – even in cases when such abortions were carried out to save the life of the mother (as should have been performed in the case of Savita Halappanavar). Burke's extreme opinions were published in the *Irish*

Independent and in the *Catholic Voice* newspaper (published every fortnight in Ireland and Britain) and probably came to the attention of some Irish politicians.[32] Burke's stance was not doctrinally sustainable[33] but, as already observed, Cardinal Brady was slow to assuage concerns about excommunication. At least one Fine Gael TD, Tom Barry, expressed deep concern about the implied threat of excommunication.[34] Despite this he was somewhat defiant, bolstered by the argument that it would be incredible hypocrisy for the Catholic hierarchy to excommunicate politicians for voting for legislation on a scheme of restrictive abortion when it did not excommunicate those who had abused children and those who covered up such abuse. It was reported that Barry requested and received assurances from both Cardinal Brady and the papal nuncio that he would not be excommunicated for supporting party policy. It is likely that the greatest pressure to vote against the government was generated at constituency level where anti-abortion activists gathered outside constituency offices, confronting their elected representatives at every opportunity.[35] Several Fine Gael TDs and senators, including Lucinda Creighton, voted against the legislation on grounds of conscience and suffered expulsion from the parliamentary party as a result.[36]

Was conflict between Catholic teaching and party loyalty on this issue inevitable? Probably not! The Catholic Church, as observed earlier, has condemned abortion unequivocally. Catholics are morally obligated to oppose all laws that are intrinsically unjust by conscientious objection and by withholding support. But what if a Bill is submitted to a national parliament that proposes a law more restrictive of abortion than a competing legislative initiative or an existing law? How should a Catholic parliamentarian vote in these circumstances? Pope John Paul II, in his encyclical *Evangelium Vitae* (1995), declared that if it was not otherwise possible to repeal or block the enactment of a pro-abortion law, Catholic parliamentarians could, in good conscience, vote for legislation that permitted some abortion but was more restrictive than the alternatives. This would be a morally acceptable means to limit the evil effects of proposed or existing legislation.[37] The central question, then, as Patrick Hannon (emeritus professor of moral theology) saw it, was whether or not the proposed legislation was intended to limit or diminish any "evil aspects" of law already in place. Hannon did not give a definitive answer. Expert opinions in the relevant disciplines were deeply divided. There was no "clean and simple solution" – too many questions remained unanswered on both sides of the debate. Catholic legislators were therefore free to act according to their conscience and could vote for or against the proposed legislation.[38]

Government politicians were very aware that they would have to contend with pro-life pressure groups in their constituencies in the course of legislating for the X Case judgment. The Pro Life Campaign (PLC) organised a National Vigil for Life in Merrion Square in Dublin, which took place on 8 June 2013. An estimated 40,000 people demonstrated their opposition to the proposed legislation. Banners and placards read: "PRO-WOMAN, PRO-LIFE, PRO-BABY" AND "WOMEN AND BABIES DESERVE BETTER THAN ABORTION".[39] Government politicians were probably more disconcerted by street rallies than by any pronouncements from the bishops.

Public statements by the Catholic bishops, both collectively and individually, urged members of the Oireachtas to vote against the legislation and criticised the imposition of party whips by the government parties.[40] The Protection of Life during Pregnancy Bill was seen as a "Trojan horse" that would clear the way for much easier access to abortion in Ireland.[41] Copies of the briefing statement issued by all the bishops were circulated to members of the Oireachtas. This document was also accessible to the public through the bishops' website. A series of *Choose Life* newsletters was published by the Catholic Communications Office to further disseminate the Church's teaching on unborn human life.[42] The right to life was seen as the most important human right because it was the basis of all other rights. The bishops asserted that abortion was not a good response to suicide ideation and that it would adversely affect the culture and practice of medicine in Ireland. The right to life of the unborn child would be, in practice, no longer equal to that of the mother. Reference was made to the General Scheme of the Protection of Life during Pregnancy Bill 2013 to make the point that moral, legal and constitutional conflicts would arise concerning freedom of conscience and religious beliefs. Medical practitioners, nurses and midwives could refuse to carry out "a lawful termination of pregnancy" or could refuse to assist such a procedure on the grounds of conscientious objection.[43] The bishops anticipated that "others" might be legally obligated to co-operate against their conscience or contrary to their religious beliefs. This was seen as a potential breach of their constitutional rights with reference to Article 44.2.3 of the Constitution, which states that: "The State shall not impose any disabilities or make any discrimination on the ground of religious profession, belief or status."[44] Another problem with conscientious objection, from the bishops' point of view, was that it was limited to individuals and did not extend to institutions, which was also seen as contrary to Article 44.[45] The party whip system in the Oireachtas in this instance was also seen as potentially unconstitutional. The legislation was open to a constitutional challenge because the legislative process itself was unconstitutional.[46]

Despite the opposition from the bishops and the PLC, the Protection of Life During Pregnancy Bill was passed by secure majorities in both houses of the Oireachtas in July 2013 and was signed into law by President Michael D. Higgins on 30 July. The word "unborn" was defined as the time from implantation to the "complete emergence of the life from the body of the woman".[47] Section 9 of the Act, which concerned the risk of suicide, was the most contentious. It would be lawful to terminate a pregnancy when there was a "real and substantial risk" of suicide and when that risk could only be averted by medical intervention to induce or bring about an abortion.[48] Sections 58 and 59 of the Offences Against the Person Act 1861 were repealed.[49] A person found guilty of illegally terminating a pregnancy could receive a prison sentence of up to 14 years.[50]

The Catholic bishops anticipated that the Protection of Life During Pregnancy Act 2013 (PLDPA) was open to challenge on a number of fronts. The PLC declared its intention to work energetically for the repeal of the Act.[51] Opinion polls indicated that a clear majority of the electorate opposed a liberal abortion regime. Nevertheless, the statistics pointed to a large percentage of Irish Catholics who held more nuanced views than their bishops.[52]

Leo Varadkar, speaking as Minister for Health, and as a medical doctor, in response to a proposal in the Dáil to repeal the Eighth Amendment, made the point that debates about abortion in Ireland had been dominated by the extremes of "pro-life" and "pro-choice". Issues of medical ethics were too complex to be addressed simply in terms of bipolar opposites of right and wrong. No abortion law could be so perfect that it would not need to be amended. Ireland was not, and is not, unique in struggling to legislate appropriately in matters of medical ethics. The frequently used terms "pro-choice" and "pro-life" failed to do justice to the complexity of the abortion issue. Varadkar declared himself "pro-life" in that he opposed abortion "on demand" and acknowledged that unborn children had rights. Still, he was critical of the Eighth Amendment because it was too restrictive. Although it served to protect the mother's right to life it failed to address elevated risks to her long-term health in cases where the threat of stroke, heart attack or epileptic seizure might result in permanent disability. Another major problem arising from the Eighth Amendment was that it provided the legal basis for compelling women to continue with their pregnancies in cases of life-limiting conditions/fatal foetal abnormalities. It had a "chilling effect" on medical doctors that impacted adversely on clinical best practice. In distressing circumstances, decisions that would otherwise be the outcome of discussions between doctors and women, couples, or next of kin in the absence of competence, were now made on the basis of legal advice.[53]

There was some support for Varadkar amongst his cabinet colleagues. Joan Burton, Tánaiste and leader of the Labour Party, expressed agreement. The Eighth Amendment did not serve women well on issues of safety and health and there was a pressing need to repeal it. Constitutional provisions were not an appropriate means to address complex and unpredictable medical cases that would arise from time to time. Pregnant women needed to see medical doctors, not lawyers, around their hospital beds.[54] There was, however, little support in government for holding a referendum to repeal Article 40.3.3. Political calculations dictated that such a risky initiative should be deferred for as long as possible.[55]

Varadkar spoke about Article 40.3.3 against the background of a tragic case of a young woman who was diagnosed brain-dead on 3 December 2014 when she was about 15 weeks pregnant and was sustained on intensive life support. Varadkar was aware of this case at the time.[56] Medical research based on case studies, internationally, indicated that the unborn baby had virtually no chance of survival. The longer the period of intensive life support the more likely it was that complications would arise from infection, heart failure, acute respiratory distress syndrome and blood clotting. All these were likely to cause the death of the foetus.[57]

The medical case in question provided compelling evidence in support of the contention that Article 40.3.3 needed to be repealed by referendum. The pregnant woman had two children. Given the hopelessness of her condition, and that of her unborn baby, the family requested her life support to be switched off. Medical personnel treating the mother wished to comply with the family's wishes, but concerns were expressed about the legality of such a course of action.[58] The PLDPA was not quite the Trojan horse for easy access to abortion so feared by pro-life campaigners. Fears were expressed by doctors about the possible fourteen-year prison sentence that could be imposed for what might be subsequently judged an illegal abortion.[59] Would switching off life support breach the constitutional rights of the foetus? Medical staff felt legally vulnerable because there was still a foetal heartbeat. Lawyers for the Health Service Executive were consulted and the case was brought before the High Court on 15 December.

Medical evidence submitted to the High Court in the *P.P. v Health Service Executive* case sheds light on the cruel irrationality that can occur when legal considerations take priority over expert medical consensus, common sense and the wishes of a distressed family in the early days of bereavement.[60] Legal counsel for the family argued that the right to life of the unborn was not "engaged" in the context of Article 40.3.3. It was not a question of intentionally terminating the life of the foetus. The words "as far as practicable" in the Article indicated that the obligation imposed on the state to defend and vindicate the right to life was not absolute. Counsel for the unborn, mindful of the death of the mother, submitted that there was no "equal right to life" to consider. The rights of the unborn took precedence over the family's wishes and the mother's entitlement to dignity in death. Yet counsel for the unborn did not argue that medical treatment should be determined by remote possibilities.[61] The "futile exercise" of sustaining life support for the mother was due to a fear of possible legal consequences. There was no medical or ethical basis for continuing with life support. Mindful that there was only "distress and death in prospect", the High Court ruled that the medical team could withdraw life support.[62] Life support was switched off shortly afterwards, on 27 December.[63]

This case was not the first of its kind. Two similar cases had occurred, in Waterford (2001) and Galway (2003). Pregnant brain-dead women had been kept on life support with virtually no prospect that the foetus in either case could be brought to viability. Medical staff were not clear about their legal obligations in circumstances that were certain to reoccur. Medical doctors had called for clear medical and legal guidelines, but nothing had been done to address this.[64] However, there should not have been a fear of prosecution when all the medical specialists agreed that there was no significant prospect of saving the foetus. There was a legal obligation to preserve unborn life only "as far as is practicable".[65]

The above cases pointed to what seemed an irrational fear among healthcare workers of terminating the life of a foetus. Was such fear irrational? It seems not. Dr Rhona Mahony, master of the National Maternity Hospital, maintained that if a woman was legally entitled to a termination of pregnancy it was very difficult to procure because the process of determination was "cumbersome and complicated". Speaking at the launch of Amnesty International's *She is Not a Criminal: The impact of Ireland's abortion law* (June 2015), she pointed out that although decisions were based on clinical judgement, these decisions were still "framed in a criminal context". A custodial sentence of up to fourteen years could be imposed on both the mother and her clinician if there was an error in clinical assessment. The risk to the life of the mother might subsequently be seen as not sufficiently substantial. And what qualified as "a substantial risk to life"? Ten per cent or 20 per cent or 80 per cent risk of death? Mahony argued that waiting for a woman to be so ill that her illness presented a risk of death was dangerous. It relied on a number of assumptions – not least that clinicians could make accurate predictions about risks to life. Some medical conditions, and complications arising from those conditions, could cause serious illness and sometimes death – but the point at which a major illness could escalate to a substantial risk of death was not "clearly marked".[66] There was considerable support within the healthcare professions in Ireland that abortion should be decriminalised on the basis that it prevented healthcare providers from delivering timely and medically-indicated care to their patients.[67]

Considerable political capital had been expended by the coalition government parties in pressing the PLDPA through parliament, which gave statutory effect to the X Case. The state had fulfilled its obligations in response to the ECHR ruling in the *A, B and C v Ireland* case. There were no plans for further legislative initiatives relating to abortion before the next general election. Therefore, when independent TD Clare Daly sought support for the Protection of Life in Pregnancy (Amendment) (Fatal Foetal Abnormalities) Bill 2013 on 6 February 2015 she met staunch resistance.[68] The Bill, if approved by the Oireachtas, would legalise abortion in circumstances where a foetus had "a fatal abnormality such that it is incompatible with life outside of the womb".[69] The Attorney General advised the government that the proposed legislation would be unconstitutional.[70] Also, there was no consensus on whether Article 40.3.3 should be amended or deleted.

Any subsequent legislation was also likely to exacerbate already deep divisions in the main political parties. The Taoiseach, Enda Kenny, was firm in his resolve that his government would not take any further legislative action for the remainder of its term in office.[71] The governing parties, with the support of many opposition TDs, easily won the Dáil vote by 104 to 20.[72] Political commentators were quick to point out that politicians, "terrified of the toxicity" of the abortion issue, would avoid addressing it if given the choice.[73]

There was (and still is) a medical and ethical complexity about "fatal" or "lethal" malformations in embryos and foetuses that stiffened the resistance of parliament to legislate. The words "fatal" or "lethal" are not strictly accurate or precise. There are at least twenty-five different congenital abnormalities, including anencephaly, trisomy 13 and trisomy 18. A study published in the *British Journal of Obstetrics and Gynaecology* found that, with the possible exception of renal agenesis, not all "lethal" conditions led inevitably to perinatal death. However, many babies died within hours or days of birth, although there were some cases where survival extended to years. But life-prolonging treatments were ethically questionable considering the "high probability of death despite treatment" and the severe nature of disabilities of infants if they survived. Was it ethical to sustain life in a biological sense if the treatment caused suffering with "little or no benefit"? An absence or severe deficit of cognitive development precluded children from forming "even minimal relationships with those around them".[74] Such cases indicated that a woman's right to choose was greater than the rights of unborn life. There was of course the risk of misdiagnosis – acknowledged by Leo Varadkar in the Dáil.[75] Yet such a risk is associated with medical practice generally.

The fears of pro-life groups that the PLDPA might open the floodgates to abortion did not seem well founded when the Department of Health published information about terminations of pregnancy carried out in 2014. There had been a total of twenty-six terminations: fourteen due to risk from physical illness; nine due to emergency from physical illness; and three arising from the risk of suicide.[76] There was no information about how advanced the pregnancies were, the illnesses, or about the time taken to reach decisions. The figure of twenty-six abortions seemed "modest" when seen against the background of an estimated 4,000 abortions carried out on Irish women each year in Britain, the unknown number of abortions induced by drugs illegally sourced through the internet, and the annual birth rate in Ireland of about 70,000.[77]

Irish society was deeply divided on the issue of abortion. Anti-abortion and pro-choice marchers confronted each other in Dublin.[78] A coalition of pro-choice organisations, the Abortion Rights Campaign, set about gathering signatures to repeal the Eighth Amendment. Tánaiste and Labour Party leader Joan Burton promised that repealing the Eighth Amendment would be a priority for her party in negotiations to form the next government. This would require holding a referendum as part of a future programme for government.[79] There was a lack of consensus across and within the main political parties on the abortion issue.[80]

The general tendency of Irish politicians to avoid addressing abortion was also evident in Northern Ireland, where access to legal abortion was much more restrictive than in the rest of the UK. There was a legal entitlement to procure an abortion if there was a significant risk to the life of the mother and if the threat to her long-term health was "probable".[81] But the guidelines for abortion were unclear. This meant that in practice women seeking abortions in cases of life-limiting conditions faced similar difficulties to those in the Republic and sometimes felt compelled to undertake the onerous journey to an abortion clinic in England. Medical staff generally tended not to terminate a pregnancy when there was legal uncertainty.[82] On 30 November 2015 the Belfast High Court delivered a landmark judgment that indicated support for abortion in Northern Ireland in cases of life-limiting conditions and in cases where a pregnancy was the result of a sexual crime. Mr Justice Mark Horner contended that legislation on abortion in Northern Ireland was contrary to Article 8 of the European Convention on Human Rights, which asserts that public authorities are obligated to respect private and family life. Even so, there were exceptions to this right, including "the protection of health or morals, or for the protection of the rights and freedoms of others".[83]

Mr Justice Horner concluded that in cases of life-limiting conditions the woman's right to choose took precedence. The foetus was "doomed": there was no life to protect; there was "nothing to weigh in the balance".[84] The Horner judgment was overturned in June 2017 by three appeal court judges in Belfast. The court ruled that changes in the law should be determined by the legislature, not by a court of law.[85] Although the Horner judgment did not change the law on abortion, it did put pressure on parliament to legislate on the issue. The Roman Catholic bishops of Northern Ireland, predictably enough, took a radically different view. Unborn children were persons, regardless of cognitive and physical impairment. Their right to life was also not diminished in cases where they were conceived as a result of a sexual crime.[86]

The Northern Ireland Assembly (at Stormont) had the power to pass legislation to broaden the grounds for abortion. In their appeal against such a possible legislative initiative the bishops questioned the appropriateness of the term "fatal" or "lethal" foetal abnormalities and highlighted the uncertainties of prognoses in these cases. Their preference was for "life-limiting conditions in pregnancy" – including anencephaly. The morally appropriate course of action was to provide resources for perinatal palliative services for terminally ill children "until natural death".[87]

The anti-abortion organisation Precious Life, the self-proclaimed largest pro-life organisation in Northern Ireland, lobbied vigorously against proposed legislation to permit abortion in cases of life-limiting conditions and where pregnancies were due to rape. It drew support from both nationalist and unionist communities – a "'holy alliance' of evangelical Protestantism and fundamentalist Catholicism".[88] Lengthy debates ensued at Stormont and shortly before the vote on 10 February 2016 it became clear that the proposed legislation would be voted down due to opposition from the Democratic Unionist Party (DUP) and the Social Democratic and Labour Party (SDLP).[89] In the aftermath of victory Precious Life declared its intention to "expose" every Assembly member who had voted for the "evil amendments".[90]

Commitment to the cause was no less intense in the opposing camp. When a Belfast woman received a three-month suspended sentence for inducing an abortion with pills bought through the internet, it provoked outrage in the Alliance for Choice. Three activists – Kitty O'Kane, Colette Devlin and Diana King – presented themselves to the Police Service of Northern Ireland (PSNI) and declared that they had illegally purchased abortion pills for women who were afraid to have the items delivered to their homes. All their packages had been delivered "by the Queen" (i.e. by the Royal Mail). The PSNI, in response, set about preparing a report for submission to the Public Prosecution Service of Northern Ireland. It was now probable that these women would be charged and convicted. They believed that they had a duty to support good law – but they also had a moral duty to oppose bad law.[91] It raised the question: Would the law become unsustainable if many women came forward with admissions of acting illegally? A post on Facebook speculated that prisons "would be filled to the brim if the law was actually enforced".[92] Although quite alarmist, this speculation raised issues of social justice and public morality. It seemed only a matter of time before women would serve time in prison for inducing abortions. These women, unable to afford abortions in Britain, were likely to come from the most vulnerable and poorest sectors of society.

It also seemed only a matter of time before prosecutions would be taken against women in the Republic. Increasing numbers of women facing crisis pregnancies were turning to abortion pills purchased through the internet.[93] It was more difficult to address the issue of abortion in the Republic than in Northern Ireland. Legal conditions were more complicated in the South because there was a constitutional dimension superimposed on the existing legislation.

As the general election drew closer in the Republic, supporters and critics of the Eighth Amendment renewed efforts to influence public opinion. Enda Kenny, evidently mindful of how even a minimalist and highly cautious legal reform initiative (i.e. the PLDPA) could seriously damage Fine Gael, spoke about setting aside the party whip – but sometime in the future. If his party – deeply divided on repeal of the Eighth Amendment – was returned to power, a citizens' assembly would be set up within six months so that abortion could be discussed in a "respectful and rational way". Fine Gael deputies would have a free vote if the assembly put forward proposals about the Eighth Amendment for consideration by the Dáil.[94] An all-party committee would also be set up to consider expert advice. Kenny emphasised the need to depoliticise the issue as much as possible.[95] The Labour Party, Sinn Féin, the Social Democrats, the Green Party, the Anti-Austerity Alliance and People Before Profit all favoured repeal of the Eighth Amendment. Although Mícheál Martin declared that Fianna Fáil would not press for repeal of the amendment, some of the party's candidates favoured such an initiative.

The PLC worked hard to make abortion a major issue during the election campaign. Leaflets were circulated widely to households, bundled together with political pamphlets, urging voters to ascertain the opinions of candidates in their constituency and to vote only for candidates who were supportive of the Eighth Amendment.[96] The initiatives of the PLC did not push abortion to centre stage in the election campaign: socio-economic matters such as public services, taxation, the housing crisis and water charges were apparently the major concerns of the electorate on 26 February 2016. It seems that the outcome of the marriage equality referendum in 2015 and recurring debates about abortion were of secondary importance.[97] An *Irish Times/* Ipsos MRBI opinion poll indicated that about 64 per cent of voters favoured repeal of the amendment to allow abortion in limited circumstances, with 25 per cent against (11 per cent had no opinion).[98] It was of course easy to exaggerate the accuracy of opinion polls. Mr Justice Mark Horner, in his judgment referred to earlier, questioned the reliability of opinion polls as indicators of public opinion. Findings could vary depending on how questions were worded, the circumstances at the time, and the sampling methodology.[99] Nevertheless, there were strong indications in this instance that the movement to repeal the Eighth Amendment was gaining momentum.

Abortion and Human Rights

The PLDPA was judged to be inadequate in terms of human rights by a number of treaty-monitoring committees of the UN. On 19 August 2014 the UN HRC expressed concern that Section 22 of the Act criminalised abortion without making exceptions for cases of fatal foetal abnormality, rape, incest and "serious risks" to the health of the mother.[100] The UN HRC recommended constitutional and legislative reforms so that abortion would be permissible in cases of fatal foetal abnormality, rape, incest and "serious risks" to the health of the mother. Ireland was urged to issue a "guidance document" without delay so that legal clarity would be in place concerning any "real and substantive risk" to the life of a pregnant woman. The third recommendation was that more channels of information should be created about options in crisis pregnancies and criminal sanctions should not be imposed on healthcare providers who gave information about safe abortion services in other jurisdictions.[101] The main observations and recommendations of the UN HRC in relation to Ireland were reiterated by the UN Committee on Economic, Social and Cultural Rights on 8 July 2015[102] and to some extent also by the UN Committee on the Rights of the Child on 1 March 2016. The latter committee recommended decriminalisation of abortion "in all circumstances". It recommended that the mandatory school curriculum for adolescents should include sexual and reproductive health education.[103]

Restricting legal access to abortion in Ireland did not of course diminish demand for it.[104] Those women who could afford to travel for abortion services did so, mainly to Britain. Many of those who could not afford to do so resorted to illegal and unsafe abortions. Pharmaceutical pills, mifepristone and misoprostol, were frequently purchased through the internet by women north and south of the border to induce abortions in the first several weeks of pregnancy. In the Republic medical doctors were not under legal obligation to report a girl or woman they suspected of having taken abortion medication. Abortion pills could sometimes cause life-threatening conditions such as excessive bleeding. The Irish Family Planning Association and Amnesty International (Ireland) pointed out the importance of assuring women (and girls) that they would not be reported to the Gardaí if they presented at an emergency department after taking abortion medication.[105] Women's lives would be put at risk in the absence of such assurances. There was also the probability that women could serve time in prison.

The merit of punishing women for induced abortions was called into question. Opposition to abortion for moral reasons did not necessarily lead to support for punitive legislation. Breda O'Brien – an *Irish Times* columnist and defender of orthodox Catholic views – argued that one could, without contradiction, abhor something without punishing the offenders. She saw little merit in the prosecution of a young woman in Northern Ireland who had been found guilty of inducing an abortion.[106] In her thought-provoking article "Abortion – we can do better than women in prison and dead babies in bins", she took the opportunity to criticise Amnesty International's advocacy of "reproductive rights" for women.[107] This led to a series of letters to the *Irish Times*. Colm O'Gorman, Executive Director of Amnesty International in Ireland, referred to the recommendations of UN human rights bodies. Access to abortion, at a minimum, should be given in cases of life-limiting conditions, rape and incest, and when there was a risk to either the life or health of the pregnant woman. Legal prohibition, rather than stopping abortion, drove it underground, and effectively denied medical advice and supervision to many women when taking abortion medication. Women's lives and health were therefore unnecessarily exposed to additional risks.[108]

Rev. Patrick G. Burke (Church of Ireland) challenged O'Gorman's contention that abortion was a right under international law. He argued that there was no explicit right to abortion in any of the UN human rights treaties. The right to abortion was an "invented right" inspired by creative interpretation, in contrast to the "actual human right" of the unborn child.[109] The distinction between the "actual" right and the "invented" right was based on the Eighth Amendment.[110] A second contributor to the *Irish Times*, Pádraig McCarthy, observed that Ireland had not signed any international human rights treaty that established a right to abortion. Human rights were established on the basis of international treaties and were not determined by UN committees publishing reports on such matters.[111]

O'Gorman responded with the observation that Ireland's "brutal" abortion laws had been condemned by the UN HRC, the UN Committee on Economic, Social and Cultural Rights, and the UN Committee on the Rights of the Child. Human rights in international treaties were stated in broad terms, leaving it to expert committees to work out interpretations and precise meanings over time. The right to abortion was made in the context of women's rights to healthcare and information about medical needs, to privacy, and to protection against cruel and degrading treatment, and the right not to be discriminated against on the basis of gender. O'Gorman pointed to a Red C opinion poll that indicated that 80 per cent of Irish people supported broader access to abortion consistent with minimum requirements for women's rights.[112]

Arguments favouring legal reforms and improved access to abortion services gathered momentum in early May 2016 as a range of human rights issues in Ireland came under critical scrutiny in the course of the Universal Periodic Review process at the UN in Geneva.[113]

There was much more to be said about abortion and human rights in the context of international law. Breda O'Brien pointed to an article in the *Human Rights Law Review* (2008) jointly written by two human rights lawyers, Christina Zampas and Jaime Todd-Gher, who later worked for Amnesty International (London). They found that the "African Women's Protocol is the only legally binding human rights instrument that explicitly addresses abortion as a human right ... however, the Protocol's reach is limited to the African region and its efficacy has yet to be tested." O'Brien added that the status of the protocol was unclear even in those African states that had ratified it – and it was certainly not applicable to Ireland.[114]

O'Brien's article provoked a response from Zampas and Todd-Gher. They believed that both their intellectual honesty and that of Amnesty International had been impugned and were determined to address what they felt were misrepresentations propagated by O'Brien. Amnesty International drew its mandate from international human rights law. Abortion, although "not an expressly stated right in human rights treaties", was "an interpreted right".[115] But it had been argued that such an inferred right was not really a human right and the contention that it was arose from biased interpretations driven by an ideological agenda. Interpreted rights could not be so easily dismissed! Zampas and Todd-Gher argued that protection from female genital mutilation and from coerced sterilisation were also interpreted rights that derived from the rights to privacy, freedom from torture and other violations. It was intended that the explicitly stated human rights in UN treaties would be applied to specific issues that needed consideration over the coming years. The authors maintained that O'Brien did not understand the development of international law. UN treaties, drafted decades ago, were:

> living instruments to be interpreted by treaty bodies, made up of experts elected by states, in light of current knowledge and understanding of the impact of states' conduct on their people.

That is how the development of international law works ... women's and girls' right to access safe and legal abortion is firmly grounded in decades of jurisprudence from a range of human rights bodies and experts.[116]

Zampas and Todd-Gher's exposition of international human rights law in this context did not impress those who were resolutely opposed to loosening restrictions on access to abortion. Rev. Burke argued that the right to life was an explicit right in human rights law – not an interpreted right – and that it took priority over what was "unstated" in international agreements.

Some ardent defenders of the Eighth Amendment sought out pro-life principles expressed in UN declarations for support. Cora Sherlock, deputy chairperson of the PLC, referred to Article 3 of the Universal Declaration on Human Rights, which upheld the right to life. In her submission to the UN HRC in Geneva on 14 July 2015 she also referred to the Convention on the Rights of the Child to make the point that "the child ... needs special safeguards and care, including appropriate legal protection, before as well as after birth."[117] However, such claims, apparently supportive of a pro-life stance, are not quite so straightforward. Although Article 3 of the Universal Declaration of Human Rights declares that everyone has a right to life, this right seems to apply only after birth: Article 1 states that "All human beings are born free and equal in dignity and rights."[118] Reference to the child "before" birth in the Convention on the Rights of the Child seemed to indicate a pro-life stance, but there is a lack of clarity about when childhood begins. The committee charged with the responsibility of interpreting and applying the principles of the convention acknowledged that the foetus had some rights. Even so, the rights of the mother superseded those of the unborn. International law broadened the basis for access to abortion consistent with the life, health and "best interests" of the mother.[119]

In early June 2016 Ireland came under renewed pressure to reform its law on abortion, especially pertaining to life-limiting conditions. Ireland was a signatory to the International Covenant on Civil and Political Rights. The UN HRC found that the state had not fulfilled its human rights obligations in the case of Amanda Jane Mellet. On 17 November 2011 Ms Mellet, who was several months pregnant, was informed that her foetus had trisomy 18 and would die in the womb or not long after birth. She decided to seek an abortion abroad. Her main reason was so that her child would be spared unnecessary suffering. The cost was high – not just financially. The committee found that Ireland, because of its legislative framework, had "subjected the author to conditions of intense physical and mental suffering". Her suffering had been exacerbated by a denial of medical care and health insurance coverage in the Irish healthcare system. She was separated from her family at a time when she needed their support. Compelled by limited financial resources, she travelled back from England while still feeling ill after the abortion procedure. She had to leave her baby's remains behind at Liverpool Women's Hospital and was further traumatised when these were later delivered to her by courier. On her return she was denied post-abortion healthcare and bereavement support by the state. She felt stigmatised by the criminalisation of abortion despite the non-viability of her foetus.[120]

Amanda Mellet's suffering was further exacerbated by the failure of healthcare professionals to provide her with appropriate information about her options. Ireland's Regulation of Information (Services Outside the State For Termination of Pregnancies) Act was found to be excessively restrictive.[121] The Act prohibited healthcare providers from promoting or advocating abortion services legally available abroad. However, there was a lack of clarity in the legislation about the distinction between "advocating" or "promoting" abortion and "supporting" a woman who expressed an intention to terminate her pregnancy. This in turn had a "chilling effect" on healthcare professionals.[122]

The UN HRC found that the balance struck between the rights of the woman and protection of the foetus, in Ireland, could not be justified. Much of the mental anguish and physical suffering experienced by Amanda Mellet could have been avoided if she had been given access to healthcare services in Ireland. The state was found to be in violation of the International Covenant on Civil and Political Rights and was reminded of its obligation as a signatory to take effective remedial action. This entailed legislative reforms and – "if necessary" – constitutional change.[123] The state had argued that Article 40.3.3 represented "the profound moral choices of the Irish people" and that it was "nuanced and proportionate" in balancing the rights of the foetus and the mother.[124] The UN HRC did not distinguish between constitutional law and legislation in this context. It concluded that the state's balancing of rights in the case of Amanda Mellet "could not be justified".[125] Whether or not the state would hold a referendum to change or delete Article 40.3.3 remained to be seen. It was under an obligation to submit information to the monitoring committee of the UN HRC within 180 days, concerning measures taken to bring its domestic law into conformity with its human rights obligations.[126]

Foetal Anomalies

Cora Sherlock dismissed the UN HRC as "a de facto lobby group for abortion". She accused it of ignoring violations of human rights in the "abortion industry" in Britain and Canada, where, in failed abortions, babies were born alive and "left to die in hospital corners". The implication was that this too could happen in Ireland if its tight restrictions on abortion were loosened. The UN HRC was now saying that children with "life-limiting" conditions were "unworthy of any legal protections" and, therefore, were of "no inherent value".[127] But this was an incorrect interpretation of the UN HRC's position. The UN HRC had criticised Ireland for not striking a morally defensible balance "between protection of the foetus and the rights of the woman". It was not a question of zero rights or absolute rights – it was about a balance of rights.

Tracy Harkin of Every Life Counts condemned the UN HRC for "pressing for abortion on disability grounds". The UN HRC had "deliberately ignored the experiences of families who had received great joy and love from carrying their babies to term".[128] This was a misrepresentation of the UN HRC's position on abortion. Abortion was not being pressed on women who wished to continue their pregnancies after diagnoses of life-limiting conditions; it was about a woman's right to choose in such circumstances. Not all women experienced "great joy" from pregnancies where there was little else but suffering and death in prospect for the foetus.

Did women who terminated their pregnancies following diagnoses of life-limiting conditions act unintentionally against their own best interests? Every Life Counts referred to an American conference paper in support of their claim that women who opted for abortion, in cases of fatal foetal abnormality, suffered more despair and depression than women who chose to continue their pregnancies. This was oversimplification to the point of misrepresentation. The paper, entitled "Pregnancy Continuation and Organizational Religious Activity Following Prenatal Diagnosis of a Lethal Foetal Defect are Associated with Improved Psychological Outcome", was presented to the National Society of Genetic Counselors (USA) in 2014. It was written by Heidi Cope and three other researchers.[129] The authors were not prescriptive and recommended that "the risks and benefits, including psychological effects, of termination and continuation of pregnancy should be discussed in detail with an effort to be as nondirective as possible." They presented their findings tentatively – "while we took great care to perform the analyses presented here, we acknowledge that limitations to the present study nonetheless do exist" – not least the limited sample size and the probability that it was not representative of the general population.[130] Key variables such as social and economic supports, and access to healthcare services, were of crucial importance and required extensive research. In the absence of these, any research findings were highly questionable.[131] However, a central point not addressed by Tracy Harkin and Every Life Counts was the element of choice for pregnant women who had received diagnoses of life-limiting conditions.

The Fine Gael-led minority government, unlike the anti-abortion lobby, did not have the option of brushing aside the UN HRC findings against Ireland. Frances Fitzgerald, Minister for Justice, acknowledged that the state, as a signatory to the International Covenant on Civil and Political Rights, had to respond "very seriously".[132] The government undertook to address the issue through the mechanism of a constitutional convention/citizens' assembly to be set up sometime within the first six months of the government's term of office. The outcome of the assembly's deliberations would be passed on for further consideration to a specially constituted Oireachtas committee. This process seemed far too slow for many opposition TDs and probably for some backbenchers.[133] It also seemed pointless. There were already two citizens' assemblies – the Dáil and the Seanad.[134] The Coalition to Repeal the Eighth Amendment and the Abortion Rights Campaign responded negatively, viewing the government's announcement as a strategy to avoid addressing the issue.[135] More significantly, it seemed that a large sector of Irish public opinion had shifted towards approval of easing restrictions on abortion in some circumstances. Irish public opinion was now more pro-choice than Irish law, although still considerably anti-abortion in an international context.[136]

Apparent shifts in public opinion did not embolden Taoiseach Enda Kenny to act decisively on the issue. Fine Gael was deeply divided on the matter. Also, the party had suffered heavy losses in the general election in February and had formed a minority coalition government with the support of nine independent TDs after protracted negotiations. Minority status in the Dáil, a divided party and a fragile coalition all indicated that he would seek the maximum political cover. A painstaking building of political consensus and outsourcing of some responsibility to a constitutional assembly and Oireachtas Committee seemed the safest way to proceed in what were highly precarious political circumstances. Any rush to hold a referendum to repeal the Eighth Amendment was doomed to fail. Furthermore, Kenny indicated his reluctance to press for reforms in abortion law when he stated that the UN HRC's findings against Ireland were not binding – unlike those of the ECHR.[137] This was a half-truth because there was a moral issue to consider.[138] Ireland had voluntarily ratified the International Covenant on Civil and Political Rights. It had signed in good faith. Ireland had accepted the competence of the UN HRC to issue authoritative interpretations when hearing cases against the state. Ireland could not invoke provisions of its domestic law as a basis for failure to comply with its international legal obligations. If the Constitution was an obstacle, the government was under an obligation to hold a referendum to remedy it. Of course, there was the possibility that such a referendum would fail to deliver change. It was counterargued that the Irish people, through the democratic process, had a right to decide its own law on this issue.[139] The Catholic Primate of All Ireland, Eamon Martin, found it unacceptable that organisations outside Ireland would dictate law on abortion.[140] From an institutional Catholic point of view, then, international human rights law was incompatible with a fundamental moral principle and might also prove incompatible with the democratic wishes of the Irish electorate.

The Fine Gael position was that, on the basis of advice from the Attorney General, legislation permitting abortion in cases of life-limiting conditions required constitutional change and therefore a referendum. Inferences drawn from the Supreme Court judgment in the *Roche v Roche* case indicated that all embryos implanted in the womb were legally protected under the terms of Article 40.3.3.[141] Some legal experts expressed a contrary opinion. It was argued that the government had the option of introducing legislation that could then be brought before the Supreme Court to determine whether or not it was compatible with the Constitution.[142]

The Protection of Life in Pregnancy amendment Bills introduced by Clare Daly TD and sponsored by Mick Wallace TD both used the term "fatal foetal abnormality" and defined it as "a medical condition suffered by a foetus such that it is incompatible with life outside the womb".[143] There was a legal difficulty with the term "fatal foetal abnormality" and with alternative terms. It was thought that termination of pregnancy could be permitted under Article 40.3.3 if there was no possibility of a live birth. If this was evident, it could be argued, in a legal context, that the right to life did not apply. But what about cases where babies might survive for a few minutes, hours or days after birth?[144] There were such cases. In some very exceptional cases, survival extended to years, even decades.

On 30 June 2016, newly appointed Minister for Health Simon Harris expressed approval of the intentions behind Wallace's Bill and regret about the state's lack of support for Amanda Mellet and other women in similar circumstances. Harris told the Dáil that he had taken legal advice from the Attorney General and medical advice from the Chief Medical Officer. The Supreme Court had reviewed the meaning of the article in the light of the Roche versus Roche case. The term protected in Article 40.3.3 was "the unborn" – not the beginning of life. If a foetus with a severe life-limiting condition was "capable of being born alive" – even if it could survive for only a very short time – it was protected by Article 40.3.3. Harris, referring to the Chief Medical Officer, told the Dáil: "It can never be said that a foetus with a fatal foetal abnormality will not be born to live for a short time, even if that is only to be minutes." Therefore, Wallace's Bill, similar to Daly's, was regarded as unconstitutional.[145] The PLDPA was the outer limit of what the government could achieve short of a referendum.

The PLC preferred the term "life-limiting conditions" and took issue with "fatal foetal abnormalities" and similar expressions. It argued that conceding to abortion in cases of life-limiting conditions would broaden the scope for legalised abortion to include disabilities such as Down syndrome and other non-terminal conditions. The emphasis on life-limiting conditions was seen by the PLC and other opponents of abortion as a Trojan horse for liberal abortion laws.[146] Breda O'Brien went so far as to write that it would be "wonderful" to discontinue the use of flawed terms like "fatal foetal abnormality" or "incompatible with life". Such terms, she believed, somehow impeded initiatives to assist families in coming to terms with distressing diagnoses without resorting to abortion.[147]

There seemed to be a preponderance of medical evidence supportive of her views. In her *Irish Times* column O'Brien referred to a research paper by consultant neonatologist and medical ethicist Professor Dominic Wilkinson and his co-authors (2012), to make the point that there was no clear definition of "fatal foetal abnormalities" (and similar terms). Neither was there a list of such abnormalities that commanded consensus amongst clinicians.[148] To bolster her argument, O'Brien referred to the newly published *National Standards for Bereavement Care Following Pregnancy Loss and Perinatal Death* (hereafter referred to as the National Standards) launched on 10 August 2016 by the Minister for Health, Simon Harris.[149]

The authors of the National Standards chose to use the term "life-limiting condition" but, as acknowledged by O'Brien, accepted that some parents did not agree with this term. Reference was made to the Wilkinson paper (2012) to observe that "there is no clear or universal term that can be used or is acceptable to most parents. Any terms used in this area are subject to conceptual and practical challenges inherent in defining such terms."[150] Therefore, it could be reasonably inferred that any term – including "life-limiting condition" – was merely a means of expression to facilitate communication. After all, the meaning of "unborn" in the Eighth Amendment was elusive for decades until it was defined (for the purposes of the Act) in the PLDPA.[151] If legislators were to use terms such as "life-limiting conditions" or "fatal foetal abnormalities", they would have to explain what they meant in a legal context. Difficulties with terminology did not, of course, undermine principles of moral philosophy applicable to abortion.

O'Brien referred to a research paper by Professor Anette Kersting and Birgit Wagner, cited by the National Standards, to make the point that termination of a pregnancy due to a foetal anomaly exposed a mother to an elevated risk of "complicated grief and mental ill-health". Kersting and Wagner found that "pathological grief was found to be particularly high in women after termination of an abnormal pregnancy."[152] O'Brien's reference to medical sources indicated that medical research favoured her moral stance. But her highly selective presentation of research findings was not only a misleading oversimplification of the Kersting and Wilkinson research papers and of the National Standards, it was a very unbalanced analysis of the tentative findings of medical research generally.[153] The National Standards cited five research papers when identifying the risk factors associated with "complicated bereavement". These risk factors included the circumstances of the death (such as that of a twin in the womb); a person's coping ability and whether or not they already had mental health or psychosocial problems; their individual circumstances (for example, whether or not they were teenagers, whether or not they had other children); the extent of social and economic supports; and access to health services.[154]

The heavy emphasis on terminology tended to obscure rather than illuminate a core issue concerning foetal anomalies – the long-term mental health of grieving mothers. O'Brien argued that pregnant women who received diagnoses of life-limiting conditions and chose to terminate their pregnancies acted against their own best interests. The implication was that the Eighth Amendment served the interests of women well by denying them the right to choose. Some mothers and fathers evidently found support and comfort from websites such as Every Life Counts and One Day More. Even so, a key point not addressed by O'Brien and other pro-life proponents was that international law favoured a woman's right to choose in cases of foetal anomalies. In many cases, such as that of Amanda Jane Mellet, termination of pregnancy was chosen so that a child would not suffer unnecessarily. Human life was not just about survival time – it needed to be much more than that.

Endnotes

————•————

1 Simon Lee, "Abortion Law: The tragic choices", *Doctrine and Life*, vol. 42 (May–June 1992), pp. 283–4.
2 For philosophical debates about the rights of human embryos and foetuses see the Appendix in this book, "Seeking Moral Boundaries: Abortion and Infanticide".
3 "Protocol annexed to the Treaty on European Union and to the treaties establishing the European Communities", Treaty on European Union (Maastricht, 7 February 1992) <http://europa.eu/eu-law/decision-making/treaties/pdf/treaty_on_european_union/treaty_on_european_union_en.pdf> accessed 17 March 2016.
4 European Court of Human Rights, Grand Chamber judgment, *A, B and C v Ireland* (application number 25579/05), 16 December 2010, paragraphs 243–68; and *Report of the Expert Group on the Judgment in A, B and C v Ireland* (November 2012), Chapter 4 <http://www.dohc.ie/publications/pdf/Judgment_ABC.pdf?direct=1>. The observations, criticisms and recommendations of the ECHR relating to Ireland were expressed by other human rights organisations, including the UN Committee Against Torture: "Consideration of reports submitted by State parties under article 19 of the Convention" (17 June 2011), paragraph 26 <http://tbinternet.ohchr.org/_layouts/treatybodyexternal/Download.aspx?symbolno=CAT/C/IRL/CO/1&Lang=E> accessed 21 May 2016.
5 *Report of the Expert Group on the Judgment in A, B and C v Ireland*, Conclusion.
6 "Winter 2012 General Meeting of the Irish Catholic Bishops' Conference", 5 December 2012 <http://www.catholicbishops.ie/2012/12/05/initial-response-report-expert-group/> accessed 14 December 2013.
7 Joan McCarthy, "Reproductive Justice in Ireland: A Feminist Analysis of the Neary and Halappanavar Cases" in Mary Donnelly and Claire Murray (eds), *Ethical and Legal Debates in Irish Healthcare: Confronting Complexities* (Manchester: Manchester University Press, 2016), pp. 19–21; "Husband: Ireland hospital denied Savita Halappanavar life saving abortion because it is a 'Catholic country'", CBS News, 14 November 2012 <http://www.cbsnews.com/news/husband-ireland-hospital-denied-savita-halappanavar-life-saving-abortion-because-it-is-a-catholic-country/> accessed 26 January 2014; RTÉ News, "Midwife confirms she told Savita Halappanavar

Ireland is a 'Catholic country'", 11 April 2013, <http://www.rte.ie/news/health/2013/0410/380613-savita-halappanavar-inquest/> accessed 28 January 2014; Jill Allison, *Motherhood and Infertility in Ireland: Understanding the Presence of Absence* (Cork: Cork University Press, 2013), p. 194.

8   Peter Boylan, *In the Shadow of the Eighth* (Penguin Ireland, 2019), pp. 87–90.

9   "Savita inquest: Jury returns verdict of medical misadventure", TheJournal.ie, 19 April 2013 <http://www.thejournal.ie/savita-inquest-jury-returns-verdict-of-medical-misadventure-876458-Apr2013/ accessed 17 March 2016). An investigation by the Health Information and Safety Authority (HIQA) found that Savita Halappanavar's death was due to "a series of failures in the management, governance and delivery of maternity services". Health Information and Quality Authority, "Patient Safety Investigation Report published by Health Information and Quality Authority", press release, 9 October 2013 <http://www.hiqa.ie/press-release/2013-10-09-patient-safety-investigation-report-published-health-information-and-qualit> accessed 1 November 2013.

10   Dr John Monaghan *et al.*, letter to the editor, *Irish Times*, 1 May 2013 <https://search-proquest-com.ucc.idm.oclc.org/docview/1346974835/8E07E88C521D44EAPQ/153?accountid=14504> accessed 11 November 2017. The views of Dr Monaghan and his colleagues were open to the same assessment of personal bias. Some of the signatories had spoken at pro-life meetings. Paul Cullen, "Obstetricians challenge Boylan evidence", *Irish Times*, 1 May 2013 <https://search-proquest-com.ucc.idm.oclc.org/docview/1346974341/A946912076344457PQ/58?accountid=14504> accessed 11 November 2017.

11   Monaghan *et al.*, letter to the editor, *Irish Times*, 1 May 2013.

12   Peter Boylan, letter to the editor, *Irish Times*, 2 May 2013 <https://search-proquest-com.ucc.idm.oclc.org/docview/1347389624/802830BBB37144DCPQ/140?accountid=14504> accessed 18 November 2019.

13   Boylan, *In the Shadow of the Eighth*, p. 89.

14   Boylan, letter to the editor, *Irish Times*, 2 May 2013. In this context it is understood that inflammation and infection are used interchangeably because inflammation is a symptom of infection.

15   Department of Health, "Government decision on ABC Expert Group option", 18 December 2012 <http://www.dohc.ie/press/releases/2012/20121218.html> accessed 25 January 2014.

16   Joint Committee on Health and Children, 8 January 2013 <https://www.oireachtas.ie/en/debates/debate/joint_committee_on_health_and_children/2013-01-08/2/#s5> accessed 7 November 2018.

17   National Collaborating Centre for Mental Health, *Induced Abortion and Mental Health* (London: December 2011), p. 8 <https://www.aomrc.org.uk/wp-content/uploads/2016/05/Induced_Abortion_Mental_Health_1211.

pdf> accessed 5 November 2018. The majority of the steering group members for the research project were psychiatrists; they included the chairperson of the perinatal section of the Royal College of Psychiatrists. The National Collaborating Centre for Mental Health in Britain was set up in 2001 by the Royal College of Psychiatrists and the British Psychological Society. Its main objective was to develop evidence-based mental health reviews and guidelines for clinical practice.

18 Joint Committee on Health and Children, 8 January 2013.

19 Ibid.

20 Ibid.

21 Ibid., 10 January 2013 <https://www.oireachtas.ie/en/debates/debate/joint_committee_on_health_and_children/2013-01-10/2/#s3> accessed 9 November 2018.

22 Pádraig McCarthy, "Caring for Mother and Child – Legislating for the X Case", *The Furrow*, vol. 64, no. 2 (February 2013), p. 117.

23 See Pádraig McCarthy, "Caring for Mother and Child", *The Furrow*, vol. 64, no. 1 (January 2013), pp. 6–7.

24 "Statement by the four Archbishops of Ireland in response to the decision today by the Government to legislate for abortion", 18 December 2012 <http://www.catholicbishops.ie/2012/12/18/statement-archbishops-ireland-response-decision-today-government-legislate-abortion/> accessed 25 January 2014.

25 "Statement by Bishop John Buckley, Bishop of Cork and Ross in response to the decision by the Government to legislate for abortion", 19 December 2012 <http://www.catholicbishops.ie/2012/12/19/statement-bishop-john-buckley-bishop-cork-ross-response-decision-government-legislate-abortion/> accessed 25 January 2014.

26 Ibid.; and "Spring 2013 General Meeting of the Irish Bishops' Conference", 6 March 2013 <http://www.catholicbishops.ie/2013/03/06/spring-2013-general-meeting-irish-bishops-conference/> accessed 14 December 2013.

27 Alex White, "Government Publishes General Scheme of the Protection of Life during Pregnancy Bill 2013", 1 May 2013 <http://alexwhitetd.wordpress.com/2013/05/01/government-publishes-general-scheme-of-the-protection-of-life-during-pregnancy-bill-2013/> accessed 15 February 2014.

28 General Scheme of the Protection of Life during Pregnancy Bill 2013, 30 April 2013, Interpretation, pp. 4–5 <http://www.merrionstreet.ie/wp-content/uploads/2013/04/Protection-of-Life-During-Pregnancy-Bill-PLP-30.04.13-10.30.pdf> accessed 19 January 2014.

29 "Preliminary response by the Catholic Bishops of Ireland to Protection of Life during Pregnancy Bill 2013", 3 May 2013 <http://www.catholicbishops.ie/2013/05/03/preliminary-response-catholic-bishops-ireland-protection-life-pregnancy-bill-2013/> accessed 19 February 2014.

30 Brian McDonald, "Cardinal keeps excommunication threat hanging over

abortion TDs", Independent.ie, 5 May 2013 <http://www.independent.ie/
irish-news/cardinal-keeps-excommunication-threat-hanging-over-abortion-
tds-29242992.html> accessed 15 February 2014.

31 Áine Ryan and Michael Commins, "Taoiseach refers Cardinal Brady
to Constitution", 7 May 2013 <http://www.mayonews.ie/index.
php?option=com_content&view=article&id=17734:taoiseach-refers-cardinal-
brady-to-constitution&catid=23:news&Itemid=46> accessed 16 February
2014.

32 Luke Byrne, "Priests told: deny communion to TDs who support abortion",
Irish Independent, 6 February 2013 <http://www.independent.ie/irish-news/
priests-told-deny-communion-to-tds-who-support-abortion-29051662.
html> accessed 24 December 2015. Cardinal Burke, speaking about the
tragic death of Savita Halappanavar, asserted that "It is, however, contrary
to right reason to hold that an innocent and defenceless human life can be
justifiably destroyed in order to save the life of the mother ... Even though,
if the reports are correct, Savita Halappanavar requested an abortion, her
request would not have made it right for the law to permit such an act which
is always and everywhere wrong." Interview of His Eminence, Raymond
Cardinal Burke, "To decriminalise abortion is a contradiction of the most
fundamental principle of the legal system", *Catholic Voice*, republished on
24 April 2014 <http://www.catholicvoice.ie/index.php/6-to-decriminalise-
abortion-is-a-contradiction-of-the-most-fundamental-principle-of-the-
legal-system?showall=&start=1> accessed 20 December 2015.

33 Bishop John Buckley (Diocese of Cork and Ross) later pointed out that
"where a seriously ill pregnant mother needs medical treatment which
may put the life of her baby at risk, such a treatment is morally acceptable
provided that every effort is made to save the life of both the mother and
the baby." "Bishop John Buckley's Homily for Mass celebrating the fiftieth
anniversary of the Church of the Holy Family, Caheragh, West Cork",
30 June 2013 <http://www.catholicbishops.ie/2013/06/30/bishop-john-
buckleys-homily-mass-celebrating-fiftieth-anniversary-church-holy-family-
caheragh-west-cork/> accessed 14 December 2013.

34 Peter Horgan, "Barry questions Cardinal: Will Government TDs be
excommunicated?", *Cork Independent*, 16 May 2013 <http://corkindependent.
com/20130516/news/barry-questions-cardinal-will-government-tds-be-
excommunicated-S65288.html> accessed 15 December 2013.

35 Claire O'Sullivan, "TD assured he will not be excommunicated for backing
abortion laws", *Irish Examiner*, 22 June 2013 <http://www.irishexaminer.com/
ireland/td-assured-he-will-not-be-excommunicated-for-backing-abortion-
laws-234822.html> accessed 15 February 2014.

36 The other parliamentarians were TDs Peter Mathews, Terence Flanagan,
Billy Timmins and Brian Walsh; and senators Paul Bradford and Fidelma
Healy Eames.

37 Pope John Paul II, *Evangelium Vitae* (25 March 1995), paragraph 73.

38 Patrick Hannon, "Abortion, Law and Morals", *Doctrine and Life*, vol. 64, no. 7–8 (July–August 2013), pp. 392–4.

39 Galway for Life, "National Vigil for Life a great success", 9 June 2013 <http://galwayforlife.blogspot.ie/2013/06/national-vigil-for-life-great-success.html> accessed 7 March 2014; and Pro Life Campaign press release, "Ireland's largest pro-life gathering ever!" <http://prolifecampaign.ie/main/well-over-40000-people-attend-national-vigil-for-life/> accessed 7 March 2014.

40 Individual statements of the bishops include: "Bishop John Buckley's Homily for Mass celebrating the fiftieth anniversary of the Church of the Holy Family, Caheragh, West Cork", 30 June 2013; "Cardinal Seán Brady raises legal and Constitutional concerns about the Protection of Life During Pregnancy Bill 2013", 1 July 2013 <http://www.catholicbishops.ie/2013/07/01/cardinal-sean-brady-raises-legal-constitutional-concerns-protection-life-pregnancy-bill-2013/> accessed 14 December 2013; "Homily of Archbishop Diarmuid Martin at Mass in Church of Saint Dominick, Dublin, 6 July 2013" <http://www.catholicbishops.ie/2013/07/06/homily-archbishop-diarmuid-martin-mass-church-saint-dominick-dublin/> accessed 14 December 2013; "Homily of Bishop Noel Treanor at Saul Mountain, Downpatrick, Diocese of Down and Connor", 7 July 2013 <http://www.catholicbishops.ie/2013/07/07/homily-bishop-noel-treanor-saul-mountain-downpatrick-diocese-connor/> accessed 14 December 2013; "Homily of Bishop Brennan, Ferns Diocese at Knock Shrine, Sunday 7 July 2013" (press release, 8 July 2013) <http://www.catholicbishops.ie/2013/07/08/homily-bishop-brennan-ferns-diocese-knock-shrine-sunday-7-july-2013/> accessed 14 December 2013; and "Homily notes of Bishop Brendan Leahy for Vigil for Life – Saint John's Cathedral, Limerick", 9 July 2013 <http://www.catholicbishops.ie/2013/07/09/homily-notes-bishop-brendan-leahy-vigil-life-saint-johns-cathedral-limerick/> accessed 14 December 2013. The papal nuncio, Archbishop Charles J. Brown, also spoke about the need to protect human life from conception to natural death and was implicitly critical of the proposed legislation: "Homily of His Excellency Archbishop Charles J Brown – Apostolic Nuncio in Ireland at Mass for Saint Oliver Plunkett", 7 July 2013 <http://www.catholicbishops.ie/2013/07/07/homily-excellency-archbishop-charles-brown-apostolic-nuncio-ireland-mass-saint-oliver-plunkett/> accessed 14 December 2013.

41 "Cardinal Seán Brady raises legal and Constitutional concerns", 1 July 2013.

42 Catholic Communications Office: "Choose Life" newsletters: 22 May 2013 <http://www.catholicbishops.ie/2013/05/22/choose-life-2013-newsletter-parishes/> accessed 26 January 2014; Issue 2, 29 May 2013 <http://www.catholicbishops.ie/2013/05/29/choose-life-2013-newsletter-issue-2/ accessed 26 January 2014); Issue 3, 6 June 2013 <http://www.catholicbishops.

ie/2013/06/06/choose-life-2013-newsletter-issue-3/> accessed 26 January 2014; Issue 4, 12 June 2013 <http://www.catholicbishops.ie/2013/06/12/choose-life-newsletter-issue-4/> accessed 26 January 2014; Issue 5, 20 June 2013 <http://www.catholicbishops.ie/2013/06/20/issue-5-choose-life-2013-newsletter/> accessed 26 January 2014; Issue 6 ("A time for clarity and truth"), 26 June 2013 <http://www.catholicbishops.ie/2013/06/26/choose-life-newsletter-issue-6-time-clarity-truth/> accessed 26 January 2014; Issue 7 3 July 2013 <http://www.catholicbishops.ie/2013/07/03/choose-life-newsletter-issue-7/> accessed 26 January 2014; Issue 8, 11 July 2013 <http://www.catholicbishops.ie/2013/07/11/issue-8-choose-life-newsletter/> accessed 15 December 2013.

43 General Scheme of the Protection of Life during Pregnancy Bill 2013, 30 April 2013, Head 12: Conscientious Objection.

44 The bishops also referred to Article 9 of the European Convention of Human Rights, which was quoted in the General Scheme. Article 9(1) states that "everyone has the right to freedom of thought, conscience and religion."

45 See General Scheme of the Protection of Life during Pregnancy Bill 2013, Head 12.

46 "Bishops' briefing note on the Protection of Life During Pregnancy Bill 2013", 8 July 2013 <http://www.catholicbishops.ie/2013/07/08/bishops-briefing-note-protection-life-pregnancy-bill-2013/> accessed 14 December 2013. The bishops anticipated that terminations of pregnancies would be contemplated in cases which were less than straightforward. What would happen when an unborn child was close to viability, for example, at 22 weeks? Would a termination of pregnancy be delayed to give the child a chance of survival? Premature delivery carried a greater risk of serious and permanent injury to the child; the bishops speculated that this would present legal problems with reference to Part 15 of the Criminal Justice Act on the Reckless Endangerment of Children.

47 Protection of Life During Pregnancy Act 2013, section 2 <http://www.oireachtas.ie/documents/bills28/acts/2013/a3513.pdf> accessed 19 January 2014.

48 Ibid., section 9.

49 Ibid., section 5.

50 Ibid., section 22.

51 Pro Life Campaign: "30.07.2013: Pro Life Campaign 'will now devote its energies to the repeal of unjust law' as president signs abortion bill into law" <http://prolifecampaign.ie/main/portfolio/detail/30th-july-2013-pro-life-campaign-will-now-devote-energies-repeal-unjust-law-president-signs-abortion-bill-law/> accessed 9 March 2014; and "14.10.2013 over 600 attend Pro Life Campaign national conference in the RDS" <http://prolifecampaign.ie/main/portfolio/detail/3723/> accessed 7 March 2014.

52 In late November 2012 a Red C poll indicated that there was an

estimated 85% support for the proposal to "Legislate for the X case, which means allowing abortion where the mother's life is threatened, including by suicide." There was 82% support for the proposal for "A constitutional amendment to extend the right to abortion to all cases where the health of the mother is seriously threatened and also in cases of rape". Support for a liberal abortion regime was found to be at 36%. "Red C poll: majority demand X case legislation", *Daily Business Post*, 1 December 2012 <http://www.businesspost.ie/#!story/Home/News/Red+C+poll%3A+majority+demand+X+case+legislation/id/78241919-150b-a2a0-577f-97741195800> accessed 11 April 2015. A survey of attitudes in April 2015 found 60% support for abortion in cases where the mother is suicidal. About 63% found abortion morally permissible in cases of "fatal foetal abnormality" (a disputed term). There was 67% support for abortion with reference to women whose pregnancies were due to rape. A large minority – 32% – believed that abortion was morally acceptable in the absence of rape, suicide or medical risks to a mother's life. Shane Doran, "Most voters back abortion if threat to mother's life", *Sunday Independent*, 12 April 2015 <http://www.independent.ie/irish-news/politics/most-voters-back-abortion-if-threat-to-mothers-life-31135407.html> accessed 12 April 2015.

53 Dáil speech by Leo Varadkar, 16 December 2014 <http://health.gov.ie/blog/speeches/speech-by-leo-varadkar-t-d-minister-for-health-thirty-fourth-amendment-of-the-constitution/> accessed 20 February 2015.

54 Fiach Kelly, "Joan Burton says abortion laws do not serve women well", *Irish Times*, 19 December 2014 <http://www.irishtimes.com/news/politics/joan-burton-says-abortion-laws-do-not-serve-women-well-1.2044589?mode=print&ot=example.AjaxPageLayout.ot> accessed 22 December 2014.

55 The minister's opinions drew criticism from Dr Ruth Cullen of the Pro Life Campaign, who saw calls for repealing the Eighth Amendment as central to initiatives to eliminate what remained of legal protection for the unborn. Iona Institute, "Varadkar attacked over abortion law comments", 17 December 2014 <http://www.ionainstitute.ie/index.php?id=3790> accessed 22 December 2014.

56 Martin Wall, "Court may decide on right of foetus in life support case", *Irish Times*, 19 December 2014 <http://www.irishtimes.com/news/ireland/irish-news/court-may-decide-on-right-of-foetus-in-life-support-case-1.2043125> accessed 22 December 2014.

57 Muiris Houston, "Key questions that arise when a pregnant woman is on life support", *Irish Times*, 18 December 2014 <http://www.irishtimes.com/opinion/key-questions-that-arise-when-a-pregnant-woman-is-on-life-support-1.2043081?mode=print&ot=example.AjaxPageLayout.ot> accessed 23 December 2014.

58 Paul Cullen and Ruadhán Mac Cormaic, "Woman on life support: medics feared legal position", *Irish Times*, 22 December 2014 <http://www.irishtimes. com/news/social-affairs/woman-on-life-support-medics-feared-legal-position-1.2045891?mode=print&ot=example.AjaxPageLayout.ot> accessed 2 January 2015.

59 Muiris Houston, "Life support case: ethical considerations a crucial part of best medical practice", *Irish Times*, 30 December 2014 <http://www. irishtimes.com/news/health/life-support-case-ethical-considerations-a-crucial-part-of-best-medical-practice-1.2051411?mode=print&ot=example. AjaxPageLayout.ot> accessed 2 January 2015; and Protection of Life During Pregnancy Act 2013, Part 3, section 22 <http://www.oireachtas.ie/documents/ bills28/acts/2013/a3513.pdf> accessed 19 January 2014.

60 The patient was sustained by mechanical ventilation. Nutrition was supplied through a nasogastric tube. The patient was under continual heavy medication for a range of conditions including multiple infections, high blood pressure and oedema. Despite intensive care the patient's condition continued to deteriorate, causing much distress to her family. There was total body oedema and "huge amounts of fluid" in the lungs. The patient's appearance was "puffy and swollen", so much so that her eyes would not close properly. Pus was oozing from the right side of her head and brain matter was extruding from a hole in the skull. Fungal infections had also taken hold. There was evidence of urinary tract infection and the lower abdominal wall was inflamed. Serious infections were arising from extensive brain decomposition and from drips, catheters and tubes in place for life support. Steroid therapy, liver dysfunction, an excessively fast heart rate and high fever all posed threats to the foetus. Toxins were pouring into the bloodstream from a "liquefying" brain. Medications were being administered for life support that were not licensed for use in pregnancy. The foetus was so far below the threshold of viability, and the mother's condition was deteriorating so fast, that the prospect of a successful delivery in the circumstances was "virtually non-existent". Judgment by Mr Justice P. Kearns, *P.P. v Health Service Executive*, Neutral Citation [2014]IEHC 622, High Court Record Number 2014 10792 P, 26 December 2014, pp. 1–9 <http:// www.courts.ie/Judgments.nsf/09859e7a3f34669680256ef3004a27de/ fb8a5c76857e08ce80257dcb003fd4e6?OpenDocument> accessed 13 January 2015. See also Boylan, *In the Shadow of the Eighth*, pp. 112–15.

61 Kearns judgment, pp. 10–11.

62 Ibid., p. 15.

63 Ruadhán Mac Cormaic, "Life support for brain-dead pregnant woman withdrawn", *Irish Times*, 28 December 2014 <http://www.irishtimes.com/ news/crime-and-law/life-support-for-brain-dead-pregnant-woman-withdrawn-1.2049636?mode=print&ot=example.AjaxPageLayout.ot> accessed 2 January 2015.

64 Ruadhán Mac Cormaic, "Medics called for guidelines after two previous cases", *Irish Times*, 22 December 2014 <http://www.irishtimes.com/news/crime-and-law/medics-called-for-guidelines-after-two-previous-cases-1.2046848?mode=print&ot=example.AjaxPageLayout.ot> accessed 23 December 2014.

65 Noel Whelan, "Why was a court ruling required to decide fate of pregnant woman on life support?", *Irish Times*, 2 January 2015 <http://www.irishtimes.com/opinion/why-was-a-court-ruling-required-to-decide-fate-of-pregnant-woman-on-life-support-1.2052877?mode=print&ot=example.AjaxPageLayout.ot> accessed 2 January 2015.

66 Mark Hilliard, "Rhona Mahony warns of legal risk to doctors in abortion cases", *Irish Times*, 9 June 2015 <http://www.irishtimes.com/news/social-affairs/rhona-mahony-warns-of-legal-risk-to-doctors-in-abortion-cases-1.2243014?mode=print&ot=example.AjaxPageLayout.ot> accessed 10 June 2015.

67 Áine McMahon, "Irish doctors call for decriminalisation of abortion", *Irish Times*, 20 November 2015 <http://www.irishtimes.com/news/social-affairs/irish-doctors-call-for-decriminalisation-of-abortion-1.2437846> accessed 8 October 2016; see also Peadar O'Grady, Maeve Ferriter and Tiernan Murray on behalf of Doctors for Choice, letter to the editor, *Irish Times*, 5 July 2016 <http://www.irishtimes.com/opinion/letters/the-eighth-amendment-1.2710201> accessed 5 July 2016.

68 Protection of Life in Pregnancy (Amendment) (Fatal Foetal Abnormalities) Bill 2013: Second Stage [Private Members], Dáil Debates, 6 February 2015 <http://oireachtasdebates.oireachtas.ie/debates%20authoring/debateswebpack.nsf/takes/dail2015020600003?opendocument#A00100> accessed 12 February 2015.

69 Protection of Life in Pregnancy (Amendment) (Fatal Foetal Abnormalities) Bill 2013, no. 115 of 2013, proposed to the Dáil by Deputy Clare Daly, 21 November 2013.

70 Constitutional lawyers in Ireland differed in their views on this issue. Ruadhán Mac Cormaic, "Legal conundrum hinges on the definition of the 'unborn'", *Irish Times*, 6 February 2015 <http://www.irishtimes.com/news/crime-and-law/legal-conundrum-hinges-on-the-definition-of-the-unborn-1.2094793> accessed 10 September 2016.

71 Stephen Collins, "Political realities shape party positions on abortion Bill", *Irish Times*, 10 February 2015 <http://www.irishtimes.com/news/politics/political-realities-shape-party-positions-on-abortion-bill-1.2098740> accessed 12 February 2015.

72 Dáil Debates, 6 February 2015 <http://oireachtasdebates.oireachtas.ie/debates%20authoring/debateswebpack.nsf/takes/dail2015021000029?opendocument#BB00300> accessed 12 February 2015.

73 "Our politicians again struggle with 'life' issues", *Irish Times*, 12 February

2015 <http://www.irishtimes.com/opinion/our-politicians-again-struggle-with-life-issues-1.2100080?mode=print&ot=example.AjaxPageLayout.ot> accessed 12 February 2015.

74 D.J.C. Wilkinson, P. Thiele, A. Watkins and L. De Crespigny, "Fatally Flawed? A review and ethical analysis of lethal congenital malformations", *British Journal of Obstetrics and Gynaecology*, vol. 119, issue 11 (October 2012), pp. 1302–8 (online, accessed 16 December 2015).

75 Dáil Debates, 6 February 2015.

76 Department of Health, *Notifications in Accordance with Section 20 of The Protection of Life During Pregnancy Act 2013*, June 2015 <http://health.gov.ie/wp-content/uploads/2015/06/annual-report-2014-Protection-of-Life-During-Pregnancy1.pdf> accessed 1 July 2015; and Ciarán D'Arcy, "Abortion policy must be reviewed, groups say", *Irish Times*, 30 June 2015 <http://www.irishtimes.com/news/social-affairs/abortion-policy-must-be-reviewed-groups-say-1.2268295?mode=print&ot=example.AjaxPageLayout.ot> accessed 1 July 2015.

77 Paul Cullen, "Analysis: Leo Varadkar's low-key report on abortion", *Irish Times*, 30 June 2015 <http://www.irishtimes.com/news/health/analysis-leo-varadkar-s-low-key-report-on-abortion-1.2267303?mode=print&ot=example.AjaxPageLayout.ot> accessed 1 July 2015.

78 Ciarán D'Arcy, "Opposing sides clash during abortion rallies in Dublin", *Irish Times*, 4 July 2015 <http://www.irishtimes.com/news/social-affairs/opposing-sides-clash-during-abortion-rallies-in-dublin-1.2273918?mode=print&ot=example.AjaxPageLayout.ot> accessed 10 July 2015; Sorcha Pollak and Carl O'Brien, "March for Choice hears call for abortion referendum", *Irish Times*, 26 September 2015 <http://www.irishtimes.com/news/social-affairs/march-for-choice-hears-call-for-abortion-referendum-1.2366549?mode=print&ot=example.AjaxPageLayout.ot> accessed 26 September 2015.

79 Niall O'Connor, "Referendum on repealing the Eighth Amendment will be Labour Party priority – Tánaiste", 26 September 2015 <http://www.independent.ie/irish-news/politics/referendum-on-repealing-eighth-amendment-will-be-labour-party-priority-tanaiste-31560276.html> accessed 27 September 2015.

80 Niall O'Connor and Philip Ryan, "Act of defiance", *Sunday Independent*, 29 November 2015, p. 1; Kevin Doyle, "Kenny gives ministers free vote on abortion campaign", *Irish Independent*, 9 January 2016 <http://www.msn.com/en-ie/news/national/kenny-gives-ministers-free-vote-on-abortion-campaign/ar-CCjcfS?ocid=spartandhp> accessed 9 January 2016; and Sarah Bardon, "Varadkar says he will not lobby FG colleagues on abortion law", *Irish Times*, 17 December 2015 <http://www.irishtimes.com/news/politics/varadkar-says-he-will-not-lobby-fg-colleagues-on-abortion-law-

1.2469855?mode=print&ot=example.AjaxPageLayout.ot> accessed 19 December 2015.

81 Juliette Jowit, "Northern Ireland's abortion laws remain restrictive and unclear", *Guardian*, 6 January 2016 <http://www.theguardian.com/world/2016/jan/06/northern-ireland-abortion-laws-restrictive-unclear-legal-women> accessed 13 February 2016.

82 Alan Erwin, "Legal action taken over guidelines on abortion in North", *Irish Times*, 12 November 2015 <http://www.irishtimes.com/news/crime-and-law/legal-action-taken-over-guidelines-on-abortion-in-north-1.2427242> accessed 2 December 2015.

83 European Court of Human Rights, Council of Europe, Article 8, European Convention on Human Rights (as amended by protocols 11 and 14, and supplemented by protocols 1, 4, 6, 7, 12 and 13) <http://www.echr.coe.int/Documents/Convention_ENG.pdf> accessed 5 March 2016.

84 "Full text of court ruling on North's abortion laws", *Irish Times*, 30 November 2015 <http://www.irishtimes.com/news/crime-and-law/full-text-of-court-ruling-on-north-s-abortion-laws-1.2448877> accessed 2 December 2015.

85 Henry McDonald, "Northern Irish appeal court refuses limited lifting of abortion ban", *Guardian*, 29 June 2017 <https://www.theguardian.com/world/2017/jun/29/northern-irish-appeal-court-refuses-limited-lifting-of-abortion-ban> accessed 30 June 2017; and Jessica Elgot and Henry McDonald, "Northern Irish women win access to free abortions as May averts rebellion", *Guardian*, 29 June 2017 <https://www.theguardian.com/world/2017/jun/29/rebel-tories-could-back-northern-ireland-abortion-amendment> accessed 30 June 2017.

86 "NI Catholic bishops respond to abortion judgment", *Irish Times*, 30 November 2015 <http://www.irishtimes.com/news/social-affairs/religion-and-beliefs/ni-catholic-bishops-respond-to-abortion-judgment-1.2449422> accessed 2 December 2015; and Gerry Moriarty, "Catholic bishops 'shocked and disturbed' by abortion ruling", *Irish Times*, 1 December 2015 <http://www.irishtimes.com/news/social-affairs/catholic-bishops-shocked-and-disturbed-by-abortion-ruling-1.2449437> accessed 2 December 2015.

87 Mark Hilliard, "Catholic bishops urge Northern politicians to reject abortion law", *Irish Times*, 9 February 2016 <http://www.irishtimes.com/news/social-affairs/catholic-bishops-urge-northern-politicians-to-reject-abortion-law-1.2528805> accessed 13 February 2016.

88 Goretti Horgan, "A Holy Alliance? Obstacles to abortion rights in Ireland North and South", in Aideen Quilty, Sinéad Kennedy, and Catherine Conlon (eds), *The Abortion Papers Ireland* Vol. 2 (Cork: Attic Press, 2015), p. 244.

89 "Bid to ease Northern Ireland abortion laws voted down", *Guardian*, 11 February 2016 <http://www.theguardian.com/uk-news/2016/feb/11/northern-ireland-abortion-laws-easing-voted-down> accessed 13 February 2016.

90 Precious Life, "Victory! Nationalists and Unionists Unite to Protect Northern Ireland's Unborn Children" <http://preciouslife.com/news/262/victory-nationalists-and-unionists-unite-to-protect-northern-irelands-unborn-children/> accessed 4 March 2016.

91 Kitty Holland, "Abortion pills trio: law making women criminals 'absolutely bad'", *Irish Times*, 25 May 2016 <http://www.irishtimes.com/news/social-affairs/abortion-pills-trio-law-making-women-criminals-absolutely-bad-1.2659395> accessed 25 May 2016.

92 Gerry Moriarty, "Women – aged 69, 68 and 71 – tell PSNI they bought abortion pills", *Irish Times*, 24 May 2016 <http://www.irishtimes.com/news/ireland/irish-news/women-aged-69-68-and-71-tell-psni-they-bought-abortion-pills-1.2658862> accessed 25 May 2016.

93 The Health Regulatory Authority, working in co-operation with customs officials, seized 28 packages in 2011 and 60 packages in 2014. Kitty Holland, "State's women face jail for taking abortion pill", *Irish Times*, 5 April 2016 <http://www.irishtimes.com/news/ireland/irish-news/state-s-women-face-jail-for-taking-abortion-pill-1.2598217> accessed 6 April 2016.

94 Marie O'Halloran, "Taoiseach pledges citizens' assembly on abortion issue", *Irish Times*, 17 December 2015 <http://www.irishtimes.com/news/politics/oireachtas/taoiseach-pledges-citizens-assembly-on-abortion-issue-1.2469135?mode=print&ot=example.AjaxPageLayout.ot> accessed 19 December 2015.

95 "'I actually struggle with this myself': Taoiseach quizzed on Eighth Amendment on TV3 couch", TheJournal.ie, 25 February 2016 <http://www.msn.com/en-ie/news/national/%e2%80%9ci-actually-struggle-with-this-myself%e2%80%9d-taoiseach-quizzed-on-eighth-amendment-on-tv3-couch/ar-BBpYyaJ?ocid=spartandhp> accessed 25 February 2016.

96 Pro Life Campaign, *General Election 2016: Ireland's pro-life laws hang in the balance* (Dublin: Pro Life Campaign).

97 See Una Mullally, "Election result is not a victory for anti-abortion lobby", *Irish Times*, 2 March 2016 <http://www.irishtimes.com/opinion/una-mullally-election-result-is-not-a-victory-for-anti-abortion-lobby-1.2557019?__vfz=c_pages%3D11000002670848> accessed 3 March 2016.

98 Stephen Collins, "Majority for repeal of Eighth Amendment, poll shows", *Irish Times*, 23 February 2016 <http://www.irishtimes.com/news/politics/majority-for-repeal-of-eighth-amendment-poll-shows-1.2544564> accessed 23 February 2016.

99 "Full text of court ruling on North's abortion laws" (see note 575).

100 There was a lack of legal and procedural clarity about what constituted a "real and substantive" risk to the life of a pregnant woman. Requirements for medical scrutiny in the cases of suicidal pregnant women were found to be excessive and were likely to exacerbate their mental distress. The Act was

deemed to be discriminatory against women who were not able to travel abroad for abortions. The committee expressed criticism of restrictions on information about crisis pregnancies under the provisions of the Regulation of Information (Services Outside the State for Termination of Pregnancies) Act 1995. Healthcare providers risked prosecution if they referred women to abortion services in another jurisdiction.

101 UN Human Rights Committee, "Concluding observations on the fourth periodic report of Ireland", 19 August 2014, paragraph 9 <http://tbinternet.ohchr.org/_layouts/treatybodyexternal/Download. aspx?symbolno=CCPR%2fC%2fIRL%2fCO%2f4&Lang=en> accessed 21 May 2016.

102 UN Committee on Economic, Social and Cultural Rights, "Concluding observations on the third periodic report on Ireland", 8 July 2015, paragraph 30 <http://tbinternet.ohchr.org/_layouts/treatybodyexternal/Download. aspx?symbolno=E%2fC.12%2fIRL%2fCO%2f3&Lang=en> accessed 21 May 2016.

103 UN Committee on the Rights of the Child, "Concluding observations on the combined third and fourth periodic reports of Ireland", 1 March 2016, paragraph 57 <http://tbinternet.ohchr.org/_layouts/treatybodyexternal/ Download.aspx?symbolno=CRC%2fC%2fIRL%2fCO%2f3-4&Lang=en> accessed 21 May 2016; and Kitty Holland, "Abortion should be decriminalised 'in all circumstances' – UN committee", *Irish Times*, 4 February 2016 <http://www.irishtimes.com/news/social-affairs/abortion-should-be-decriminalised-in-all-circumstances-un-committee-1.2522911> accessed 7 February 2016.

104 There was a demand for access to abortion even at the height of the Catholic Church's influence in independent Ireland. Irish women preferred to ingest oral substances instead of choosing a surgical procedure. Cara Delay, "Pills, Potions, and Purgatives: Women and abortion methods in Ireland, 1900–1950", *Women's History Review*, vol. 28, no. 3 (2019), pp. 479–99.

105 Kitty Holland, "Women who take abortion pill 'should not be reported'", *Irish Times*, 6 April 2016 <http://www.irishtimes.com/news/social-affairs/women-who-take-abortion-pills-should-not-be-reported-1.2599522> accessed 6 April 2016.

106 In April 2016 a woman in Northern Ireland was found guilty of such an offence under the provisions of the Offences Against the Person Act 1861 and was sentenced in Belfast Crown Court to three months in prison, which was suspended. The young woman did not have the financial means to procure a legal abortion in Britain. Her housemates had informed the PSNI after they discovered a foetus of 10 to 12 weeks' gestation in a refuse bin. Mark Breslin, director of the Family Planning Association (Northern Ireland), expressed outrage that the woman had, in effect, been punished for lacking financial or other resources to travel to England for a legal and

safe abortion. Kitty Holland, "Woman's conviction for buying abortion pills is 'outrageous'", *Irish Times*, 5 April 2016. A second case was pending in Northern Ireland against a mother who had imported abortion pills for her teenage daughter. It was clear that other similar cases would arise in the future.

107 Breda O'Brien, "Abortion – we can do better than women in prison and dead babies in bins", *Irish Times*, 9 April 2016 <http://www.irishtimes.com/opinion/breda-o-brien-abortion-we-can-do-better-than-women-in-prison-and-dead-babies-in-bins-1.2603648> accessed 17 May 2016.

108 Colm O'Gorman, letter to the editor, *Irish Times*, 15 April 2016 <http://www.irishtimes.com/opinion/letters/amnesty-international-and-abortion-1.2610994> accessed 16 May 2016.

109 Patrick G. Burke, "Amnesty International and abortion", letter to the editor, *Irish Times*, 21 April 2016 <http://www.irishtimes.com/opinion/letters/amnesty-and-abortion-1.2617913> accessed 16 May 2016.

110 Ibid.

111 Pádraig McCarthy, "Amnesty International and abortion", letter to the editor, *Irish Times*, 21 April 2016 <http://www.irishtimes.com/opinion/letters/amnesty-and-abortion-1.2617913> accessed 16 May 2016.

112 Colm O'Gorman, letter to the editor, *Irish Times*, 20 April 2016 <http://www.irishtimes.com/opinion/letters/amnesty-international-and-abortion-1.2616426> accessed 16 May 2016.

113 Kitty Holland, "Many states question Irish record on abortion at UN", *Irish Times*, 12 May 2016 <http://www.irishtimes.com/news/social-affairs/many-states-question-irish-record-on-abortion-at-un-1.2644354> accessed 12 May 2016.

114 Breda O'Brien, "Amnesty abandons values of Seán MacBride", *Irish Times*, 23 April 2016 <http://www.irishtimes.com/opinion/amnesty-abandons-values-of-se%C3%A1n-macbride-1.2621162> accessed 16 May 2016.

115 Jaime Todd-Gher and Christiana Zampas, letter to the editor, *Irish Times*, 28 April 2016 <http://www.irishtimes.com/opinion/letters/amnesty-and-abortion-1.2626655> accessed 16 May 2016.

116 Ibid.

117 Pro Life Campaign, "Pro Life Campaign addresses UN human rights committee in Geneva today", 14 July 2015 <http://prolifecampaign.ie/main/portfolio/detail/14-07-2015-pro-life-campaign-addresses-un-human-rights-committee-in-geneva-today/> accessed 7 June 2016; and UN General Assembly, Declaration of the Rights of the Child, 20 November 1959 <http://www.unicef.org/malaysia/1959-Declaration-of-the-Rights-of-the-Child.pdf> accessed 6 June 2016. The declaration was the basis of the Convention on the Rights of the Child.

118 UN General Assembly, Universal Declaration of Human Rights, 10 December 1948 <http://www.ohchr.org/EN/UDHR/Documents/UDHR_

Translations/eng.pdf> accessed 6 June 2016.

119 See Abby F. Janoff, "Rights of the Pregnant Child vs. Rights of the Unborn under the Convention on the Rights of the Child", *Boston University International Law Journal*, vol. 22, no. 1 (2004), pp. 163–88 <http://www. bu.edu/law/journals-archive/international/volume22n1/documents/163-188. pdf> accessed 6 June 2016. The UN Committee on the Rights of the Child, as observed earlier, recommended the decriminalisation of abortion in Ireland.

120 UN Human Rights Committee, "Views adopted by the Committee under article 5(4) of the Optional Protocol, concerning communication No. 2324/2013", 9 June 2016, paragraph 7.4 <http://tbinternet.ohchr. org/_layouts/treatybodyexternal/Download.aspx?symbolno=CCPR/C/116/ D/2324/2013&Lang=en> accessed 10 June 2016.

121 Ibid., paragraph 7.5.

122 Ibid., paragraph 3.10, claims submitted to the committee; see also footnote 3.

123 Ibid., paragraphs 7.8; 8; 9.

124 Ibid., paragraph 4.2

125 Ibid., paragraph 7.4.

126 Ibid., paragraph 10.

127 Pro Life Campaign, "UN committee has become a de facto lobby group for abortion" <http://prolifecampaign.ie/main/portfolio/detail/09-06-16-un-committee-become-de-facto-lobby-group-abortion-plc/> accessed 12 June 2016.

128 Susan Gately, "Every Life Counts questions UN committee abortion ruling", CatholicIreland.net, 10 June 2016 <http://www.catholicireland.net/every-life-counts-questions-un-committee-abortion-ruling/> accessed 12 June 2016.

129 Every Life Counts failed to mention that the conference paper was later published in the science journal *Prenatal Diagnosis*. The original research work was limited to anencephaly – a lethal neural tube defect.

130 Although the authors concluded that "there appears to be a psychological benefit to women to continue the pregnancy following prenatal diagnosis of a lethal foetal defect", they also found that "when termination is chosen, procedures performed earlier in gestation are certainly advantageous physically, but there may be a psychological benefit as well." Heidi Cope, Melanie E. Garrett, Simon G. Gregory and Allison E. Ashley-Koch, "Pregnancy Continuation and Organizational Religious Activity Following Prenatal Diagnosis of a Lethal Fetal Defect is Associated with Improved Psychological Outcome", *Prenatal Diagnosis*, vol. 35, no. 8 (April 2015) <https://www.researchgate.net/publication/274967787_Pregnancy_continuation_and_organizational_religious_activity_following_prenatal_diagnosis_of_a_lethal_fetal_defect_is_associated_with_improved_psychological_outcome_Psychological_outcome_following_pre> accessed 12 June 2016.

131 It is probable that correlation will be confused with causation in narrowly

focused studies of limited sample size and when variables of central importance are not researched or are inadequately researched.

132 Suzanne Lynch, Elaine Edwards and Sarah Bardon, "Fitzgerald promises to address highly critical UN report on Irish abortion law", *Irish Times*, 10 June 2016, p. 3.

133 Paul Cullen, "Latest criticism ratchets up international pressure for change", *Irish Times*, 10 June 2016, p. 3.

134 Marie O'Halloran, "Abortion assembly a 'pointless exercise' in democracy", *Irish Times*, 15 July 2016 <http://www.irishtimes.com/news/politics/oireachtas/abortion-assembly-a-pointless-exercise-in-democracy-1.2723792> accessed 4 August 2016.

135 Gráinne Griffin, Orla O'Connor, Ailbhe Smyth and Alison O'Connor, *It's a Yes! How Together for Yes Repealed the Eighth and Transformed Irish Society* (Dublin: Orpen Press, 2019).

136 Pat Leahy: "Middle ground has shifted on abortion, but will politicians shift with it?", *Irish Times*, 15 June 2016, p. 4; and "Majority support repeal of Eighth Amendment, poll shows", *Irish Times*, 8 July 2016 <http://www.irishtimes.com/news/politics/majority-support-repeal-of-eighth-amendment-poll-shows-1.2714191> accessed 8 July 2016.

137 Pat Leahy, "Kenny says UN abortion ruling not binding", *Irish Times*, 15 June 2016, p. 1.

138 For compelling legal arguments in support of this, see "The UN and the Eighth Amendment", letter to the editor (61 signatories), *Irish Times*, 23 June 2016 <http://www.irishtimes.com/opinion/letters/the-un-and-the-eighth-amendment-1.2695139> accessed 23 June 2016. The majority of the signatories were university law lecturers, most outside Ireland.

139 Rev. Patrick G. Burke, "The UN and the Eighth Amendment", letter to the editor, *Irish Times*, 24 June 2016 <http://www.irishtimes.com/opinion/letters/the-un-and-the-eighth-amendment-1.2696826> accessed 24 June 2016.

140 Lynch, Edwards and Bardon, op. cit.

141 In this context, it is important to observe that when the state advanced its case in *D v Ireland* the Supreme Court had not delivered its judgment in *Roche v Roche*. Eileen Barrington, "Article 40.3.3 of the Constitution and Fatal Foetal Abnormalities", Citizens' Assembly, 7 January 2017 <https://www.citizensassembly.ie/en/Meetings/Eileen-Barrington-Paper.pdf> accessed 9 January 2017.

142 See, for example, Fiona de Londras (professor of global legal studies, School of Law, University of Birmingham), "UN move confirms law on abortion is unsustainable", *Irish Times*, 10 June 2016, p. 16.

143 Protection of Life in Pregnancy (Amendment) (Fatal Foetal Abnormalities) Bill 2013, introduced by Clare Daly TD, 21 November 2013 <https://www.oireachtas.ie/documents/bills28/bills/2013/11513/b11513d.pdf> accessed 10 September 2016; and Protection of Life in Pregnancy (Amendment)

(Fatal Foetal Abnormalities) (No. 2) Bill 2013, sponsored by Mick Wallace TD, 28 November 2013 <https://www.oireachtas.ie/documents/bills28/bills/2013/12213/b12213d.pdf> accessed 10 September 2016.

144 Mac Cormaic, "Legal conundrum".

145 "Speech by Simon Harris TD, Minister for Health – Protection of Life during Pregnancy (Amendment) (Fatal Foetal Abnormalities) (No 2) Bill 2013", 30 June 2016, Department of Health website <http://health.gov.ie/blog/speeches/speech-by-simon-harris-t-d-minister-for-health-protection-of-life-during-pregnancy-amendment-fatal-foetal-abnormalities-no-2-bill-2013/> accessed 4 February 2017.

146 Pro Life Campaign: "Babies diagnosed with life-limiting conditions" (2015) <http://prolifecampaign.ie/main/portfolio/detail/the-hard-cases-explained/> accessed 14 September 2016; and "Misinformation at heart of Wallace abortion bill, says PLC" (1 July 2016) <http://prolifecampaign.ie/main/portfolio/detail/01-07-16-misinformation-heart-wallace-abortion-bill-says-plc/> accessed 14 September 2016.

147 Breda O'Brien, "Why terminology matters when it comes to pregnancy loss", *Irish Times*, 20 August 2016 <http://www.irishtimes.com/opinion/breda-o-brien-why-terminology-matters-when-it-comes-to-pregnancy-loss-1.2761949> accessed 20 August 2016.

148 See D.J.C. Wilkinson *et al.*, "Fatally Flawed?"

149 Simon Harris, when officially launching the National Standards, prudently referred to diagnoses of "life-limiting or fatal foetal anomaly". Health Service Executive, *National Standards for Bereavement Care following Pregnancy Loss*, 10 August 2016 <http://www.hse.ie/eng/services/news/media/pressrel/%20NationalStandardsBereavementCare%20.html> accessed 20 August 2016.

150 Health Service Executive, *National Standards for Bereavement Care Following Pregnancy Loss and Perinatal Death*, Version 1.15, 10 August 2016 <http://www.hse.ie/eng/about/Who/acute/bereavementcare/standardsBereavementCarePregnancyLoss.pdf> accessed 20 August 2016.

151 In his paper read before the Citizens' Assembly (4 March 2017), John O'Dowd (lecturer in the School of Law, University College Dublin), observed that the definition of the unborn in the Protection of Life During Pregnancy Act 2013 was "given for the purposes of that Act only, so it could also be that the Act is intended merely to confine the protection given by the criminal law so that it applies to one category of the unborn only, even if that concept is in fact wider under the Constitution." John O'Dowd, "The Unborn, Within and Beyond the Eighth Amendment", paper read to the Citizens' Assembly, 4 March 2017 <https://www.citizensassembly.ie/en/Meetings/John-O-Dowd-Paper.pdf> accessed 11 March 2017.

152 Anette Kersting and Birgit Wagner, "Complicated Grief after Perinatal Loss", *Dialogues in Clinical Neuroscience*, vol. 14, no. 2 (June 2012), pp. 187–

94 <http://www.ncbi.nlm.nih.gov/pmc/articles/PMC3384447/> accessed 20 August 2016.

153 On the general point of research about "complicated grief", Kersting and Wagner concluded that "there is a substantial lack of randomized controlled trials in this field of research" (ibid.). Breda O'Brien made no reference to some points of fundamental importance made by Professor Dominic Wilkinson and his co-researchers which she cited in pursuit of correct terminology. Professor Wilkinson and his co-authors, mindful of limited research data and uncertainties in prognosis, argued that a woman's autonomy should be respected. They acknowledged that there were genuine ethical arguments against prolonging life in cases of severe congenital malformations regardless of whether or not the term "lethal" was deemed appropriate. Wilkinson *et al.*, "Fatally Flawed?".

154 Health Service Executive, *National Standards for Bereavement Care Following Pregnancy Loss*, p. 46.

CHAPTER EIGHT

———•———

Challenges to the Catholic Ethos

Healthcare Services and the Catholic Ethos

PLANS TO RELOCATE THE NATIONAL MATERNITY HOSPITAL (NMH) in Dublin from Holles Street to the St Vincent's Hospital site at Elm Park sparked an outcry in April 2017, not only because a hospital built at taxpayers' expense would be privately owned, but also because some services, such as tubal ligations and vasectomies, would not be provided due to Catholic teaching on sexual morality. Concern about the Catholic ethos in healthcare requires some explanation, which in turn will benefit from a brief historical account.

St Vincent's Hospital, set up in 1834 by the Religious Sisters of Charity, was the first hospital in Ireland established by a Catholic religious order that was dedicated specifically to the care of the Catholic population. The Sisters of Mercy reinforced the trend of religious contributions to healthcare when they opened the Mercy Hospital in Cork (1857), the Mater Misercordiae Hospital in Dublin (1861), and the Mater in Belfast (1883). In the following decades hospitals became increasingly dependent for staff on nuns, especially the Sisters of Mercy.[1] There was a sectarian element in the drive to provide hospital services managed and staffed by Catholics, for Catholics.[2]

By the time the Irish Free State was set up in 1922, religious involvement and management of health services was well established. The power of the Church in southern Irish society did not arise simply because of its large majority (over 90 per cent of the population). The historian J.H. Whyte observed that other states, such as Italy, Spain,

Portugal, and some Latin American countries, probably had larger Catholic majorities. Even so, it did not follow that Church influence in these states was greater than in Ireland. Ireland was unusual, not so much for its large Catholic majority, but for the very high proportion of Catholics who were practising and firmly committed to their faith.[3] This, together with heavy Church involvement in education, social welfare services and healthcare services, gave the Catholic Church enormous power in matters of public policy in Ireland. It was not in the interests of any politician or political party to challenge such power – disapproval from the Church would cost votes.[4] Yet it was not simply that Irish politicians were afraid to challenge the power of the Church. Most of them shared the conservative outlook of their priests and bishops.[5] A notable exception was Dr Noël Browne, Minister for Health in the first Inter-Party Government (1948–1951). His attempts to implement the Mother and Child Scheme, originally drafted by the previous Fianna Fáil government, met with robust opposition from the Catholic hierarchy and the Irish Medical Association. Browne received little support from his cabinet colleagues and the scheme was abandoned in April 1951. The scheme was subsequently revived and amended, with the objections of the bishops in mind, and was given legislative effect in the Health Act 1953.

The Catholic Church robustly defended its domain in health and education. In matters of health, it vigorously opposed Catholic patients being treated by Protestant doctors. The publication of the papal encyclical *Casti Connubii* (1930) and the proceedings of the Anglican Church's Lambeth Conference (1930) crystallised doctrinal differences on issues such as birth control. There was some concern among Catholic bishops that Protestant doctors would prescribe contraceptives to Catholic women. Both Church and state saw the ban on contraceptives as an issue of public morality and prioritised it over the health of women.[6]

Tom Inglis observed in his *Moral Monopoly: The Rise and Fall of the Catholic Church in Ireland* (1998) that twenty-six of the sixty-three hospitals in the state were Catholic voluntary hospitals. Orders of nuns and brothers owned and managed, not just hospitals, but nursing homes, hospices and homes for the disabled. The ownership and control of hospitals by religious orders, and their representation on the boards of management of public hospitals, gave the Church considerable influence over the practice of medicine in Ireland.[7] The Church provided a range of social, health and educational services that the state was unable or unwilling to provide. Therefore, the relationship between church and state suited both.

The Lourdes Hospital (Drogheda), run by the Medical Missionaries of Mary until 1997, in common with other Catholic hospitals, prohibited all forms of artificial contraception. The only approved birth control method in the hospital was the highly unreliable Billings method based on calculations of the infertile phase of the menstrual cycle. Sterilisations – tubal ligations and vasectomies – were prohibited, even in circumstances where another pregnancy would be dangerous. However, "the Catholic ethos" did permit "indirect sterilisation": it was permissible to remove a diseased organ such as a uterus even though the woman would then be incapable of having a baby. In such cases the intention was to preserve the health of the woman, not to prevent future pregnancies.[8] In the Lourdes Hospital inquiry (2006) Judge Maureen Harding Clark found "much evidence" that the prohibition on sterilisations gave rise to the practice of "compassionate hysterectomies" in hospitals with a Catholic ethos – "an unspoken Irish solution to an Irish question". Surgeons' clinical judgement was not questioned in such cases. Tubal ligations were a different matter, especially in the Lourdes Hospital. A rigid adherence to conservative Catholic doctrine gave rise to the performance of sterilisations by hysterectomy when tubal ligations would have been more appropriate. Hysterectomy was far more invasive and traumatic for the patient and there was a likelihood of adverse psychological consequences.[9] Even so, religious ideology overruled clinical judgement and best medical practice – the welfare of women was of secondary importance.[10]

Can a similar judgement be made on the issue of symphysiotomies? A detailed historical analysis will not be undertaken here, but it is important to make a few observations in the context of examining contemporary attitudes in Ireland towards Catholic medical ethics, and specifically in relation to objections to the proposed plan to place the state-funded National Maternity Hospital in the ownership of a Catholic organisation.

Pubic symphysiotomy is a surgical procedure to enlarge the delivery capacity of the mother's pelvis when the baby is too large to pass through. It entailed cutting the fibrous cartilage of the pubic symphysis that joins the pubic bones at the front of the pelvis. The procedure was sometimes used as an alternative to caesarean section. It was widely reported that the majority of women who underwent this surgery experienced lifelong pain, incontinence and difficulties in walking.[11] The procedure was described in such terms as "brutal", and "butchered genitals", and was associated with a subservience to Catholic orthodoxy.[12] Two reports commissioned by consecutive Ministers of Health, Dr James Reilly and Dr Leo Varadkar, indicated a need for a radical change in narrative. Judge Yvonne Murphy (11 March 2014) pointed to a number of medical reasons why in some cases symphysiotomy was carried out in preference to caesarean section. It was found that the maternal mortality rate was higher in cases of caesarean sections than with symphysiotomy.[13] In some cases a caesarean was not possible and a symphysiotomy had to be performed to save the life of the baby.[14] Symphysiotomy was rarely performed in obstetric practice in Ireland, occurring in less than 0.05 per cent of deliveries between 1940 and 1985.[15] It can be inferred from the Murphy Report that Catholic ethics did exert, to some extent, a detrimental effect on best clinical practice, considering that the practice of symphysiotomy continued in Our Lady of Lourdes Hospital up to 1984, by which time it had almost completely ceased in the Dublin maternity hospitals. Symphysiotomy was performed less frequently from the early 1960s because of improved techniques for caesarean sections, improved techniques for diagnosing pelvic disproportion, better management of labour, and better management of infections in cases of caesarean delivery.[16]

Medical research indicated that some patients suffered long-term effects arising from symphysiotomy, including constant back pain, urinary incontinence, and higher-grade sacroiliac joint osteoarthritis. Yet it seemed that in rare cases there might still be a role for symphysiotomy, for example in a breech presentation when the baby's head is obstructed.[17]

Years of activism by women who had undergone symphysiotomy, Dr Oonagh Walsh's historical study of *Symphysiotomy in Ireland 1944 to 1984* (2013), and the Murphy Report (2014) influenced the government to set up a redress scheme for women who had undergone symphysiotomy between 1940 and 1990 – regardless of why the surgery was performed. The terms of the Surgical Symphysiotomy Payment Scheme were framed on "widespread assumptions" that symphysiotomy almost certainly caused lifelong suffering and that Irish obstetricians were guided by Catholic doctrine on contraception rather than by best clinical practice.[18] In her report (19 October 2016) to the Minister for Health (Simon Harris), Judge Clark failed to find evidence of a religious motive overriding obstetric considerations for the performance of symphysiotomies in "available" medical records. Yet it cannot be simply inferred from this finding that the Catholic ethos did not exert any influence. Symphysiotomies were carried out to avoid the need for repeat caesarean sections in a jurisdiction where artificial contraceptives were disapproved of by most Catholics and were illegal. Sterilisation was legal, but it was not performed in any of the maternity hospitals in Dublin at the time.[19] Furthermore, Clark found some evidence of religious motivation in the National Maternity Hospital Annual Report (1949).

Two masters of the National Maternity Hospital, Alex Spain and Arthur Barry, were known for their support for Catholic beliefs about contraception and sterilisation, and for their advocacy of symphysiotomy as a means of circumventing demands by their patients for sterilisation or contraception. Clark acknowledged that there is much uncertainty about assessing the impact of the Catholic ethos on the professional judgements of those obstetricians who supported the case for symphysiotomies in the 1940s. Symphysiotomies were also carried out at the Rotunda and Erinville – both of which were non-Catholic hospitals and were unlikely to have been influenced by Roman Catholic doctrine.[20]

Judge Clark concluded from her research that the lives of many babies had been saved by symphysiotomy.[21] Alleged suffering and disabilities had been greatly exaggerated.[22] Judge Clark's findings were nuanced, reflecting the complexity of interacting medical, social and religious influences. This meticulous scrutiny of the evidence contrasted with reports in some sections of the media who preferred "the more lurid and unfounded accounts projected by some activists and bloggers". Clark was not confident that standards of reporting by these media sources would improve.[23] The symphysiotomy issue, despite the exaggerations, inaccuracies and oversimplifications, served to stiffen opposition to any extension of Catholic moral teaching that might impinge on access to healthcare services relating to sterilisation, assisted reproduction – and abortion if legal grounds for it were extended.

In a broader context, Catholic medical ethics had suffered reputational damage. A case in point is the Church's stance against the use of condoms, not only for birth control but also for reducing the risk of sexually transmitted diseases (STDs) such as Acquired Immunodeficiency Syndrome (AIDS).[24] In the early 1990s fears about the spread of AIDS influenced politicians to pass legislation that lifted restrictions on access to non-medical contraceptives. In 1993 official figures pointed to: 1,368 cases HIV positive, 341 cases of AIDS, and 150 dead.[25] The orthodox Catholic stance was morally questionable and naive. It still insisted that sexual intercourse was morally permissible only within marriage. The safest sex possible was with one partner in a faithful relationship. This was all very well but when people were falling ill and dying from AIDS there was a pressing need to emphasise that if one failed to be virtuous, there was still a much greater moral obligation to be safe and not to endanger another person's life or health. The Methodist minister Rev. Graham Hamilton advised those who did not comply with the Christian concept of marriage, and who were sexually active, that they should at least "practise safe sex using a condom".[26] It was, from a realistic and Christian perspective, the lesser of two evils – something the Catholic Church generally failed to grasp[27] and which sometimes frustrated the initiatives of those who sought to disseminate information about the prevention of STDs.[28]

A number of other issues served to heighten concerns about how the Catholic ethos might impede or obstruct the delivery of healthcare services in some hospitals in receipt of state funding. A case in point is the delay in the commencement of a drug trial for the treatment of lung cancer at the Mater Hospital. Pregnancy had to be avoided by women undergoing treatment with Tarceva because of concerns that the new drug could harm an unborn child. Although abstinence was acknowledged in the leaflet issued by the manufacturers of the drug (Roche Ireland), the emphasis on artificial contraception provoked criticism and led to delays.[29] The matter was eventually resolved after some protests by medical specialists and a decision by the Mater Hospital board to grant permission for the drug trial to commence.[30] This controversy, although short-lived, brought into focus the difficulties that can arise when a religious ethos conflicts with what is generally regarded as best medical practice.

In the late twentieth century, the decline of Church influence in healthcare services became increasingly evident. Declining vocations meant that the Church was unable to place brothers and nuns in key positions to influence policy and the training of doctors and nurses. Sterilisation procedures (tubal ligations and vasectomies) became available in the 1980s.[31] The power of the institutional Church was not what it once was – yet it wasn't negligible. Hundreds of millions of euros worth of health service assets in Ireland were controlled by religious orders, especially by the Sisters of Bon Secours, the Religious Sisters of Charity, and the Sisters of Mercy. Ireland was not unusual in this context. The Roman Catholic Church was the largest non-governmental provider of healthcare services internationally and issues of public concern were sometimes raised when decisions had to be made about institutions against the background of ageing and shrinking memberships.[32] Religious orders were less and less able to directly manage the hospitals their predecessors had founded. New managerial structures were required. The Religious Sisters of Charity were among those orders who felt compelled to adapt to changing conditions.[33]

In 2003 St Vincent's Healthcare Group Limited (SVHG) was formed and St Vincent's University Hospital (affiliated to University College Dublin since 1999) was transferred to the company. The Religious Sisters of Charity became the shareholders and two of the Sisters were members of the board of directors. The SVHG constitution required the hospital to function in compliance with the Religious Sisters of Charity's Health Service Philosophy and Ethical Code. It was reported that some services that were legally permissible, such as the morning-after pill and sterilisations, were not permitted procedures in the hospital.[34] This ethical code became a focus of controversy in April 2017.

The National Maternity Hospital Controversy

The NMH came under increasing pressure to relocate from its old premises in Holles Street to a new building more suited to the needs of modern medicine. There was also a need for co-location with a general hospital. Women experiencing complicated and sometimes life-threatening pregnancies needed timely access to a range of specialist care facilities. Options for co-location were very limited. Protests against the planned relocation to the St Vincent's Hospital campus (first announced in 2013) almost certainly shocked the Religious Sisters of Charity. They had provided nursing and medical care to thousands of Irish patients over generations. Precedents had been set over many decades where hospitals and schools had been built by the state on Church lands and were owned by the Church or by its religious orders. Nevertheless, goodwill and trust from the public was not forthcoming, for reasons which have already received attention. Further to this, the historical legacy of the Religious Sisters of Charity was tainted by the scandalous abuse and exploitation of women in the Magdalene Laundries (also known as Magdalene Asylums). This was exacerbated by the refusal of the Religious Sisters of Charity, and three other religious orders, to contribute to a redress scheme for several hundred survivors.[35]

A small project might have escaped public attention, but the massive scale of the NMH relocation plan did not facilitate business as usual. The estimated cost of the new hospital was €300 million. There was widespread consternation that such a huge investment of taxpayers' money was intended for a hospital that would not be owned by the state. Within days of the controversy breaking, 85,000 people had signed an online petition expressing opposition to ownership by the Sisters of Charity.[36] On 18 April 2017 the Department of Health assured the public that the identity and ethos of the NMH would be retained. The new hospital would have full operational, clinical, financial and budgetary independence. This independence would be underpinned by the "reserved powers" specified in the agreement and by a "golden share" held by the Minister for Health.[37] Dr Rhona Mahony, master of the NMH at Holles Street, spoke to Seán O'Rourke on RTÉ, reassuring the listeners that the new hospital would have complete clinical independence, free of a Catholic ethos. Ownership was not her concern – control was the issue.[38] The new NMH was to be operated by a new company and would be managed in conformity with national maternity policy. This did little to calm public concerns. Doubts persisted about whether or not ownership of the hospital could be neatly separated from control of the hospital.

Differences of opinion were expressed about the extent to which Catholic ethics would impact on the provision of healthcare services. Professor Michael Keane, a clinical director at St Vincent's Hospital, dismissed concerns about the Catholic ethos as misleading. Sterilisations were carried out at St Vincent's when indicated for medical reasons, such as cancer, as distinct from elective reasons. Seventy Mirena coils – long-term contraceptive devices – had been fitted by hospital staff in 2016.[39] Columnist and broadcaster Sarah Carey observed in the *Sunday Independent* that the NMH at Holles Street was a "voluntary hospital" (i.e. not owned by the state) whose chairperson (of the executive committee) was the Catholic Archbishop of Dublin. Despite this, the clinical director acted independently. Medical procedures such as sterilisations and legal abortions were carried out without interference from the Church. Archbishop Diarmuid Martin did not attend meetings, regarding it as inappropriate. Neither was there any evidence of interference from nuns or priests. Carey saw ownership, and the financial implications arising from it, as the central issues. The Religious Sisters of Charity were paid a €1.2 million rental fee per year by St Vincent's Healthcare Group (SVHG) for their land. The nuns were dying out. In the long term, beneficiaries from this and other similar revenue streams were likely to be businesspeople, investment managers, property managers and lawyers.[40] Consultants, with a foot in both the private hospitals and the public hospitals, also stood to gain from a malfunctional hybrid system of the public and private sectors.[41]

The chairmanship of the executive committee of St Vincent's was reserved for the Archbishop of Dublin under the terms of the National Maternity Hospital Dublin (Charter Amendment) Act 1936. He was also chairman of the board of governors. Archbishop Martin considered his automatic appointment "anachronistic" and had requested two ministers for health to remedy this. He did not wish to be chairman and had not attended or chaired board meetings. The deputy chairperson carried out that function instead.[42] There seemed to be little reason for concern about Church interference in the running of the hospital. But any optimism that fears about Church intervention would recede was dashed when Bishop Kevin Doran, chairman of the Bishops' Committee for Bioethics, asserted that any healthcare organisation regarding itself as Catholic had "a special responsibility" to uphold the Church's teachings about human life and dignity. This responsibility was not diminished or negated by receipt of public funding. Canon law imposed a duty on a hospital that was on Church land to operate in accordance with the rules of the Church. Doran added that he was initially speaking "in general terms" and did not know the details of the legal relationship between the Religious Sisters of Charity and SVHG.[43] These comments could only have given weight to the objections of Dr Peter Boylan and others who opposed the proposed handing over of a publicly funded hospital to a private sector organisation.

Boylan's concerns about clinical independence could not be easily dismissed. He was a former master of the NMH (1991–1997) and chairman of the executive council of the Institute of Obstetricians and Gynaecologists at the Royal College of Physicians of Ireland. He was not without influential supporters when he expressed criticism about plans for the new NMH. Two former masters of the Rotunda Hospital, Professor Sam Coulter-Smith and Dr Michael Darling, expressed opposition to the proposed transfer of the NMH to the ownership of the Religious Sisters of Charity.[44] Dr Chris Fitzpatrick, a former master of the Coombe Hospital, believed that the transfer of the NMH to a religiously owned property would lead to a conflict of interests between medical doctors and the Catholic Church. It was also "deeply insensitive" in view of "the chequered history" of the Catholic Church in Ireland in matters relating to female reproductive health. He believed that the owners of the St Vincent's site should hand over the property at no cost to the NMH in the interests of women and babies, which would be in the national interest.[45] His resignation from the project board of the NMH in support of Boylan on 28 April was a considerable blow to the credibility of the agreement that would have handed ownership of the NMH to St Vincent's.[46]

Dr Rhona Mahony pointed out, in an interview on RTÉ's *Morning Ireland*, that the nuns did not wish to run the hospital and that the hospital would continue to offer contraception services, in vitro fertilisation, and terminations of pregnancy when there is a risk to the life of the mother.[47] Mahony's confidence in the clinical independence of the new hospital won majority support in the NMH's board of management. Boylan (her brother-in-law) expressed his opinions at several board meetings, to no avail. On 27 April he resigned from the executive committee of the NMH in protest against the decision to transfer sole ownership of the NMH to the Religious Sisters of Charity. Boylan pointed out that hospitals on Church land were obliged to regulate medical procedures and practices in accordance with the teachings of the Church. The company running the hospital was owned by the Religious Sisters of Charity. The belief that Catholic rules would not apply was "naive and delusional". An issue of major concern was that all women who needed specialist care would be transferred through an interconnecting corridor to the adjacent general hospital, where Catholic ethics definitely applied. Boylan believed that the structure of the board of management was "fatally flawed", was weighted in favour of the Religious Sisters of Charity and was "a recipe for conflict".[48]

Boylan's understanding of the Catholic ethos applying in Catholic hospitals was at variance with that of Michael Keane referred to earlier. There was an element of ambiguity in Keane's argument that indicated that doctors at St Vincent's were sidestepping or avoiding the issue. He acknowledged that some medical professionals might "assume" that they should not perform sterilisation procedures, but this was "a historical thing".[49] The fitting of Mirena coils (intrauterine devices) implied that there was some tolerance by the religious authorities of contraceptive methods that were incompatible with Church teaching. Tolerance was extended, it seems, when contraception and sterilisation procedures were for "medical reasons" rather than elective. Boylan informed Paul Cullen of the *Irish Times* that it was common knowledge that GPs did not refer their patients for elective sterilisations to St Vincent's because such procedures were not facilitated by the hospital. He observed that "No GP would send a woman for an elective tubal ligation to St Vincent's ... You can put in a Mirena coil but you say it's for heavy periods."[50]

Deception, in such circumstances, was a prerequisite for best medical practice.

Concerns that the provision of healthcare services would be adversely impacted by the imposition of Catholic ethics were not dissipated by government assurances. On Sunday 7 May 2017 over 1,500 people marched in protest in Dublin, demanding that the government not grant ownership of the future NMH to the Religious Sisters of Charity. An online petition opposed to such a plan was signed by over 100,000 people.[51] As protests for a change of plan gathered momentum the nuns responded with a landmark decision on 29 May 2017. The Religious Sisters of Charity disclosed their intention to end their involvement in the SVHG (which included St Vincent's University Hospital, St Vincent's Private Hospital and St Michael's Hospital, Dun Laoghaire) and would not play any role in the new NMH. Ownership of the SVHG would be transferred to a new company with charitable status, to be named St Vincent's. The Sisters were not to have any involvement with this company and would not be shareholders. The requirement in the SVHG constitution to manage and maintain clinical facilities, in compliance with the Religious Sisters of Charity Health Service Philosophy and Ethical Code, was to be amended so that the company would function in "compliance with national and international best practice guidelines on medical ethics and the laws of the Republic of Ireland".[52]

A number of contentious issues still needed to be addressed. For example, the NMH and St Vincent's were both voluntary hospitals, outside state ownership, and were to remain outside state ownership, despite being state-funded. Canon James Moriarty (Dublin) observed that ownership of the NMH was to be "transferred from a known group with a known set of values to an unknown group with an unknown set of values. It remains to be seen whether this can be called progress."[53] The hospital, as matters stood, would be handed over to an "unaccountable private healthcare company".[54] Concern was also expressed that the NMH would come under the control of the much larger adjacent general hospital in St Vincent's.[55] But concerns about religious control had been assuaged. Public and press interest subsided.

The SVHG was not in a position to simply hand over the site at Elm Park to the state because it was deep in debt and the land had been used as collateral for borrowings to build St Vincent's Private Hospital. *Sunday Independent* columnist Dearbhail McDonald argued that the main issue was commercial, not religious.[56] John McManus, writing in the *Irish Times*, went so far as to argue that the disagreement about St

Vincent's and the NMH "was never about the nuns and their Catholic ethos".[57] Diametrically opposite opinions were expressed by leading medical professionals. Dr Declan Keane (clinical director at the NMH, and consultant obstetrician and gynaecologist at both the NMH and St Vincent's) maintained that the new NMH would not be subject to the Catholic ethos.[58] Boylan acknowledged that the Catholic ethos had little impact on general medicine and surgery. The same could not be said in relation to obstetrics and gynaecology, which were "fraught with difficulties".[59]

The religious dimension in the controversy was clearly evident – although it can be overstated. Professor Chris Fitzpatrick saw "unfortunate resonances of Dr Noël Browne versus archbishop John Charles McQuaid and the Mother and Child Scheme controversy" in the debate about the NMH.[60] However, there are some major differences between the two controversies. For example, the interventionist and authoritarian traits of McQuaid were not discernible in Archbishop Diarmuid Martin. As already observed, Archbishop Martin did not wish to be chairman of the Executive Committee of the NMH. He had informed Mary Harney, then Minister of Health, that he did not wish to be chairman.[61] Another major difference was that, in contrast to the 1950s, the bishops could not issue instructions to the government with the expectation that it would meekly comply. The bishops, almost certainly aware of their diminished influence, said little as events unfolded. Furthermore, it seems that some priests were not supportive of Bishop Doran's assertion about the Catholic ethos and the NMH. Fr Gabriel Daly (Order of St. Augustine) criticised Doran's "careless intervention" in the context of a Church in which the aspirations and anticipated reforms of the Second Vatican Council had been frustrated.[62]

The Association of Catholic Priests accepted "the principle that a National Maternity Hospital must be in full compliance with the laws of the land, and that no group or religious affiliation can dictate what is or is not permissible therein … where public money is being used to build and fund the hospital, it is important that it is in the ownership of the state."[63] This latter point, although sound in principle, was not as straightforward as it seemed. This was not just in the case of the NMH but in the broader context of healthcare services and education, where state funding and private ownership had become entangled over decades. James Menton, chairman of the SVHG, pointed out that both St Vincent's and the NMH "were making substantial contributions" to the new hospital – the Elm Park site and the proceeds of the sale of the

Holles Street property from St Vincent's and the NMH respectively.[64] Therefore, the project was far from entirely state-funded.

The Religious Sisters of Charity were put in a difficult position not of their own making. They were duty-bound to apply Catholic ethics to institutions they owned, even when those institutions were state-funded. Patsy McGarry, religious affairs columnist with the *Irish Times*, observed that they were not oblivious to the difficult circumstances in which they found themselves in relation to the laws of the state, which were increasingly diverging from Catholic ethics in matters relating to human reproduction. Denying a legally permissible treatment in a state-funded hospital could not be easily brushed aside as if there was no ethical issue to address.[65]

The entanglement of Church and state in the provision of public services carried considerable risks. It was reported that the Religious Sisters of Charity could have transferred their ownership of the Elm Park site to the Vatican if they were "hell-bent on locking" down the Catholic ethos in perpetuity. This option may have been considered by other religious orders.[66] Consolidating the Catholic ethos was seen as especially important in traditionalist Catholic circles in relation to abortion, which might become more easily available if the Eighth Amendment was repealed. Fr Kevin O'Reilly, philosopher and theologian at Rome's Pontifical University of St Thomas Aquinas (the Angelicum) informed the *Irish Catholic* that, under canon law, Irish religious organisations could not sell or donate their properties without permission from the Vatican if such properties were valued at more than €3.5 million. All disposals of assets in this category were subject to scrutiny by the Congregation for Institutes of Consecrated Life and Societies of Apostolic Life. Approval would not be granted without at least receiving agreement from the local bishop or archbishop – in this instance Archbishop Diarmuid Martin. However, O'Reilly believed that in this case the Vatican authorities should overrule the Religious Sisters of Charity, otherwise their decision would ultimately facilitate "direct" abortions in the new hospital.[67] It is unlikely that O'Reilly received any support from Diarmuid Martin. The archbishop told Patsy McGarry of the *Irish Times* that the NMH was not a Catholic hospital and he was not aware of demands that the new NMH should be a Catholic hospital.[68]

O'Reilly observed that the Religious Sisters of Charity had been subjected to unrelenting criticism before making their decision to withdraw from St Vincent's. He saw this as setting a dangerous precedent where religious orders would capitulate under pressure and co-operate with "the culture of death".[69] He renewed his criticism of the Sisters in the *Irish Times*. Anyone with "some degree of moral common sense" could see that the nuns' decision would facilitate legal abortions sometime in the future. There was more than a hint of moral superiority in O'Reilly's critique of the beleaguered congregation. If an unethical medical procedure was performed in the new NMH, no nun who had participated in the congregation's decision could claim that it had been unpredictable. He then urged the representatives of the Sisters "to display courage by withdrawing from any deal that is ordered to the destruction of human life".[70]

O'Reilly had raised an interesting point about the possibility of property transfer to the Vatican. A decision by a religious order to hand over ownership of hospitals or schools to the Vatican to preserve their Catholic ethos would probably generate popular resentment and outrage. Massive transfers of assets to another state – in large part created and developed through revenues derived from taxpayers and voluntary subscriptions – would hardly be in the best interests of the Church in Ireland. A probable outcome would be a greater awareness of the misdeeds of religious orders and a lack of due recognition of their contributions to a wide range of public services that were not being met by the state.

In early December 2018, controversy arose about the lack of progress in relocating the NMH. This was about eighteen months after the Religious Sisters of Charity had disclosed their intention to withdraw from the SVHG. The *Irish Catholic* reported that the Archdiocese of Dublin had been "left in the dark" about developments – if any – in setting up a completely secular St Vincent's charity. A canon lawyer, speaking on condition of anonymity, speculated that the nuns might have failed to take account of their obligations under canon law when they announced their withdrawal from the SVHG.[71] Construction work had commenced at Elm Park despite the lack of progress in transitioning from the religious to the secular. Further investment was stalled until the matter of secular ownership had been resolved. In November 2019, Peter Boylan expressed his concerns about the Elm Park development in the course of radio interviews and in his book, *In the Shadow of the Eighth*. Hospitals built on Catholic land were subject to canon law and Catholic ethics. He anticipated that the Vatican would not agree to the "alienation" of the Elm Park site from Church ownership considering that abortions, IVF and other procedures prohibited by Catholic teaching would be carried out at the hospital.[72] Boylan was well informed about how the Catholic ethos had restricted women's access to reproductive healthcare internationally, especially in the USA.[73]

On 21 November 2019 the *Irish Catholic* published a statement by the Religious Sisters of Charity. Archbishop Diarmuid Martin had consented to their decision to withdraw from the SVHG and recommended approval to the Vatican. But the repeal of the Eighth Amendment in 2018 was not well received in Rome. Fr O'Reilly believed that Ireland now had "an extremely liberal abortion regime". Fr Vincent Twomey SVD urged the Vatican to resist pressure by the Irish government on the issue. Despite this, the nuns were confident of "a positive outcome shortly".[74] On 8 May 2020 they disclosed that they had received approval from the Holy See to transfer ownership of the SVHG Group. This in turn would facilitate the transfer of the SVHG site to a new and independent charitable organisation to be named St Vincent's Holdings CLG (SVH CLG). However, this fell short of public ownership and raised important questions.[75] For example, who would own SVH CLG? What precise area of land was being transferred? Issues concerning ownership and governance of the NMH still needed to be resolved.[76]

The Vatican, through the mechanism of canon law, can still impede access in Church-owned hospitals to healthcare services that are deemed to be unethical. It can act as a brake on progress but this is likely to cause resentment against the Church in Ireland, which would ultimately prove counterproductive. Irish society has radically changed since *Humanae Vitae*. The institutional Church has failed to adapt – in so many ways. It clung tenaciously to the precepts of a medieval theology which were clearly not acceptable to most Catholics. It rejected calls for the right of priests to marry and for the rights of women to join the priesthood. All these contributed greatly to the continuous fall in religious vocations which have eroded, and will continue to erode, the power of the institutional Church in matters of public policy relating to health and education.

Endnotes

———•———

1   Maria Luddy, "'Angels of Mercy': Nuns as Workhouse Nurses, 1861–1898" in Elizabeth Malcolm and Greta Jones (eds), *Medicine, Disease and the State in Ireland, 1650–1940* (Cork: Cork University Press, 1999), pp. 102–3.

2   In the cases of St Vincent's and the Mater Misercordiae, sectarian divisions played an important role in the creation of hospital services at a time when the boards and medical staff of Dublin's voluntary hospitals were mainly Protestant. Mary E. Daly, "'An Atmosphere of Sturdy Independence': The State and the Dublin Hospitals in the 1930s" in Malcolm and Jones, op. cit., p. 236.

3   J.H. Whyte, *Church and State in Modern Ireland 1923–1979* (Dublin: Gill and Macmillan, 1984 (2nd edn)), pp. 3–4.

4   Louise Fuller, *Irish Catholicism Since 1950: The Undoing of a Culture* (Dublin: Gill and Macmillan, 2002), p. 4.

5   See Dermot Keogh, *Twentieth-Century Ireland: Nation and State* (Dublin: Gill and Macmillan, 1994), pp. 29–30, 209.

6   Sandra L. McAvoy, "Regulation of Sexuality in the Irish Free State" in Malcolm and Jones, op. cit., pp. 256–7.

7   Tom Inglis, *Moral Monopoly: The Rise and Fall of the Catholic Church in Ireland* (University College Dublin Press, 1998), pp. 226–7.

8   Judge Maureen Harding Clark, *The Lourdes Hospital Inquiry: An Inquiry into peripartum hysterectomy at Our Lady of Lourdes Hospital, Drogheda* (Dublin: Government Publications, January 2006) <http://health.gov.ie/wp-content/uploads/2014/05/lourdes.pdf> accessed 7 February 2018, p. 42. For Church teaching about "indirect sterilisation" see also Fr Dermot Hurley, *Billings Ovulation Method: A Pastoral Approach for Priests and Other Parish Workers* (London: Catholic Truth Society, 1994), p. 12.

9   Clark, *The Lourdes Hospital Inquiry*, op. cit., pp. 236, 243–7.

10 In the late 1990s it became clear to the Medical Missionaries of Mary that they would no longer have the personnel from their own ranks to continue running the hospital. They sold it to the North Eastern Health Board. Shortly thereafter a range of contraceptive services were made available and tubal ligations were undertaken. Clark, *The Lourdes Hospital Inquiry*, op. cit., pp. 43, 305. See also Joan McCarthy, "Reproductive Justice in Ireland: A Feminist Analysis of the Neary and Halappanavar Cases" in Mary Donnelly and Claire Murray (eds), *Ethical and Legal Debates in Irish Healthcare: Confronting*

Complexities (Manchester: Manchester University Press, 2016), pp. 9–23.

11 For example, Ronit Lentin, "After Savita: Migrant mothers and the politics of birth in Ireland" in Aideen Quilty, Sinéad Kennedy and Catherine Conlon (eds), *The Abortion Papers Ireland* Vol. 2 (Cork: Attic Press, 2015), p. 180.

12 Marie O'Connor, "Mutilated by brutal 'surgery of last resort'", *Sunday Independent*, 7 September 2008 <https://www.pressreader.com/ireland/sunday-independent-ireland/20080907/282071977702278> accessed 7 February 2018; and Anthea McTeirnan, "Speech for Abortion Papers Symposium, June 2013" in Quilty, Kennedy and Conlon (eds), op. cit., p. 65.

13 Judge Yvonne Murphy, *Independent Review of Issues relating to Symphysiotomy*, 11 March 2014 <http://health.gov.ie/wp-content/uploads/2014/07/Scanned-Murphy-report-redacted-version1.pdf> accessed 8 February 2018.

14 Ibid., p. 4; see also p. 5.

15 Ibid., p. 7.

16 Ibid., pp. 5, 7, 12.

17 Ibid., pp. 14–16.

18 Judge Maureen Harding Clark, *The Surgical Symphysiotomy Ex Gratia Payment Scheme*, 19 October 2016 <http://health.gov.ie/wp-content/uploads/2016/11/The-Surgical-Symphysiotomy-Ex-Gratia-Payment-Scheme-Report.pdf> accessed 8 February 2018, p. 5.

19 Ibid., pp. 15–16.

20 Ibid., pp. 20–21.

21 Ibid., pp. 10, 159.

22 Nearly 600 applications were received under the *ex gratia* payment scheme; 399 received awards – 142 for having suffered "significant disability" (ibid., pp. 10–11). In 173 cases claimants had failed to establish that they had undergone a symphysiotomy or pubiotomy (pp. 13–14). Judge Clark found that "the evidence did not confirm that symphysiotomy inevitably leads to lifelong pain or disability ... the majority of applicants who underwent a symphysiotomy made a good recovery and went on to have normal pregnancies and deliveries and to lead a full life" (p. 12).

23 Ibid., p. 34. See also Paul Cullen, "Symphysiotomy: the whitewash that never was", *Irish Times*, 23 November 2016 <https://www.irishtimes.com/opinion/symphysiotomy-the-whitewash-that-never-was-1.2878271> accessed 8 February 2018.

24 The infective organism is the human immunodeficiency virus (HIV). AIDS – acquired immunodeficiency syndrome – refers to the symptoms caused by the virus. The immune system is weakened to the point that it can no longer defend the body against infections and the disease. AIDS will cause death if left untreated.

25 Chrystel Hug, *The Politics of Sexual Morality in Ireland* (London: Macmillan Press, 1999), pp. 130–2.

26 Ibid., p. 124.

27 For an exception to this see Ann Nolan and Shane Butler, "AIDS, Sexual Health, and the Catholic Church in 1980s Ireland: A Public Health Paradox?" *American Journal of Public Health*, vol. 108, no. 7 (2018), pp. 908–13.

28 In 1994 the Mater Hospital, mindful of its Catholic ethos, banned HIV prevention leaflets and posters from its AIDS unit. Claire Hogan, "Catholic Church's influence over Irish hospital medicine persists", *Irish Times*, 28 April 2016 <http://www.irishtimes.com/opinion/catholic-church-s-influence-over-irish-hospital-medicine-persists-1.2626856> accessed 16 May 2016.

29 "Mater advisory group deferred cancer drug trial", *Irish Times*, 6 October 2005 <https://www.irishtimes.com/news/mater-advisory-group-deferred-cancer-drug-trial-1.501647> accessed 15 February 2018.

30 Eithne Donnellan, "A clash of cultures", *Irish Times*, 8 October 2005 <https://www.irishtimes.com/news/a-clash-of-cultures-1.503193> accessed 14 February 2018; and Eilish O'Regan, "Mater does U-turn on cancer trial", Independent.ie, 19 October 2005 <https://www.independent.ie/irish-news/mater-does-uturn-on-cancer-trial-25962301.html> accessed 14 February 2018.

31 Fuller, *Irish Catholicism Since 1950*, p. 260.

32 Colm Keena, "Religious congregations control health service assets worth hundreds of millions", *Irish Times*, 2 May 2017 <http://0-search.proquest.com.library.ucc.ie/docview/1893721953/fulltext/18EE7F22E2394B63PQ/31?accountid=14504> accessed 15 May 2017.

33 In 2009 there were 264 Religious Sisters of Charity. Only 15 of these were aged under 60. Their institutions included hospitals, hospices, nursing homes and counselling services, controlled through ten different companies, the biggest of which was St Vincent's Healthcare Group. Maeve Sheehan, "Hospital deal hanging in the balance as row rages about Church and State", *Sunday Independent*, 23 April 2017, p. 16.

34 Patsy McGarry, "IVF, sterilisation and morning-after pill banned by Sisters of Charity", *Irish Times*, 28 April 2017 <http://www.irishtimes.com/news/social-affairs/religion-and-beliefs/ivf-sterilisation-and-morning-after-pill-banned-by-sisters-of-charity-1.3064123> accessed 28 April 2017.

35 Families were urged to commit women or girls who were pregnant outside wedlock to these institutions. Girls and women deemed at risk suffered the same fate. Conservative religious attitudes and state collusion facilitated the admission of thousands of women to the Magdalene Laundries. The last Magdalene Laundry in Ireland closed in 1996. Several hundred women were entitled to compensation, from both the state and the religious orders. The four religious orders were the Sisters of Mercy, the Sisters of Charity, the Good Shepherd Sisters and the Sisters of Our Lady of Charity. In February 2013 the Taoiseach, Enda Kenny, issued an apology on behalf of the state and declared that the government would put in place a scheme for payment,

and other supports such as medical cards, psychological and counselling services, and other welfare needs. By November 2017 the state had paid out €25.7 million as part of a redress scheme for 682 women. Conall Ó Fátharta, "Flanagan: €25.7m paid out to 682 Magdalene Laundry survivors", *Irish Examiner*, 13 November 2017 <https://www.irishexaminer.com/ireland/flanagan-257m-paid-out-to-682-magdalene-laundry-survivors-462711.html> accessed 6 February 2018. The religious orders, including the Sisters of Charity, refused demands from the Irish government, the UN Committee on the Rights of the Child, and the UN Committee Against Torture to contribute to a redress scheme for the survivors. This was widely reported in the media. See for example, Cahir O'Doherty, "Irish religious orders confirm they will not pay Magdalene Laundry victims", *Irish Central* <https://www.irishcentral.com/news/irish-nuns-orders-confirm-they-will-not-pay-magdalene-laundry-victims> accessed 5 February 2017; and RTÉ. ie, "UN criticises religious orders over refusal to contribute to Magdalene redress fund", 23 May 2014 <https://www.rte.ie/news/2014/0523/619228-magdalene-redress/> accessed 5 February 2018.

36 Maeve Sheehan and Philip Ryan, "Revealed: the deal to curb nuns' role", *Sunday Independent*, 23 April 2017, pp. 1, 4.

37 Department of Health, "Statement from the Department of Health regarding the Governance arrangements in relation to the new National Maternity Hospital", 18 April 2017 <http://health.gov.ie/blog/press-release/statement-from-the-department-of-health-regarding-the-governance-arrangements-in-relation-to-the-new-national-maternity-hospital/>.

38 Vivienne Clarke, "National Maternity Hospital 'will be completely independent' – Mahony", *Irish Times*, 20 April 2017 <http://www.irishtimes.com/news/health/national-maternity-hospital-will-be-completely-independent-mahony-1.3055036> accessed 4 May 2017.

39 Paul Cullen, "Catholic ethos 'a red herring' for maternity hospital, says doctor", *Irish Times*, 10 May 2016 <http://www.irishtimes.com/news/health/catholic-ethos-a-red-herring-for-maternity-hospital-says-doctor-1.2641390> accessed 31 May 2017.

40 Sarah Carey, "Maternity hospital row should be over money – not the politics of fertility", *Sunday Independent*, 23 April 2017, p. 29.

41 John McManus, "Vincent's should be split up while there is a chance: The maternity hospital row was never about nuns or their Catholic ethos", *Irish Times*, 31 May 2017 <http://0-search.proquest.com.library.ucc.ie/docview/1903657551/1AD98059EE834B2DPQ/80?accountid=14504> accessed 31 May 2017. For an extensive critique of Ireland's healthcare system, see Liam Kirwan, *An Unholy Trinity: Medicine, Politics and Religion in Ireland* (Dublin: Liffey Press, 2016).

42 Patsy McGarry, "Archbishop Martin seeks removal from chair at Holles Street", *Irish Times*, 27 April 2017, p. 2. Three local parish priests were ex

officio members of the board of governors.

43   Justine McCarthy, "Bishop says new hospital must obey the church",
     Sunday Times, 23 April 2017 <https://search-proquest-com.ucc.idm.oclc.
     org/docview/1890741404/170D4D30DC054ACFPQ/2?accountid=14504>
     accessed 22 April 2018; Ciarán D'Arcy, "Catholic bishop clarifies weekend
     comments on National Maternity Hospital", *Irish Times*, 25 April 2017
     <http://www.irishtimes.com/news/health/catholic-bishop-clarifies-
     weekend-comments-on-national-maternity-hospital-1.3060692> accessed
     28 April 2017; and Órla Ryan, "Bishop says new maternity hospital should
     obey rules of Catholic Church", TheJournal.ie, 23 April 2017 <http://www.
     thejournal.ie/new-maternity-hospital-3354182-Apr2017/> accessed 28 April
     2017.

44   Ronan McGreevy and Paul Cullen, "Board of National Maternity Hospital
     reaffirms move to St Vincent's campus", *Irish Times*, 27 April 2017, p. 2;
     and Justine McCarthy and Colin Coyle, "Third master raises NMH fears",
     Sunday Times, 30 April 2017, p. 4.

45   Paul Cullen, "Nuns should hand over maternity hospital site – Coombe
     ex-master", *Irish Times*, 26 April 2017 <http://www.irishtimes.com/
     news/health/nuns-should-hand-over-maternity-hospital-site-coombe-ex-
     master-1.3061247> accessed 28 April 2017.

46   Paul Cullen, "National Maternity Hospital relocation planner resigns",
     Irish Times, 28 April 2017 <http://www.irishtimes.com/news/health/
     national-maternity-hospital-relocation-planner-resigns-1.3064217>
     accessed 28 April 2017; and "Senior doctor calls for absolute separation
     of church and medicine", RTÉ News, 2 May 2017 <https://www.rte.ie/
     news/2017/0428/871017-national-maternity-hospital/> accessed 17 February
     2018.

47   McGreevy and Cullen, op. cit.

48   Text of letter from Dr Peter Boylan to the deputy chairman of the executive
     committee of the National Maternity Hospital, 27 April 2017, accessed
     through an internet link to Paul Cullen's article, "Peter Boylan: 'I've
     been vilified by a lot of people'", *Irish Times*, 28 April 2017 <http://www.
     irishtimes.com/news/health/peter-boylan-i-ve-been-vilified-by-a-lot-of-
     people-1.3064091> accessed 28 April 2017.

49   Cullen, "Catholic ethos a 'red herring'".

50   Cullen, "Peter Boylan: 'I've been vilified by a lot of people'".

51   Kitty Holland, "Crowds protest religious ownership of new maternity
     hospital", *Irish Times*, 9 May 2017 <http://www.irishtimes.com/news/
     social-affairs/crowds-protest-religious-ownership-of-new-maternity-
     hospital-1.3074668> accessed 9 May 2017.

52   "Statement by Sr Mary Christian, Congregational Leader of the Religious
     Sisters of Charity", 31 May 2017 <https://www.associationofcatholicpriests.
     ie/2017/05/the-new-national-maternity-hospital-and-the-religious-

sisters-of-charity/> accessed 19 February 2018; and <https://static.rasset. ie/documents/news/statement-by-sr-mary-christian.pdf> accessed 24 February 2018.

53 Canon James Moriarty, letter to the editor, *Irish Times*, 30 May 2017.

54 Eoin Kelleher, letter to the editor, *Irish Times*, 30 May 2017.

55 Paul Cullen, "St Vincent's hospitals to drop Catholic guidelines", and "Decision marks a huge victory for people power", *Irish Times*, 30 May 2017, pp. 1 and 3.

56 Dearbhail McDonald, "In the name of God, we cannot let this maternity deal collapse", *Sunday Independent*, 23 April 2017, p. 29.

57 McManus, "Vincent's should be split up while there is a chance".

58 Declan Keane (clinical director at the NMH), "Maternity hospital must move with the times – so please stop misstating facts", *Irish Times*, 4 June 2017, p. 12.

59 Peter Boylan, "Big problems remain over NMH structure", *Irish Times*, 3 June 2017 <http://www.irishtimes.com/opinion/peter-boylan-big-problems-remain-over-new-nmh-structure-1.3105640> accessed 3 June 2017.

60 Cullen, "National Maternity Hospital relocation planner resigns".

61 Patsy McGarry, "Catholic archbishop has no wish to be chair of National Maternity Hospital", *Irish Times*, 1 June 2017 <http://www.irishtimes. com/news/social-affairs/religion-and-beliefs/catholic-archbishop-has-no-wish-to-be-chair-of-national-maternity-hospital-1.3104383> accessed 2 June 2017.

62 Gabriel Daly (OSA), "Catholic Ethos and Other Mysteries", Association of Catholic Priests website, 7 May 2017 <https://www. associationofcatholicpriests.ie/2017/05/catholic-ethos-and-other-mysteries/> accessed 27 February 2018.

63 Association of Catholic Priests, "The National Maternity Hospital", 10 May 2017 <https://www.associationofcatholicpriests.ie/2017/05/the-national-maternity-hospital/> accessed 27 May 2017; and Patsy McGarry, "Leading priest supports Dr Peter Boylan on new maternity hospital", *Irish Times*, 29 May 2017 <http://www.irishtimes.com/news/social-affairs/religion-and-beliefs/leading-priest-supports-dr-peter-boylan-on-new-maternity-hospital-1.3099455?mode=print&ot=example.AjaxPageLayout. ot> accessed 29 May 2017.

64 Paul Cullen, "St Vincent's must retain ownership of new maternity hospital, says chairman", *Irish Times*, 30 May 2017, p. 3.

65 Patsy McGarry, "Surprise move recognises more diverse Ireland", *Irish Times*, 30 May 2017, p. 3.

66 Dearbhail McDonald, "Don't throw baby out with the bathwater", *Sunday Independent*, 4 June 2017, p. 12.

67 Greg Daly, "Vatican urged to block hospital plan", *Irish Catholic*, 8 June

2017 <http://www.irishcatholic.ie/article/vatican-urged-block-hospital-plan> accessed 8 June 2017.

68 Patsy McGarry, "Catholic archbishop has no wish to be chair of National Maternity Hospital".

69 Daly, "Vatican urged to block hospital plan", op. cit.

70 Fr. Kevin E. O'Reilly, "Sisters of Charity must reject any NMH deal that will destroy innocent life", *Irish Times*, 13 June 2017 <http://www.irishtimes.com/opinion/sisters-of-charity-must-reject-any-nmh-deal-that-will-destroy-innocent-life-1.3117120> accessed 13 June 2017. O'Reilly's published comments were motivated by an *Irish Times* editorial which he quoted in his article. The editor had observed that "St Vincent's" – the new independent voluntary company – would be guided by "national and international best practice guidelines on medical ethics and the laws of the Republic of Ireland". He then commented that this "should allay fears that medical procedures allowed by law would not be carried out in the new NMH at St Vincent's where these may be in conflict with the teachings of the Catholic Church". Editorial: "A watershed moment", *Irish Times*, 30 May 2017, p. 13.

71 Greg Daly, "Archbishop in the dark on nuns' maternity hospital plans", *Irish Catholic*, 6 December 2018 <https://www.irishcatholic.com/archbishop-in-the-dark-on-nuns-maternity-hospital-plans/> accessed 21 November 2019.

72 "Site for new maternity hospital still under religious control – Boylan", RTE.ie, 9 November 2019 <https://www.rte.ie/news/ireland/2019/1109/1089729-national-maternity-hospital/> accessed 9 November 2019; and Boylan, *In the Shadow of the Eighth*, Chapter 21.

73 See Boylan, *In the Shadow of the Eighth*, pp. 122–3. There is a large volume of published research supportive of Boylan in relation to restrictions imposed on women's access to reproductive healthcare in Catholic-managed hospitals. See, for example: Angel M. Foster, Amanda Dennis and Fiona Smith, "Do Religious Restrictions Influence Ectopic Pregnancy Management? A National Qualitative Study", *Women's Health Issues*, issues 21–22 (2011), pp. 104–9; Lois Uttley, Sheila Reynertson, Lorraine Kenny and Louise Melling, *Miscarriage of Medicine: The Growth of Catholic Hospitals and the Threat to Reproductive Health Care* (New York: American Civil Liberties Union, and MergerWatch, 2013) <https://www.aclu.org/report/miscarriage-medicine> accessed 30 September 2019; Lori R. Freedman, and Debra B. Stulberg, "The Research Consortium on Religious Healthcare Institutions: Studying the impact of religious restrictions on women's reproductive health", *Contraception*, vol. 94 (2016), pp. 6–10.

74 Michael Kelly, "Vatican urged to block nuns' hospital transfer", *Irish Catholic*, 21 November 2019 <https://www.irishcatholic.com/vatican-urged-to-block-nuns-hospital-transfer/> accessed 22 November 2019.

75 Religious Sisters of Charity, "Religious Sisters of Charity to Gift to People of Ireland Lands at St Vincent's Healthcare Group to the Value of €200 million"

/https://rsccaritas.com/index.php/rscnews/1112-gift-to-people-of-ireland/ accessed 9 May 2020. The text of the announcement, despite its title, does not indicate a transfer of lands owned by the SVHG to public ownership.

76 Patsy McGarry, "Mixed reaction to announcement of Rome assent to transfer of site at St Vincent's", *The Irish Times*, 8 May 2020 /https:// www.irishtimes.com/news/social-affairs/religion-and-beliefs/mixed-reaction-to-announcement-of-rome-assent-to-transfer-of-site-at-st-vincent-s-1.4248635/ accessed 8 May 2020.

CHAPTER NINE

———•———

Debates About the Eighth Amendment

2016–2017

Abortion and Women's Mental Health

THREE MONTHS BEFORE THE GENERAL ELECTION IN February 2016, Enda Kenny promised that Fine Gael, if returned to power, would set up a citizens' assembly to thoroughly examine the Eighth Amendment. Any recommendations by the assembly would then be considered by the Oireachtas. Fine Gael TDs and senators would be allowed a free vote.[1] Kenny was re-elected Taoiseach on 6 May 2016 and his minority government, supported by nine independent TDs, set up the Citizens' Assembly to examine the Eighth Amendment, fixed-term parliaments, climate change and an ageing population.[2] The Eighth Amendment was addressed first. The conclusions and recommendations of the assembly were to be submitted to the Oireachtas for further debate. The assembly comprised 100 citizens including the chairperson, Supreme Court judge Ms Justice Mary Laffoy. The members, none of whom were politicians or members of advocacy groups, were selected to be broadly representative of society and entitled to vote in a referendum.

The inaugural meeting of the Citizens' Assembly was held on 15 October 2016. The Pro Life Campaign (PLC) lost no time in expressing its disapproval. The "clear purpose" of the assembly was to "pave the way for a referendum that will strip the unborn child of his or her right to life".[3] In its written submission to the assembly on 12 December 2016, the PLC warned that repeal of the Eighth Amendment would deprive the unborn of "all meaningful protections".[4] This ignored the restrictions imposed by the Protection of Life During Pregnancy Act 2013 and the probability that there were implied rights in other clauses in the Constitution that might offer some degree of protection of unborn human life.

The PLC believed that "restrictive" abortion would inevitably lead to abortion "on demand". There seemed to be many examples based on abortion trends in other countries. One in five pregnancies were aborted in the UK, France and Spain. This was thought to be about 300 per cent more than the Irish rate. Laws shaped behaviour. This was evident in, for example, wearing safety belts and not smoking in pubs and workplaces. The PLC was concerned not only to protect the right to life of the unborn but also to protect women experiencing crisis pregnancies who might make decisions that they would later come to regret.[5] The PLC argued that there was a "systemic denialism" at the centre of the repeal campaign about "the extent and strength of the peer reviewed research debunking claims" that access to abortion was beneficial to the mental health of women. The PLC stated that:

> Many peer-reviewed studies … confirm the testimony of post-abortive women that abortion itself heightens the risk of future mental health problems. And there is comprehensive longitudinal research showing that women who have abortions are more likely to commit suicide compared to all women of reproductive age.[6]

This claim, if accepted as true, would have undermined the case for repealing the Eighth Amendment. It is therefore critically important to examine the PLC's assertion in some detail on this point.

An extensive survey of published research by the Task Force on Mental Health and Abortion, set up by the American Psychological Association, found that adult women who had a legal, single, first-trimester abortion of an unwanted pregnancy for non-therapeutic reasons were not at greater risk of mental health problems than women who delivered an unwanted pregnancy. Most adult women who terminated a pregnancy did not suffer mental ill-health. The relative risk of mental health problems among women who terminated a wanted pregnancy because of foetal abnormality was no greater than that of women who miscarried a wanted pregnancy or experienced a stillbirth or the death of a newborn. Claims that mental health problems were caused by abortion were not supported by research findings. There were many complicating variables, such as "life circumstances" and personality traits, that had negative and long-term impacts regardless of how a pregnancy was resolved. Several research teams had attempted to "control for many of these factors" but frequently found it impossible to achieve this. In the USA, research pointed to negative psychological consequences following first-trimester abortion due to perceptions of stigma, the perceived need for secrecy about abortion decisions, and low social support for the abortion decision. The strongest predictor of mental ill-health following abortion was a history of mental health problems before the pregnancy.[7] The Task Force found methodological flaws – "often severe in nature" – in most of the research papers in its extensive survey.[8]

Did the PLC find any evidence from medical journals that gave reason to re-evaluate the evidence about abortion and mental health? The PLC referred to five research papers about the impact of abortion on women's mental health in its paper "The Eighth Amendment – A Life-Saving Beacon of Hope", which it submitted to the Citizens' Assembly on 16 December 2016. The research data in these papers did not give any reason for drawing different conclusions from those of the Task Force of the American Psychological Association.[9] For example, the research of Professor David Fergusson and his co-authors (2006) found that "abortion in young women may be associated with increased risks of mental health problems" – although the cause and effect link had not been established. In other words, correlation of statistical data on abortion and mental health issues did not establish a causal linkage. The authors acknowledged the major difficulty of "uncontrolled confounding", such as socio-economic conditions, family circumstances and pre-abortion mental health problems. They concluded that:

> [T]he issue of whether or not abortion has harmful effects on mental health remains to be fully resolved … There is a clear need for further well-controlled studies to examine this issue before strong conclusions can be drawn about the extent to which exposure to abortion has harmful effects on the mental health of young women.[10]

The PLC's observation associating abortion with higher suicide rates was misleading when reference was made to the research findings of Dr Mika Gissler and his co-researchers. In 2005 they concluded: "It is unlikely that induced abortion itself causes death due to injury; instead, it is more likely that induced abortions and deaths due to injury share common risk factors."[11] In 2015 Gissler and his co-researchers found that women in the aftermath of an induced abortion were exposed to a two-fold risk of suicide relative to all women of reproductive age. However, they did not interpret the data to mean that induced abortion *per se* caused a deterioration in mental health and increased suicide risk. Research data indicated that the risks for homicide and accidental death also increased after induced abortion. Furthermore, single women and those in lower socio-economic positions were over-represented among women who committed suicide or who died from other external causes after induced abortion. Statistical data did not support the hypothesis that abortion caused suicides. Gissler and his co-authors thought it more likely that the increased risk of suicide after an induced abortion was due to an external cause common to both induced abortion and suicide.[12]

It would be reasonable to assume that the PLC carefully selected scientific research papers supportive of its stance that induced abortions clearly and significantly elevated the risks of mental health and suicide. The case it made based on its selection does not withstand scrutiny. This indicates that there was not a clear and significant causal linkage between induced abortion and mental health problems.[13]

The issue of whether or not to use the term "life-limiting conditions" instead of "fatal foetal abnormalities" was a recurring theme. The PLC, and the Irish Catholic bishops, criticised the use of "fatal foetal abnormalities" in the assembly's deliberations, observing that those who used it were seeking to "normalise abortion". Medical evidence submitted to the Citizens' Assembly favoured their critique of "fatal foetal abnormalities". Dr Peter McParland (National Maternity Hospital), in his presentation to the Citizens' Assembly, stated that he and his medical colleagues avoided using the term. The word "fatal" in this context was not precisely definable. Furthermore, prenatal diagnosis in some cases gave rise to inaccurate diagnoses of anatomical abnormalities. Ultrasound, for example, could sometimes be "fuzzy."[14]

The frequency of "major" congenital abnormalities (i.e. resulting in death, severe disabilities, or in need of major surgery) was about 1–1.5 per cent. The "vast majority" of women in Ireland who received such diagnoses chose to continue their pregnancies. However, there was an increasing minority of women in these circumstances who were choosing abortion. Ongoing and anticipated advances in non-invasive prenatal testing, lower costs, and greater accessibility to such services, indicated strongly that more pregnancies in future years would be diagnosed with foetal abnormalities (such as Down syndrome, Patau syndrome and Edwards syndrome).[15]

Ms Justice Mary Laffoy acknowledged that terminology created difficulties for the assembly and that many medical practitioners did not use the term "fatal foetal abnormality" when speaking to a woman about a diagnosis. Nevertheless, the assembly would not discourage use of the term because it featured in common discourse.[16] At the same time, the assembly was aware that "life-limiting conditions" was more medically accurate. In a legal context, this was highly significant. Eileen Barrington (senior counsel) informed the assembly that the term "fatal foetal abnormalities" was open to challenge because in most, if not all, of these conditions a baby might be born alive. Although there were legal arguments to the contrary, Article 40.3.3 almost certainly precluded terminations of pregnancy in cases of fatal foetal abnormalities.[17]

A major problem with Article 40.3.3 was that it did not reflect societal consensus. There was no societal consensus on the status of human embryos and foetuses and there was not likely to be. In the absence of such consensus, how then should the legal status of embryos and foetuses be determined? Bobbie Farsides (professor of clinical and biomedical ethics, Brighton and Sussex Medical School) argued that the current legal position was problematic because it was excessively restrictive. It upheld only the most conservative sector of public opinion. The merit of changing the law in favour of a pro-choice position was that it would facilitate a broad spectrum of opinion. Those who felt strongly against abortion, many for religious reasons, were free to decline options that would be inconsistent with their moral convictions. Those who did not share such convictions would be free to choose in accordance with what they believed to be necessary and morally permissible.[18]

The assembly could choose to retain, amend or repeal Article 40.3.3. The second weekend of discussions on 7–8 January 2018 indicated that the assembly was leaning towards constitutional change.[19] The PLC accused the assembly of pursuing a biased agenda. It complained that the assembly had neglected to give due attention to the positive impact of the Eighth Amendment: thousands of lives had been saved; many parents who had considered abortion changed their minds; their children were alive because of the Eighth Amendment. Anecdotal evidence did not receive the "prominent airing" it deserved. Instead, there was undue emphasis on abortion in cases of life-limiting conditions and rape, and on criticism of the Eighth Amendment from international organisations. The PLC expressed concern about what it saw as an imbalance of speakers, objecting especially to the assembly's invitations to the British Pregnancy Advisory Service and the Guttmacher Institute (New York) – both of which had "deep roots in the abortion industry".

Credibility could only be restored if those administering the programme of the assembly focused almost entirely on the benefits of the Eighth Amendment relating to the protection of human life and dignity.[20] The word "industry" in this context was, of course, highly offensive to those who saw abortion as a healthcare service for women experiencing crisis pregnancies.[21]

The assembly's fourth weekend meeting on 4–5 March 2017 was carefully structured to give equal representation to advocacy groups and representative organisations on both sides of the abortion debate. For example, the first public session provided a platform for Doctors for Life Ireland and Doctors for Choice. The fourth public session facilitated the Pro Life Campaign, the Iona Institute, Amnesty International and the Coalition to Repeal the Eighth Amendment.

Doctors for Life Ireland invoked the first principle of medical practice – "above all … do no harm" (*primum non nocere*). In pregnancy there are two patients. Termination of pregnancy was ethically permissible only in exceptional circumstances when it was necessary to save the life of the mother. Reference was made to the *Guide to Professional Conduct and Ethics for Registered Medical Practitioners*, which states: "You have an ethical duty to make every reasonable effort to protect the life and health of pregnant women and their unborn babies." In cases where there were diagnoses of life-limiting conditions the appropriate response was palliative care, similar to cases where "other people" were terminally ill.[22]

Doctors for Choice Ireland, as the name implied, took the opposite stance, advocating the repeal of the Eighth Amendment and the decriminalisation of abortion. They saw "harm" in a different light. Article 40.3.3 harmed both women and children. Any rights attaching to unborn human life were not addressed. Doctors for Choice were "advocates" for their patients, who evidently did not include the unborn. They believed that it was unethical for a girl or woman to be compelled to sustain a pregnancy against her wishes. Furthermore, it was also unethical for a doctor to be influenced by religious beliefs when providing healthcare.

Doctors for Choice argued that legal sanctions against abortion did not prevent abortion taking place. Reference was made to an earlier presentation to the Citizens' Assembly by Dr Gilda Sedgh of the Guttmacher Institute. She and her fellow researchers found that the lowest abortion rates occurred in states with liberal abortion laws. The largest declines in abortion rates occurred in countries where abortion was "broadly" legal. This research was published in the leading peer-reviewed medical journal *The Lancet*.[23] Sedgh and her co-authors also found that limited access to contraception was an important contributory factor to abortion rates. This inverse relationship between access to contraception and the frequency of abortion also applied to states with restrictive abortion laws.

In the case of Ireland, abortion was accessible in the sense that thousands of Irish residents each year travelled abroad for terminations of pregnancy or used abortion pills in the early weeks of pregnancy. Abortion was available to women who: (1) had the financial means to travel abroad to avail of such services (most frequently to Britain); (2) were healthy enough to travel; (3) had the security of EU or Irish citizenship to travel unimpeded; or (4) were able to procure abortion pills. It was argued that Irish law promoted inequality of access to healthcare by discriminating against women who were too poor or too ill to travel, or were refugees (as in the Y Case, 2014).[24]

Doctors for Choice told the Citizens' Assembly that, internationally, there was a higher frequency of depression during pregnancy than at any other time in life. In cases of unwanted pregnancy there was a 50 per cent greater probability of postnatal depression.[25] Women were at greater risk of psychological ill health in states where abortion was stigmatised. Risks to physical health were evident when abortion pills (mifepristone and misoprostol) were taken outside carefully regulated clinical environments. Women's lives were sometimes exposed to elevated risks in hospitals because Article 40.3.3 imposed unsafe medical practices arising from legal uncertainties about when it was permissible to terminate a pregnancy.

Doctors for Choice argued, with reference to the tragic death of Savita Halappanavar, that Article 40.3.3 imposed unsafe medical practices on medical doctors in Ireland. Misinformation about abortion was a major concern – for example, that abortion increases the risk of breast cancer or elevates the risks of severe mental health problems and suicide. Peer-reviewed research papers were frequently misquoted to mislead readers and listeners. In this context Doctors for Choice referred to research papers authored by Professor David Fergusson, Dr Mika Gissler, and their collaborators (examined above).[26]

The need for a cautious and nuanced interpretation of research data made no discernible impact on the pro-life advocacy groups (such as Youth Defence) at the Citizens' Assembly.[27] Every Life Counts continually oversimplified and presented an imbalanced interpretation of scientific research in relation to diagnoses of severe foetal abnormalities. For example, it referred to the work of Astrid Guttman and her co-researchers to make the point that parents "should not be deprived of the love and joy" experienced in the usually short survival time of babies with life-limiting conditions.[28] The Guttman paper was a study of survival and surgical interventions for children diagnosed with trisomy 13 and 18. Early mortality occurred in most cases; only 10–13 per cent survived for ten years. There was very little published research data about neurocognitive development. Surgeries were "controversial". Guttman and her co-authors acknowledged several limitations to their study, the most important being "the lack of quality-of-life measures to add important context to the survival data". Information about quality of life issues was very limited and most of what was available was sourced from parental reporting. The study provided information about survival duration, but the authors observed that "measurement of quality of life in the context of major surgeries will be important to help families and clinicians balance the risks and benefits of interventions."[29]

The misrepresentation of scientific research by Every Life Counts was especially evident in the case of a paper published by Cork-based researchers Orla A. Houlihan and Keelin O'Donoghue. The advocacy group stated, in reference to Houlihan and O'Donoghue, that "96% of parents continued with the pregnancy after a diagnosis of trisomy 13 or 18."[30] The authors did indeed find that in most cases there was a tendency to continue pregnancy after diagnosis. But this should be seen in context. There was a lack of prenatal screening and anomaly scans. Diagnosis, on average, occurred at 20.5 weeks for trisomy 13, and 22 weeks for trisomy 18. Detailed second-trimester structural anomaly scans were carried out in only about 33 per cent of the cases studied. Not surprisingly the authors found that, in a "relatively high number" of cases, diagnosis of trisomy 13 and trisomy 18 occurred after birth. There was a high rate of caesarean and emergency deliveries. The authors contrasted their findings with international studies that found that up to 78 per cent of women chose elective termination after diagnosis.[31] Considering the costs, increased risks to health, and psychological stress of travelling abroad for an elective termination (as in the cases of Amanda Mellet and Siobhán Whelan), it should not be surprising that many women who had received diagnoses of trisomy 13 and 18 "chose" to continue their pregnancies.[32]

Every Life Counts pointed to two research papers to make the point that nearly 90 per cent of parents who continued their pregnancy after receiving a diagnosis of trisomy 13 or trisomy 18 experienced a "positive" outcome. Ninety-eight per cent of parents described their surviving children as "happy" and reported that these children had a positive impact on their lives and on the lives of their families.[33] The leading author of both research papers was neonatologist and clinical ethicist Dr Annie Janvier.[34] In the first paper Janvier and her colleagues acknowledged the very substantial limitations of their research. They stated that their survey was "not a representative sample of children born with T13–18". They did not collect any data about women who had chosen to terminate their pregnancy, nor on couples who had suffered foetal loss. Another limitation was that information had been obtained through self-reporting questionnaires, which were, as the authors acknowledged, inherently biased. Finally, the authors acknowledged that most women with trisomy 13 and trisomy 18 diagnoses chose to terminate their pregnancies and that their decisions were probably consistent with the opinions of many physicians.[35] In the second paper Janvier and her co-researchers acknowledged similar limitations. Their findings, therefore, were to be interpreted "with caution". Furthermore, they recommended that prenatal counselling should be informative and non-directive to help parents make decisions in accordance with their values.[36]

Scientific research, when closely examined, was not supportive of arguments that Article 40.3.3 served to protect the health of pregnant women. A survey of literature cited by pro-life advocacy groups revealed tentative findings, uncertainties and complexities that pointed to the need for further extensive research before any reliable conclusions could be reached.

The Iona Institute approached science from a different angle from that of Every Life Counts. It observed that those who sought to legalise abortion refused to "acknowledge the humanity of the child" and were wilfully ignorant of what science could reveal. The "baby in the womb" was a human being. It was undeniably human – apparently a source of unease for those who sought to liberalise abortion law. But was it a person? The Iona Institute argued that definitions of "personhood" were all too frequently proposed to exclude unborn human life. Having raised this important point, the institute summarily dismissed personhood as a "subjective concept". The "human" property of unborn life was "much more objective" and was deemed sufficient to elevate it to a level deserving of "fundamental rights" and therefore worthy of constitutional protection. It followed from this that it was wrong to hold a referendum to remove Article 40.3.3 from the Constitution.[37] But was the right to life of embryos and foetuses a fundamental right? If the will of the majority was to be overturned because of the need to defend fundamental rights it led to the question: What institution or sector of society has the moral credentials or status to define such rights? The Iona Institute did not address this question.

A consequence of addressing the issue of abortion in terms of fundamental rights rather than seeking to balance competing rights was that it tended to close off debate rather than enhance it. It was both conceptually neat and philosophically weak. A similar approach was taken with the biomedical sciences, which were, in effect, marginalised. Science was invoked to emphasise that the embryo or foetus was human and was then dismissed. There was no ethical discussion in relation to the gradual development of neural networks, brainwaves, sentience, or the gradual emergence of mental faculties.[38]

The Iona Institute expressed the view that the expert testimonies of invited speakers had pushed the Citizens' Assembly towards an emphasis on the "supposed problems" of Article 40.3.3 and the rights of women – with little consideration given to the rights of the unborn. Questions put to the delegates exacerbated this tendency. The Iona Institute's presentation to the Citizens' Assembly was very much in harmony with that of the Irish Catholic bishops. The bishops too spoke about the "fundamental right" to life of the unborn arising from his or her status as a person. Although the state did not have the power to "give" a right to life, Article 40.3.3 was important because it prevented parliament from enacting legislation that would diminish or eliminate the benefits of such a right. The bishops maintained that Article 40.3.3 upheld an appropriate balance of rights between the mother and her unborn child.[39]

Archbishop Eamon Martin, Primate of All Ireland, assured his audience at an Iona Institute conference that the Catholic Church did not wish to create a theocratic state in Ireland. What the Church did wish for was an important role in a pluralist democratic state. Faith would be impoverished if it was compartmentalised and confined to the private sphere. Exclusion of faith from "the public square" would not serve society well because the concept of the common good and the understanding of human nature would both be diminished. Catholics and all people of goodwill were called upon to speak out in public debate about abortion and several other issues relating to social justice and human rights.[40]

There was no reason to doubt the goodwill of all members of the Citizens' Assembly. The majority were probably Roman Catholic – even so, they were not swayed by the bishops or by the Iona Institute when they voted on a series of recommendations on 22–23 April 2017. An overwhelming majority – 87 per cent – voted that "Article 40.3.3 should not be retained in full." Fifty-seven per cent voted in favour of replacing Article 40.3.3 with a constitutional provision that would explicitly enable the Oireachtas to legislate to address terminations of pregnancy, any rights of pregnant women, and any rights of the unborn. A majority of members approved of twelve reasons for the legal termination of pregnancy.[41] The outcome of the assembly's deliberations was surprisingly liberal.

It was highly questionable whether the assembly was representative of public opinion. An *Irish Times*/Ipsos MRBI opinion poll of 1,200 voters at 100 sampling points, and in all constituencies, indicated that only 16 per cent were against repeal or replacement of Article 40.3.3. However, it also indicated that any change to the Constitution would have to be very restrictive if it was to be carried in a referendum.[42] Another *Irish Times*/Ipsos MRBI poll, published on 27 May, indicated strong majorities in favour of abortion legislation for cases when there was a serious threat to the physical and mental health of the mother, and in cases of rape or diagnoses of "fatal" foetal abnormality. The opinion poll indicated a large gap between the assembly's recommendations and the opinions of voters.

Divergences between public opinion and the assembly's findings were open to exploitation by defenders of the Eighth Amendment, who could point to "the slippery slope" leading to increasing liberalisation. If campaigners for repeal were to succeed they needed to avoid pressing their demands too far. Attention needed to be given to nuanced opinions. Furthermore, firm assurances from government were required on the scope of intended legislation.[43] The outcome of a referendum to retain, amend or repeal Article 40.3.3 depended very much on how each side responded to the concerns of "middle ground" voters. A contributor to the *Irish Times* observed that the central question about abortion was: At what point in gestation did the unborn become "a person with the right to life"? Pro-life extremists, mainly conservative Catholics, saw the right to life from conception onwards. Pro-choice extremists focused entirely on the rights of women, ignored the rights of the unborn or were dismissive of such rights. Most people, it seemed, believed that the right to life was applicable sometime after conception and at some point before birth.[44] The Citizens' Assembly had conceded much to the pro-choice movement. It seemed that any proposals by the government for constitutional and legislative changes would have to be more restrictive than the assembly's recommendations.[45]

Medical Evidence against the Eighth Amendment

The Joint Committee on the Eighth Amendment of the Constitution was set up to review the recommendations of the Citizens' Assembly. Its 22 members comprised sixteen TDs and six senators. The chairperson was Senator Catherine Noone of Fine Gael. The committee worked to a tight schedule and it met in public session from September to December 2017. In addition to considering the recommendations of the Citizens' Assembly, the committee received written and oral submissions from medical and legal experts and from advocacy groups including the Center for Reproductive Rights (based in New York) and One Day More. Attention here will be given to the medical expertise informing the committee's deliberations because it is of crucial importance in considering the balance of rights between mothers and foetuses.

Professor Fergal Malone, Master of the Rotunda Hospital (Dublin) and consultant obstetrician, attended to give evidence on 11 October 2017. He also represented the Royal College of Surgeons in Ireland as chairman of its department of obstetrics and gynaecology. Although he told the committee that he was not an advocate for "pro-choice" or "pro-life", his evidence clearly pointed towards the need to repeal the Eighth Amendment. When parents were given a diagnosis of a fatal foetal abnormality they had the option of continuing the pregnancy with access to perinatal palliative care. Those who chose to terminate their pregnancy had to travel to another jurisdiction. These patients did not enjoy continuity of care and were therefore exposed to increased risks to health while travelling, especially arising from haemorrhage and infection. One patient had already died on such a journey to Britain.[46]

Malone expressed a belief widely held by doctors that they should be able to provide appropriate healthcare for their patients without having to consider the possibility of a criminal conviction in cases of termination of pregnancy. He advised politicians against simple legislative initiatives. It was not advisable to draw up a list of foetal anomalies as grounds for termination. Lists of foetal diagnoses would change over time. An individual abnormality that might not be considered "lethal" might frequently be fatal when associated with other abnormalities.[47] Multiple abnormalities were sometimes diagnosed. Malone also advised against specifying precise gestational age limits in legislation. Viability was not precisely predictable and it was likely to change over time. In view of the complexity and variability that arose from one patient to another, Malone believed that decisions about termination were best left to patients and their doctors and should not be restricted by arbitrary legal cut-off points.

Malone's evidence was followed by that of Dr Rhona Mahony, then master of the National Maternity Hospital, one of the largest maternity hospitals in Europe. She pointed to the adverse impact of the law on clinical decision-making arising from the Eighth Amendment. Her reference to the *P.P. v Health Service Executive* case (2014) supported her point that medico-legal interpretations of the Eighth Amendment distorted or obstructed clinical judgement and could do so again.[48] Termination of pregnancy was legal if there was a substantial risk to the life of the mother which could be eliminated only by terminating the pregnancy. Clinicians and their patients were exposed to the risk of a custodial sentence of up to fourteen years if there was an error in clinical judgement. The process of determining whether or not a termination should be carried out was too "cumbersome and complicated". There was an underlying assumption that risks of maternal death could be predicted with precision – this was not true. Mahony argued that doctors should be allowed to err on the side of caution to ensure the safety of women. It was not good medical practice to allow a woman to become so ill that she was clearly at risk of dying before a termination of pregnancy could be carried out.[49]

Women were sometimes exposed to avoidable risk because of legal considerations. For example, if the waters around a foetus break at about fourteen weeks' gestation, the baby is very unlikely to survive. But doctors were required to wait until infection or chorioamnionitis developed before they could intervene. Termination was carried out when the risk of maternal death, due to infection, rose to a level deemed "significant". Another example of avoidable risk was in the case of conjoined twins where "significant organs" were shared and there was no prospect of survival. In such cases, where pregnancies were allowed to proceed, high-risk caesarean surgery was unavoidable. Mahony's evidence to the committee probably represented mainstream thinking amongst obstetricians and gynaecologists. She informed the committee that the council of the Royal College of Obstetricians and Gynaecologists voted strongly in support of removing criminal sanctions associated with abortion in Britain. Termination of pregnancy should be subject to regulatory and professional standards, in common with other medical procedures.[50]

Senator Rónán Mullen, well known for his pro-life views, was sceptical about the weight of medical evidence against the Eighth Amendment. Even in Britain, criminal law was in place to restrict abortion. The case for a harsh legal deterrent seemed to be justified to protect society against rogue doctors. No doctor had been prosecuted for carrying out an illegal abortion in Ireland. Senator Mullen then argued that, if Malone and Mahony could not find any cases where doctors had been prosecuted, it seemed that the law was well balanced in relation to the management of risks in clinical practice. But Mullen misunderstood the conditions under which medical doctors had to make decisions. Both Mahony and Malone argued that clinicians were constrained by law from acting in the best interests of their patients. The reason why no doctor had been prosecuted was because doctors generally worked within the law, even when it was contrary to their clinical judgement.[51] Mullen, despite the weight of medical evidence, did not concede that the Eighth Amendment was excessively restrictive on the judgement of doctors.

The assessment of risk was not just a matter for doctors – it was an issue for doctors in consultation with parents. Dr Peter Boylan, chairman of the Institute of Obstetricians and Gynaecologists, emphasised the importance of the woman's role in the management of pregnancy. It was their lives that were at risk. Some women would accept high risks to continue a pregnancy. A mother of four children might not wish to sustain a pregnancy if doing so would exacerbate her diabetes, which would in turn cause further irreversible damage to her eyes and kidneys. A woman who, after years of IVF, is pregnant for the first time, might be willing to accept that risk. The doctor's clinical assessment of risk was not all that mattered. It was also critically important to consider the woman's assessment of the risk for her personally.[52]

Boylan believed that Article 40.3.3 presented major difficulties for doctors, which in turn worked against the best interests of their patients. He had served as an independent expert witness for the coroner in the inquest into the death of Savita Halappanavar and had been an expert witness for the family in the case of *P.P. v Health Service Executive* (2014). These cases were presented as examples to make the point that doctors were inappropriately put in a position where they had to interpret the Constitution in the course of treating their patients. Boylan acknowledged that there were deficiencies in the care of Savita Halappanavar. But if her request for a termination of pregnancy in the first few days of her admission to hospital had been acceded to, she would not have died of sepsis and septic shock.

Professor Sabaratnam Arulkumaran's evidence was supportive of Boylan's. He was certain that, in the Halappanavar case, legal considerations delayed termination, despite all the medical indications pointing towards the need to terminate without delay to save the mother. Arulkumaran was president-elect of the International Federation of Obstetrics and Gynaecology and the leading author of a Health Service Executive report (June 2013) on the death of Savita Halappanavar. He acknowledged Ireland's excellent record concerning low maternal mortality rates. This point had frequently been made by defenders of the Eighth Amendment to bolster their case that it did not unduly restrict doctors in caring for their patients. However, Arulkumaran pointed to the thousands of Irish women who travelled abroad every year as an important factor in Ireland's ranking of sixth in the world for low maternal mortality rates. If Irish women were unable to procure legal abortions in Britain, a probable increase in illegal abortions might result in a global ranking of twentieth or fortieth for Ireland.[53]

Three of the committee's twenty-two members – Senator Rónán Mullen, Mattie McGrath TD (independent) and Peter Fitzpatrick TD (Fine Gael) were strong advocates for the retention of the Eighth Amendment. McGrath referred to the research paper by Heidi Cope and her colleagues in *Prenatal Diagnosis* (see Chapter 7) to make the point that women who chose abortion after a diagnosis of anencephaly were more likely to suffer depression than those women who chose to continue their pregnancy.[54] He asked Professor Malone if he was familiar with this study and if it influenced his clinical practice. Malone, an experienced researcher and author of many research papers, replied that he had read the article and was not impressed by its findings: the research methodology was flawed; and sufficient care had not been taken to avoid bias in the recruitment of patients for the study.[55]

The medical evidence submitted to the committee persuaded most of its members that Article 40.3.3 was an impediment to best medical practice. On 18 October 2017 they agreed "in principle" that "Article 40.3.3 should not be retained in full." Irish law on abortion was not fit for purpose.[56] This recommendation was almost inevitable and reflected public opinion.[57] The committee members had considered medical and legal evidence in relation to: (1) the adverse impact of Article 40.3.3 on the provision of medical services to pregnant women, especially in relation to the timing of critical clinical decisions where women's lives were at risk; (2) the Mellet and Whelan cases in which the UN Human

Rights Committee had found Ireland to be in breach of its obligations under the International Covenant on Civil and Political Rights; and (3) the reality of abortion where thousands of Irish women were travelling to Britain every year or were inducing abortion at home through the use of abortion pills without medical supervision and support.[58]

Mullen described the committee's proceedings as "a farcical and cynical process". A clear indication of bias was the "thorough preponderance of witnesses-invitees in favour of abortion".[59] However, it seems that both Mullen and McGrath were less than co-operative with their fellow committee members in the selection of witnesses.[60] Members were asked to propose witnesses, but they were required to justify their choice and provide evidence of expertise, including published research work. Further justification had to be offered if the person was travelling from abroad. Professor Monique Chireau, an obstetrician–gynaecologist at Duke University Medical Center, North Carolina, was proposed by McGrath. Yet it seems that neither McGrath nor Mullen provided any justification for the attendance of Chireau, despite several requests from Senator Noone. Furthermore, they informed the *Irish Times* that it was not their role to select witnesses – it was the role of the chairperson and the committee staff.[61]

Claims of bias were made against the committee by Mullen and McGrath.[62] Bishop Kevin Doran of Elphin (chairman of the Catholic Bishops' Consultative Group on Bioethics) expressed support for those who declined to speak before a committee that had apparently already reached a decision on the issue under discussion.[63] The committee was under pressure to complete its work by 20 December at the latest.[64] Senator Noone acknowledged that the committee was experiencing difficulties in finding pro-life experts to attend as witnesses.[65] Pro-life experts were found, but persuading them to attend seems to have been the main problem. Patricia Casey (professor of psychiatry, University College Dublin, and consultant psychiatrist at the Mater Misericordiae University Hospital) received an invitation from the committee but made a decision not to attend before the vote on Article 40.3.3. She was applauded for her decision at a conference entitled *Abortion, Disability and the Law*, jointly organised by the Anscombe Bioethics Centre (UK) and the Consultative Group on Bioethics of the Irish Catholic Bishops' Conference.[66]

The vote not to retain Article 40.3.3 "in full" is significant in the above context. Gerry Whyte, professor of law at Trinity College Dublin, was one of three main speakers at the *Abortion, Disability and the Law* conference. He pointed out that repealing the word "equal" in the clause would remove the equivalence between the right to life of the mother and the right to life of the unborn. This would have a lesser impact than full deletion. Some constitutional rights of the unborn would still be retained. He pointed out that the joint Oireachtas committee was considering the option of replacing the text in Article 40.3.3 with text providing for abortion on a broader basis and/or giving expression to a rebalancing of rights.[67] It was not as if the committee had closed off options for meaningful discussion. And yet there seemed to be a persistent misunderstanding on this point, referred to by both Senator Noone and Billy Kelleher TD (Fianna Fáil) at the committee meeting on 8 November 2017. They emphasised the difference between repealing the Eighth Amendment and not retaining it in full, against a background where the credibility of the committee was continually called into question from outside, and from within its own ranks by McGrath and Mullen.[68]

Pro-life activists persisted in their attempts to undermine the credibility of the committee, taking advantage of its difficulties in persuading pro-life witnesses to attend. It is likely that they contributed to the committee's problem of balancing pro-life and pro-choice speakers by discouraging attendance of pro-life witnesses. Potential speakers who were pro-life would be less likely to attend a committee meeting if they thought that it was heavily biased towards pro-choice. Cora Sherlock of the Pro Life Campaign (PLC) claimed that the committee had invited twenty-four "abortion advocates" and only four "pro-life" speakers. This bias was compounded by the committee's vote not to fully retain the Eighth Amendment "before they had even heard from half of their invited witnesses". The committee had "voted for abortion with no intention of reconsidering its stance". It then "scrambled to invite pro-life witnesses … in an attempt to create a false perception of balance". Sherlock concluded that potential pro-life witnesses were aware of duplicity at the heart of the committee's proceedings and would not facilitate it. The committee's reputation was ruined beyond repair.[69]

Assertions of bias elicited an angry response. Committee member Senator Lynn Ruane said, "If all the evidence is stacked against you, the easiest thing to claim is bias. It does not mean it is true. This is part of an orchestrated campaign to undermine the work of the committee."[70] The committee indicated in its report that it had not reached an irrevocable decision on 18 October when it stated that no evidence adduced in the course of its later deliberations persuaded it to change its opinion about the need for constitutional reform.[71]

Some medical evidence – or perhaps the lack of it, depending on one's perspective – did seem to favour arguments put forward by senators Mullen and McGrath. McGrath questioned Dr Mahony on exactly how the Eighth Amendment restricted doctors in providing the best care for their patients. The fear of prosecution by doctors, it seemed, had been exaggerated. The proceedings of the Joint Committee on Health and Children (8 January 2013), of which McGrath was a member, indicated that Mahony and "other obstetricians" were, at that meeting, unable to refer to any case where an avoidable maternal death had occurred when doctors had felt unable to intervene to save the mother's life due to Article 40.3.3. Fifteen obstetricians who had practised in Ireland wrote to the committee strongly disagreeing with Mahony about doctors' fears of prosecution.[72] A balanced reference to Mahony's evidence to the Joint Committee would have taken account of her concerns about the lack of accurate data, especially in relation to the many thousands of undocumented cases of women travelling abroad for terminations of pregnancy. Mahony had also referred to the inadequacies of sections 58 and 59 of the Offences Against the Person Act 1861, which was the operative law at the time.[73] Also, there was strong medical evidence to indicate that Michelle Harte, diagnosed with a malignant melanoma and in the early stages of pregnancy in 2010, might have survived if there had been no legal impediment to the continuance of her cancer treatment in Ireland.[74]

Protagonists on both sides of the debate agreed that the tragic case of Savita Halappanavar was an avoidable maternal death but disagreed on whether or not Article 40.3.3 was a contributing factor. Boylan wrote to the committee on 25 October 2017 pointing out that Mullen had made "several assertions at odds with the facts". Mullen had claimed that Halappanavar's consultant obstetrician, Dr Katherine Astbury, "was in no way constrained by the Eighth Amendment" – contrary to the evidence by both Professor Sabaratnam Arulkumaran and Boylan himself. He then referred to the transcript of the inquest (third day) into Halappanavar's death, which seemed to support this point.[75] Boylan referred to questions 176 to 179 inclusive. It is clear from Astbury's responses that she did indeed feel constrained by Irish law and was unable to facilitate Halappanavar's request for a termination.[76] But Mullen counterargued with reference to the same text of the inquest. Dr Astbury, unaware of some of the patient's symptoms which had been observed earlier, believed that Halappanavar was "not physically unwell".[77] Termination was illegal in the absence of a threat to the mother's life.[78] Apparently, the failure to save Halappanavar was due to deficiencies in her medical care – not due to Irish law.

It seemed also that the opinions of Dr Boylan had been over-rated. Mullen referred to the letter published in the *Irish Times* on 1 May 2013 signed by eleven medical consultants (including eight obstetricians) who had been critical of Boylan's expert testimony in the Halappanavar case. It is difficult to avoid the conclusion here that Mullen's intention was to mislead the committee by a deliberate omission of evidence when he failed to take account of Boylan's response to his critics on 2 May 2013 (see Chapter 7).

Some key findings in the Halappanavar case were not given due emphasis. Medical evidence to the committee left little doubt that Irish law had contributed to the death of Savita Halappanavar.[79] Arulkumaran told the committee on 18 October that it was "very clear" to him in the course of the enquiry that

> [T]he thing preventing the physician from proceeding was the legal issue because she repeatedly said she was concerned about the legal issue … the mother was sick. There was no question about that. Even at the last minute they were using a hand probe to see whether the baby's heartbeat was present or not. Any junior doctor would have said it was a serious condition and they must terminate. They were just keeping her going because of the mere fact that the heartbeat was there. The legislation played a major role in making a decision.[80]

Mullen, in his reply to Boylan, did not address the points raised by Arulkumaran's evidence to the committee. Arulkumaran was chairman of a team that had investigated the death of Savita Halappanavar and was the leading author of a subsequent report published by the Health Services Executive in June 2013. In that report Arulkumaran and his co-authors strongly recommended that members of the Oireachtas should consider changes to the law, including constitutional change, concerning the management of inevitable miscarriages in the early second trimester of pregnancy, especially in relation to ruptures of the chorion and amnion (membranes that surround the foetus).[81]

Risks to the mental health of pregnant women received attention from the committee on 25 October. Veronica O'Keane (professor of clinical psychiatry at Trinity College Dublin and consultant psychiatrist at Tallaght Hospital) observed that the majority of Irish voters had upheld the risk of suicide as a legitimate reason for abortion in 1992 and in 2002. She expressed approval of the decision by the Citizens' Assembly not to distinguish between mental and physical health. She agreed with the assembly's finding that Irish law should allow for the unpredictability of risks associated with psychiatric and obstetric care and concluded that the Eighth Amendment needed to be removed from the Constitution. However, her opinion that "the mental health of everybody in Ireland is being damaged by the eighth amendment because we are all shamed by the current situation" was clearly unsustainable. Mattie McGrath pointed to the thousands of people who had marched in Dublin in support of the Eighth Amendment and whose mental health was clearly not harmed. The implication, of course, was that a much larger number of Irish voters, who did not openly express their intentions to vote for retention, did not suffer any ill-health due to the Eighth Amendment. Still, McGrath failed to challenge O'Keane on the important issues she raised in support of repeal.[82]

The issue of terminating pregnancies in cases of rape was one of the major arguments for repealing or amending Article 40.3.3. Rape as grounds for the right to abortion was fraught with intractable legal difficulties. Tom O'Malley (senior lecturer in law at the National University of Ireland, Galway) had elaborated on these in his submission to the Citizens' Assembly on 4 February 2017. For example, prosecution proceedings were far too long. It was not uncommon for two or three years to elapse between the occurrence of an alleged offence and the final verdict in a criminal trial. What standard of proof would be required? Should the Gardaí be involved?[83] On 25 October 2015 O'Malley informed the Oireachtas Committee that some jurisdictions did allow abortion in cases of rape. The legal complexities that might otherwise arise were avoided because of a general access to abortion in the early months of pregnancy in many of these jurisdictions.[84]

Evidence presented to the committee on the issue of rape pointed to a pressing need to broaden access to abortion. Dr Maeve Eogan (consultant obstetrician and gynaecologist at the Rotunda Hospital, Dublin) informed the committee that about 5 per cent of women who attended an Irish Rape Crisis Centre in 2015 became pregnant as a result of rape. Many victims of sexual violence did not tell anyone about it for a broad range of reasons, including shame, self-blame, fear of judgement and lack of information. In cases where women did report rape shortly after the offence there was no physical examination that reliably demonstrated the absence of consent.[85] Dr Eogan's evidence to the committee was corroborated by that of Ms Noeline Blackwell, chief executive of the Dublin Rape Crisis Centre. Reporting rape to access abortion was not as straightforward as it seemed. There was a "massive under-reporting of rape". Many women who contacted the Dublin Rape Crisis Centre were not ready to inform the Gardaí "for a long time, if ever". Imposing a requirement to report rape to access abortion presented a risk of re-traumatising and re-victimising a woman. It placed them in vulnerable circumstances where they had to convince someone that their account of events justified access to support.

As observed earlier, the committee was due to report to both Houses of the Oireachtas by 20 December in compliance with its terms of reference. On 13 December it voted on various aspects of the abortion issue. The vote to simply repeal the Eighth Amendment (repeal *simpliciter*, i.e. with no replacement text) was passed by fourteen votes to six.[86] The Citizens' Assembly, in contrast, had voted that "Article 40.3.3 should not be retained in full" and that a new constitutional provision should enable the Oireachtas to legislate for the termination of pregnancy. The *Report of the Joint Committee on the Eighth Amendment of the Constitution* (December 2017) clearly indicates that the committee was very much influenced by the evidence from experts in healthcare and law. For example, the committee did not differentiate between the life and health of the mother because medical evidence presented to the committee pointed to the difficulties medical specialists experienced in defining when a threat to health escalated to become a threat to life. Therefore, the committee recommended that termination of pregnancy should be legally permissible when the life or health of the woman is at risk and that no distinction should be drawn between the mental and physical health of the woman.[87]

The committee acknowledged that, in cases of pregnancy caused by rape "or other sexual assault", the requirement for evidence would present major difficulties and might be unworkable in practice. The under-reporting of rape and the need to avoid the further traumatisation of victims were strong influencing factors. The committee therefore recommended that termination of pregnancy should be lawful "with no restriction as to reason" through a GP-led service with a gestational limit of 12 weeks.[88] This recommendation was also put forward in response to the unsupervised use of abortion pills procured through the internet and to address the needs of women who for financial or domestic reasons, or due to immigration status, were unable to procure abortion pills through the internet, or could not travel.[89]

The committee had heard medical evidence from Professor Fergal Malone on 11 October, and from Mr Peter Thompson, a consultant in foetal medicine at Birmingham's Women's and Children's Hospital (UK) on 29 November. Thompson, in common with Malone, urged the committee not to make a list of "fatal" or "lethal" conditions. There was no consensus among medical experts about what "lethal" means. Furthermore, ongoing progress in the medical sciences would require regular adjustments to the list. Generally, a diagnosis was not "a binary state of affairs" but rather a medical assessment of risks and probabilities. Most of the foetal anomalies were chromosomal or were abnormalities of the central nervous system. There was a strong case to be made for the exclusion of gestational limits if abortion was legally permitted. Many diagnoses were made very late in pregnancies. Anomaly scans were carried out at about 20 weeks' gestation. Sometimes an additional "local" scan was carried out to confirm a specific diagnosis. Also, women needed time to come to terms with the information and make their decisions.

Thompson informed the committee that, in Britain, Clause E of the Abortion Act 1967 permitted termination of pregnancies in cases where "there is a substantial risk that if the child were born it would suffer from such physical or mental abnormalities as to be seriously handicapped". The medical profession was given discretion to decide the meaning of "substantial" and "serious". In 2016 an estimated 140 women from Ireland (from a total of 3,265) had terminations under Clause E of the Act.[90] The committee was clearly guided by the evidence of Malone and Thompson when it recommended that "it shall be lawful to terminate a pregnancy without gestational limit where the child has a foetal abnormality that is likely to result in death before or shortly after birth."[91]

The committee reached a different conclusion about foetal abnormalities that were not likely to cause death before or shortly after birth, such as Down syndrome.[92] Unlike the Citizens' Assembly, the committee recommended against the termination of pregnancy in cases where "significant" foetal abnormalities were not likely to lead to death.[93] Another point of difference with the Citizens' Assembly was the recommendation by the committee that termination of pregnancy, for socio-economic reasons, should not be lawful after 12 weeks.[94]

The Pro Life Campaign was blunt – and misleading – in its condemnation of the recommendations of the Oireachtas Committee. The committee's recommendations were presented simply as an advocacy for "abortion on demand". Its objection against abortion "up to birth on health grounds that are not and cannot be defined" took no account of the medical evidence submitted concerning assessments of risks to patients and the threat of prosecution hanging over doctors which sometimes proved inimical to best clinical practice.[95] The government, of course, was not bound to accept the committee's report, but it had indicated that it would be guided by the recommendations.

Undermining the credibility of the Citizens' Assembly and the Oireachtas Committee would have been a major victory for the pro-life campaign. In late February 2018 a recruitment anomaly relating to the Citizens' Assembly came to light when the polling company Red C carried out an internal audit and suspended one of its employees. Niamh Uí Bhriain, representing Save the 8th, viewed the assembly as "an unrepresentative sham". Cora Sherlock, speaking for the Pro Life Campaign, called for an independent audit of how members were recruited and claimed that there was an issue of public confidence to be addressed. However, the concerns of Uí Bhriain and Sherlock were groundless. Ms Justice Mary Laffoy observed that the anomaly in question had occurred after the assembly had submitted its report on the Eighth Amendment to the Oireachtas.[96]

Allegations of bias were levelled against the Oireachtas Committee on the basis that no medical expert had attended the proceedings to argue against abortion. Senator Catherine Noone informed the *Irish Times* that GPs and consultants were contacted by the committee membership and secretariat to make the case for retention of the Eighth Amendment on medical grounds. Not one of them was willing to come forward![97] The failure to persuade any pro-life doctor to appear before the committee lent credence to the assertion that the committee was biased. A contributor to the *Irish Times* found it "astonishing" that no doctor in favour of retaining the status quo had attended the committee's proceedings, considering that Dr Orla Halpenny gave a presentation to the Citizens' Assembly on behalf of Irish Doctors for Life.[98] A substantial number of doctors were clearly opposed to repealing the Eighth Amendment.[99] The problem was not finding such doctors – it was persuading them to attend the committee's proceedings. Dr Orla Halpenny wrote to the *Irish Times* on 24 February confirming this. Doctors for Life had received an invitation but had declined to attend on the basis that the committee had already voted to "recommend repealing the Eighth Amendment".[100] This was almost certainly untrue.[101] The committee, as observed earlier, had voted on 18 October 2017 to recommend that "Article 40.3.3 should not be retained in full" – a far less radical proposal than simple repeal. It voted to recommend simple repeal on 13 December – only seven days before the completion of its report.

Allegations of bias against both the Citizens' Assembly and the Oireachtas Committee did not impact significantly on public opinion. A much more important question in early 2018 was whether or not their recommendations were more than a step too far for most of the electorate, who seemed to favour constitutional and legal reforms only in favour of "hard cases".

Endnotes

—————•—————

1   RTÉ, "Taoiseach would call forum on abortion if re-elected", 27 November 2015 <https://www.rte.ie/news/2015/1127/749698-abortion/> accessed 4 December 2018.

2   For a study of the Citizens' Assembly in the context of deliberative democracy and referendums, see David M. Farrell, Jane Suiter, and Clodagh Harris, "'Systematizing' Constitutional Deliberation: The 2016–18 citizens' assembly in Ireland, *Irish Political Studies*, vol. 34, issue 1 (2019), pp. 113–23.

3   Pro Life Campaign, "PLC will mount reasoned and robust defence of 8th Amendment" <http://prolifecampaign.ie/main/portfolio/detail/15-10-16-plc-will-mount-reasoned-robust-defence-8th-amendment/> accessed 19 February 2017.

4   Pro Life Campaign, "The Eighth Amendment – A Life-Saving Beacon of Hope: Submission to the Citizens' Assembly" 16 December 2016 <https://www.citizensassembly.ie/en/Submissions/Submissions-Received/> accessed 14 March 2017.

5   Pro Life Campaign: "PLC submission highlights lives saved by the Eighth Amendment" <http://prolifecampaign.ie/main/portfolio/detail/16-12-16-plc-submission-highlights-lives-saved-eighth-amendment/> accessed 19 February 2017; and "The Eighth Amendment – A Life-Saving Beacon of Hope".

6   Pro Life Campaign, "The Eighth Amendment – A Life-Saving Beacon of Hope".

7   Brenda Major *et al.*, "Abortion and Mental Health: Evaluating the evidence", *American Psychologist*, vol. 64, issue 9 (2009) <http://web.a.ebscohost.com.ucc.idm.oclc.org/ehost/detail/detail?vid=3&sid=79664021-f9b0-4e81-87a5-2972aa6ae1bd%40sessionmgr4007&bdata=JnNpdGU9ZWhvc3QtbGl2ZQ%3d%3d#AN=2009-23092-001&db=pdh> accessed 5 May 2018; and American Psychological Association, "Mental Health and Abortion: Overview" <http://www.apa.org/pi/women/programs/abortion/index.aspx> accessed 2 May 2018.

8   *Report of the APA Task Force on Mental Health and Abortion*, American Psychological Association, 2008 <http://www.apa.org/pi/women/programs/abortion/mental-health.pdf> accessed 2 May 2018; and "Mental Health and Abortion: Overview".

9   The research papers referred to by the PLC were published in the years

2005–2015. The paper by Heidi Cope *et al.* has already been commented on in the previous chapter in relation to the pro-life organisation Every Life Counts. Heidi Cope, Melanie E. Garrett, Simon G. Gregory, and Allison E. Ashley-Koch, "Pregnancy Continuation and Organizational Religious Activity Following Prenatal Diagnosis of a Lethal Fetal Defect is Associated with Improved Psychological Outcome", *Prenatal Diagnosis*, vol. 35, no. 8 (April 2015).

10   David M. Fergusson, John Horwood and Elizabeth M. Ridder, "Abortion in Young Women and Subsequent Mental Health", *Journal of Child Psychology and Psychiatry*, vol. 47, no. 1 (2006), quotations from pp. 16 and 23. In a more extensive longitudinal study Professor Fergusson and his fellow researchers concluded that: "Although the weight of evidence favours the view that abortion has a small causal effect on mental health problems, other explanations remain possible. In particular it could be suggested that the small association between abortion and mental health found in this study could be explained by uncontrolled residual confounding." David M. Fergusson, John Horwood and Joseph M. Boden, "Abortion and Mental Health Disorders: Evidence from a 30-year longitudinal study", *British Journal of Psychiatry*, vol. 193 (2008), quotations from p. 450. Furthermore, they took care to emphasise that their research findings did "not support strong pro-life positions that claim that abortion has large and devastating effects on the mental health of women". Neither was their research supportive of strong pro-choice opinions that discounted any impact on mental health. The strongest inference that could be drawn from the data was that abortion, for "some women", presented a "modestly increased risk of a range of common mental health problems" (p. 450).

11   Mika Gissler, Cynthia Berg, Marie-Hélène Bouvier-Colle and Pierre Buekens, "Injury Deaths, Suicides and Homicides Associated with Pregnancy, Finland 1987–2000", *European Journal of Public Health*, vol. 15, no. 5 (2005), p. 462.

12   Mika Gissler, Elina Karalis and Veli-Matti Ulander, "Decreased Suicide Rate after Induced Abortion, after the Current Care Guidelines in Finland 1987–2012", *Scandinavian Journal of Public Health*, vol. 43 (2015), pp. 99–101 <http://journals.sagepub.com/doi/full/10.1177/1403494814560844> accessed 16 March 2017.

13   Furthermore, its claim of "comprehensive longitudinal research" supportive of such a linkage is difficult to reconcile with its quotation from the Gissler research paper (2015) where the authors emphasised: "Neither were our data suitable for investigating whether an increased suicide rate after induced abortion is caused by common risk factors or by causality." The quotation from page 101 of Gissler *et al.* (2015) is in the PLC's "The Eighth Amendment – A Life-Saving Beacon of Hope", note 10.

14   "Citizens' Assembly will continue to use the 'contentious' term fatal foetal

abnormality", Independent.ie <http://www.independent.ie/irish-news/
citizens-assembly-will-continue-to-use-the-contentious-term-fatal-foetal-
abnormality-35348988.html> accessed 9 January 2017.

15 Peter McParland, "Antenatal Diagnosis and Management of Fetal
Abnormalities", Citizens' Assembly, 7 January 2017 <https://www.
citizensassembly.ie/en/Meetings/Dr-Peter-McParland-Paper.pdf> accessed 9
September 2017.

16 "Citizens' Assembly will continue to use the 'contentious' term fatal foetal
abnormality", Independent.ie.

17 Eileen Barrington, "Article 40.3.3 of the Constitution and Fatal Foetal
Abnormalities", Citizens' Assembly, 7 January 2017 <https://www.
citizensassembly.ie/en/Meetings/Eileen-Barrington-Paper.pdf> accessed 9
January 2017.

18 Bobbie Farsides, "The Moral Status of the Human Fetus: A Pro-
choice Approach", Citizens' Assembly, 7 January 2017 <https://www.
citizensassembly.ie/en/Meetings/Professor-Bobbie-Farsides-Paper.pdf>
accessed 5 March 2017.

19 Ruadhán Mac Cormaic, "Citizens' Assembly leans towards change in
Ireland's abortion laws", *Irish Times*, 8 January 2017 <http://www.irishtimes.
com/news/social-affairs/citizens-assembly-leans-towards-change-in-ireland-
s-abortion-laws-1.2929372?mode=print&ot=example.AjaxPageLayout.ot>
accessed 9 January 2017.

20 Pro Life Campaign, "PLC challenges Citizens' Assembly to redress
'unacceptable imbalance' in speakers" <http://prolifecampaign.ie/main/
portfolio/detail/04-11-17-plc-challenges-citizens-assembly-redress-
unacceptable-imbalance-speakers/> accessed 19 February 2017. Breda
O'Brien, writing in the *Irish Times*, expressed misgivings about the
assembly and saw it as deeply flawed. She argued, with reference to the Yale
psychologist Irving L. Janis, that group discussions and conclusions could be
easily manipulated by the choice of speakers and the wording of session titles:
"Signs are not good from Citizens' Assembly", *Irish Times*, 11 February 2017,
p. 14.

21 The pejorative term "abortion industry" was sometimes used by those
who supported the retention of the Eighth Amendment; for example, the
pamphlet: "My heart has been beating since I was 21 days old: am I a choice
or a child?" (Dublin: Youth Defence, circa 2017).

22 Doctors for Life Ireland, "Presentation on the Eighth Amendment to the
Citizens' Assembly 2017", 5 March 2017 <https://www.citizensassembly.ie/
en/Meetings/Doctors-for-Life-Paper.pdf> accessed 7 March 2017. Reference
was made to the *Guide to Professional Conduct and Ethics for Registered Medical
Practitioners*, 8th edn, 2016, no. 48.1.

23 Gilda Sedgh (Guttmacher Institute), "Key Facts, on Abortion Worldwide",
Citizens' Assembly, 4 February 2017 <https://www.citizensassembly.ie/en/
Meetings/Gilda-Sedgh-Paper.pdf> accessed 6 March 2017; in reference to

Gilda Sedgh *et al.*, "Abortion Incidence between 1990 and 2014: Global, regional and subregional levels and trends", *The Lancet* 388.10041 (2016): 258–67.

24 Miss Y, a young immigrant, arrived in Ireland in March 2014 and sought asylum. Shortly afterwards she discovered that she was pregnant. She revealed that she had been raped in her own country. She was so distressed about her pregnancy that she expressed a wish to die. She was denied an abortion in Ireland. Financial costs and her status as an asylum seeker prevented her from procuring an abortion in Britain. Her son was delivered (at about 25 weeks' gestation) by caesarean section in August 2014.

25 Doctors for Choice Ireland, PowerPoint presentation, Citizens' Assembly, 5 March 2017 <https://www.citizensassembly.ie/en/Meetings/Doctors-for-Choice-Powerpoint.pdf> accessed 7 March 2017.

26 Doctors for Choice Ireland, "Doctors for Choice Position Paper for Citizens' Assembly, 23 February 2017", presented to the Citizens' Assembly, session 1 on 5 March 2017 <https://www.citizensassembly.ie/en/Meetings/Doctors-for-Choice-s-Paper.pdf> accessed 7 March 2017.

27 Youth Defence gave an inaccurate and imbalanced interpretation of the research findings in the Fergusson (2008) and Gissler (2005) papers discussed earlier. Youth Defence, Paper presented to the Citizens' Assembly, 5 March 2017 <https://www.citizensassembly.ie/en/Meetings/Youth-Defence-s-Paper.pdf> accessed 23 March 2017. For another example of misinterpretation see Bernadette Goulding, "I Will Not Remain Silent" in Conor O'Riordan (ed.), *Debating the Eighth: Repeal or Retain?* (Dublin: Orpen Press, 2018), p. 47. Goulding stated, in reference to the Fergusson paper (2006), that a research project in New Zealand had "confirmed that young women who have abortions subsequently experience elevated rates of suicidal behaviours, depression, substance abuse, anxiety and other mental health problems". See earlier discussion of the research work of David Fergusson and his co-authors (2006 and 2008).

28 Every Life Counts, Paper presented to the Citizens' Assembly, 5 March 2017 <https://www.citizensassembly.ie/en/Meetings/Every-Life-Counts-Paper.pdf> accessed 25 March 2017.

29 Katherine E. Nelson, Laura C. Rosella, Sanjay Mahant and Astrid Guttmann, "Survival and Surgical Interventions for Children with Trisomy 13 and 18", *Journal of the American Medical Association*, vol. 316, no. 4 (2016), pp. 420–8. The second paper referred to by Every Life Counts, in the same context, is M. Jaquier, A. Klein and E. Boltshauser, "Spontaneous Pregnancy Outcome after Prenatal Diagnosis of Anencephaly", *British Journal of Obstetrics and Gynaecology*, vol. 113, no. 8 (August 2006), pp. 951–3. The sample size for the Boltshauser paper was 211 pregnancies in cases of anencephaly. Information about the pregnancies was very limited and was collected from parents through the medium of two internet home pages. The authors acknowledged

that a selection bias towards families with access to the internet was likely. The researchers did not receive approval from an institutional research committee. Boltshauser and his colleagues avoided discussion of the ethical aspect of managing pregnancies in cases of anencephaly.

30 Every Life Counts, Paper presented to the Citizens' Assembly, 5 March 2017. The sample size was 70. Elective terminations (outside the Republic of Ireland) occurred in four cases. This gives a figure of 94.3% – not 96% – of parents who "continued" the pregnancy.

31 Orla A. Houlihan and Keelin O'Donoghue, "The Natural History of Pregnancies with a Diagnosis of Trisomy 18 or Trisomy 13: A retrospective case series", *BMC Pregnancy and Childbirth*, vol. 13 (November 2013) <http://bmcpregnancychildbirth.biomedcentral.com/articles/10.1186/1471-2393-13-209> accessed 25 March 2017.

32 For the harrowing details of the case of Siobhán Whelan, see Paul Cullen, "Irish abortion law violated woman's human rights, says UN" and "She left Ireland feeling like 'a criminal leaving her country'", *Irish Times*, 14 June 2017, p. 5

33 Every Life Counts, Paper presented to the Citizens' Assembly, 5 March 2017.

34 Annie Janvier is listed last in the second paper but her leading role is indicated in both papers by contact details for correspondence.

35 Annie Janvier, Barbara Farlow and Benjamin S. Wilfond, "The Experience of Families with Children with Trisomy 13 and 18 in Social Networks", *Pediatrics*, vol. 130, no. 2 (August 2012), p. 297.

36 Jennifer Guon, Benjamin S. Wilfond, Barbara Farlow, Tracy Brazg and Annie Janvier, "Our Children are Not a Diagnosis: The experience of parents who continue their pregnancy after a prenatal diagnosis of trisomy 13 or 18", *American Journal of Medical Genetics*, Part A 164A (2013), pp. 308–18.

37 Iona Institute, Presentation about Article 40.3.3 to the Citizens' Assembly, 5 March 2017 <https://www.citizensassembly.ie/en/Meetings/The-Iona-Institute-s-Paper.pdf> accessed 9 March 2017.

38 For arguments based on neural development and the emergence of personhood see, for example, Paul S. Penner and Richard T. Hull, "The Beginning of Individual Human Personhood", *Journal of Medicine and Philosophy*, vol. 33 (2008), pp. 174–82. For a broader philosophical analysis, with reference to neuroscience, see the Appendix to this book ("Seeking Moral Boundaries: Abortion and Infanticide").

39 Irish Catholic Bishops' Conference, Presentation to the Citizens' Assembly, 5 March 2017 <https://www.citizensassembly.ie/en/Meetings/ICBC-s-Paper.pdf> accessed 9 March 2017.

40 Irish Catholic Bishops' Conference, "The importance of speaking in the public square – address by Archbishop Eamon Martin", 25 March 2017

<http://www.catholicbishops.ie/2017/03/25/the-importance-of-speaking-in-the-public-square-address-by-archbishop-eamon-martin/> accessed 29 March 2017.

41 Gestational limits, if any, were specified for each of these reasons, giving three categories: 12 weeks, 22 weeks, and no gestational limits. Termination of pregnancy for socio-economic reasons was supported by 72%. In this sector of the vote 40% agreed with the gestational limit of up to 12 weeks only, 50% for up to 22 weeks only, and 10% for no restriction as to gestational age. There were stronger levels of support for terminations in cases of substantial risks to the life of the mother (including by suicide), "serious risk" or "risk" to both the physical and mental health of the mother; pregnancy caused by rape; foetal abnormality likely to result in death either before or shortly after birth; and a significant abnormality not likely to result in death before or shortly after birth. A clear majority – 72% (excluding those who did not express an opinion) – voted that no distinction should be made between the physical and mental health of the mother. *First Report and Recommendations of the Citizens' Assembly: The Eighth Amendment of the Constitution*, 29 June 2017 <https://www.citizensassembly.ie/en/The-Eighth-Amendment-of-the-Constitution/Final-Report-on-the-Eighth-Amendment-of-the-Constitution/Final-Report-incl-Appendix-A-D.pdf> accessed 27 January 2018, pp. 3–4, 12–13, 16, 23, 32–6.

42 Pat Leahy, "Irish Times/Ipsos MRBI poll: replace constitutional control on abortion", *Irish Times*, 3 March 2017 <http://www.irishtimes.com/news/social-affairs/irish-times-ipsos-mrbi-poll-replace-constitutional-control-on-abortion-1.2995968> accessed 3 March 2017; and "Poll shows public support for abortion is cautious and conditional", *Irish Times*, 3 March 2017 <http://www.irishtimes.com/news/social-affairs/poll-shows-public-support-for-abortion-is-cautious-and-conditional-1.2995696> accessed 3 March 2017.

43 "Ipsos MRBI poll: abortion, voters and nuance", *Irish Times*, 27 May 2017 <http://www.irishtimes.com/opinion/editorial/ipsos-mrbi-poll-abortion-voters-and-nuance-1.3097371?mode=print&ot=example.AjaxPageLayout.ot> accessed 26 June 2017.

44 See Denis McCarthy, letter to the editor, *Irish Times*, 26 June 2017 <http://www.irishtimes.com/opinion/letters/the-eighth-amendment-1.3131441?mode=print&ot=example.AjaxPageLayout.ot> accessed 26 June 2017. McCarthy was writing with the *Irish Times*/MRBI poll of 27 May in mind.

45 Pat Leahy, "Bitter abortion ballot campaign on the horizon: Dáil must decide if they should frame a workable abortion referendum", *Irish Times*, 30 June 2017 <http://0-search.proquest.com.library.ucc.ie/docview/1914683154/2E43CE9A9A6E41A0PQ/96?accountid=14504> accessed 30 June 2017; Pat Leahy and Sarah Bardon, "FG ministers believe only restrictive abortion law will pass: cabinet members reluctant

to put forward referendum on changes they do not endorse", *Irish Times*, 28 September 2017 <https://search-proquest-com.ucc.idm.oclc.org/docview/1943388380/8469DAF548564E09PQ/2?accountid=14504> accessed 28 September 2017.

46 Joint Committee on the Eighth Amendment of the Constitution, 11 October 2017, Houses of the Oireachtas website <https://www.oireachtas.ie/en/debates/debate/joint_committee_on_the_eighth_amendment_of_the_constitution/2017-10-11/3/> accessed 26 October 2017.

47 Professor Malone gave hypoplastic left heart syndrome as an example of a foetal abnormality which is very severe but not necessarily fatal. However, if the foetus is also diagnosed with severe growth restriction and a major intracranial abnormality, the combined effect of all these abnormalities could eliminate any significant prospect of survival.

48 See Chapter 7 for details about the *P.P. v Health Service Executive* High Court case (2014).

49 Dr Meabh Ní Bhuinneáin, obstetrician and gynaecologist at Mayo University Hospital, informed the committee (18 October 2017) that medical practice was very much about assessing probabilities. Contrary to the terminology of the Citizens' Assembly, precise differentiation between serious risk to health and serious risk to life could not be supported by definition.

50 Joint Committee on the Eighth Amendment of the Constitution, 11 October 2017, Houses of the Oireachtas website.

51 Professor Malone gave the example of a patient with ruptured membranes, vulnerable to infection. At 14–16 weeks' gestation there might be infection but yet no clinical signs (sub-clinical chorioamnionitis). There is no prospect of delivering a viable baby in these circumstances. Doctors were not permitted to intervene, notwithstanding that there is no justification for exposing the patient to risk when there is no prospect of delivering a live baby. However, a patient in consultation with her doctor may well decide to accept the risk if the foetus is close to viability, at about 23 weeks.

52 Joint Committee on the Eighth Amendment of the Constitution, 18 October 2017, Houses of the Oireachtas website <https://www.oireachtas.ie/en/debates/debate/joint_committee_on_the_eighth_amendment_of_the_constitution/2017-10-18/3/> accessed 20 October 2017.

53 Ibid.

54 Heidi Cope, Melanie E. Garrett, Simon G. Gregory and Allison E. Ashley-Koch, "Pregnancy Continuation and Organizational Religious Activity following Prenatal Diagnosis of a Lethal Fetal Defect is Associated with Improved Psychological Outcome", *Prenatal Diagnosis*, vol. 35, no. 8 (April 2015).

55 Joint Committee on the Eighth Amendment of the Constitution, 11 October 2017, Houses of the Oireachtas website.

56 *Report of the Joint Committee on the Eighth Amendment of the*

Constitution (Houses of the Oireachtas, December 2017), section
1.7 <http://www.oireachtas.ie/parliament/media/committees/
eighthamendmentoftheconstitution/Report-of-the-Joint-Committee-on-
the-Eighth-Amendment-web-version.pdf> accessed 22 December 2017.

57 See Pat Leahy, "Reconciling positions on abortion is a political debate",
Irish Times, 21 October 2017 <https://search-proquest-com.ucc.idm.oclc.
org/docview/1953294531/4E0D4C9BF246E0PQ/88?accountid=14504>
accessed 21 October 2017.

58 *Report of the Joint Committee on the Eighth Amendment of the Constitution*
(Houses of the Oireachtas, December 2017), section 1.8.

59 Joint Committee on the Eighth Amendment of the Constitution, 18
October 2017, Houses of the Oireachtas website <https://www.oireachtas.
ie/en/debates/debate/joint_committee_on_the_eighth_amendment_of_the_
constitution/2017-10-18/4/> accessed 2 August 2018.

60 The committee met on 11 July to discuss a draft scheme for completing its
work within three months of its first public session in September. Selection of
witnesses was discussed. Agreement was reached that a final decision on the
list of witnesses would be made at the meeting scheduled for 13 September.
Joint Oireachtas Committee on the Eighth Amendment, press release,
12 July 2017 <https://webarchive.oireachtas.ie/parliament/mediazone/
pressreleases/2017/name-43149-en.html> accessed 2 July 2018.

61 Initially, it was decided to exclude advocacy groups, but the committee
later reversed its decision on this matter. Mullen submitted three requests:
Caroline Simons, legal adviser to the Pro Life Campaign; Professor M.J.
McCaffrey, professor of paediatrics and perinatal medicine at the University
of North Carolina; and Martin and Sinead McBreen, parents of a girl with
Down syndrome. McGrath requested Professor William Binchy, an expert on
constitutional law well known for his support for the Eighth Amendment;
Liz McDermott, a representative of One Day More; and Professor Monique
V. Chireau, Duke University Medical Centre, North Carolina. There was
no positive outcome to Mullen's proposals. Two of McGrath's requests
succeeded: William Binchy and Liz McDermott attended. Sarah Bardon,
"Eighth Amendment Committee comes under tough scrutiny", *Irish
Times*, 20 October 2017 <https://search-proquest-com.ucc.idm.oclc.org/
docview/1952920900/8B6789A6B32D480BPQ/36?accountid=14504>
accessed 21 October 2017. Professor M.J. McCaffrey wrote to the committee
informing the members that he had received his invitation to attend on 26
October – several days after the vote. McCaffrey was a professor of paediatrics
at the University of North Carolina with expertise in foetal anomalies,
especially trisomy 13, trisomy 18 and anencephaly. He expressed concern
that the proceedings of the committee were "deeply biased in favour of
repeal". He was aware of the vote taken on 18 October and believed that the
committee's invitation was "a retrospective effort to ... offer some illusion of

balance to the Oireachtas hearings". McCaffrey had followed the proceedings of the committee – especially the medical evidence – on its website and he observed that no medical expert had spoken in favour of retaining the Eighth Amendment. He claimed that surgical abortion increased the risk of pre-term births for mothers in future pregnancies – especially "very preterm" births (26 weeks to less than 32 weeks). No other medical expert had informed the committee of the link between surgical abortion and pre-term births. McCaffrey declined the committee's invitation to attend on the basis that to do so would be to "participate in a charade with a preordained conclusion". By limiting his contribution to a written submission he relieved himself of the "daunting" task of presenting medical research findings to "such a biased group". M.J. McCaffrey, letter to the Joint Oireachtas Committee on the Eighth Amendment, 7 November 2017 <https://webarchive.oireachtas.ie/ parliament/media/committees/eighthamendmentoftheconstitution/JCEA-55RC---Response-from-Dr.-Marty-McCaffrey.pdf> accessed 2 July 2018. A problem with McCaffrey's decision was that it devalued his evidence because the committee was deprived of the opportunity of questioning him on his submission, especially on his claim of a causal association between abortion and elevated risks of pre-term births for future pregnancies.

62 Colm Keena, "Claims of abortion committee bias rejected", *Irish Times*, 23 November 2017 <https://search-proquest-com.ucc.idm.oclc.org/ docview/1967208927/730CF42E2CA64593PQ/54?accountid=14504> accessed 23 November 2017.

63 Patsy McGarry, "Oireachtas Committee 'appears' to have made up mind, says bishop", *Irish Times*, 21 October 2017 <https://search-proquest-com.ucc.idm. oclc.org/docview/1953295123/4E0D4C9BF246E0PQ/31?accountid=14504> accessed 21 October 2017.

64 To comply with its terms of reference, the commission was under the obligation to report its conclusions and recommendations to the Dáil and Seanad within three months of its first public meeting – which was held on 20 September. Establishment of a Special Committee on the Eighth Amendment of the Constitution, 4 April 2017, Dáil Éireann <https://www. oireachtas.ie/en/debates/debate/dail/2017-04-04/8/> accessed 5 July 2018. The Dáil motion to set up the committee was followed by that of Seanad Éireann on 13 April.

65 Pat Leahy, "National Women's Council targets middle ground with abortion campaign", *Irish Times*, 13 November 2017 <https://search-proquest-com.ucc.idm.oclc.org/ docview/1963034940/41897DB437EC4D54PQ/35?accountid=14504> accessed 13 November 2017.

66 Patsy McGarry, "Repealing Eighth Amendment 'removes' constitutional protection for unborn", *Irish Times*, 21 October 2017 <https://search-proquest-com.ucc.idm.oclc.org/

docview/1953294526/4E0D4C9BF246E0PQ/32?accountid=14504>
accessed 21 October 2017.

67 Address by Gerry Whyte, "Repeal or Replace? The legal implications of
amending Article 40.3.3" at *Abortion, Disability and the Law* conference,
jointly hosted by the Anscombe Bioethics Centre and the Consultative
Group on Bioethics of the Irish Catholic Bishops' Conference, 20
October 2017, Irish Catholic Bishops' Conference website <https://www.
catholicbishops.ie/2017/10/20/papers-delivered-at-the-conference-abortion-
disability-and-the-law/> accessed 5 July 2018.

68 Joint Committee on the Eighth Amendment of the Constitution, 8
November 2017, Houses of the Oireachtas website <https://www.oireachtas.
ie/en/debates/debate/joint_committee_on_the_eighth_amendment_of_the_
constitution/2017-11-08/2/> accessed 24 August 2018.

69 Pro Life Campaign, "PLC accuses Noone of making 'highly misleading'
statements about committee", 13 November 2017 <http://prolifecampaign.
ie/main/portfolio/detail/13-11-17-plc-accuses-noone-making-highly-
misleading-statements-committee/> accessed 15 November 2017. See also
Pro Life Campaign, "Senator Noone has new excuse every day for why her
committee is so biased", 4 December 2017 <http://prolifecampaign.ie/main/
portfolio/detail/04-12-17-senator-noone-new-excuse-every-day-committee-
biased-plc/> accessed 15 December 2017.

70 Bardon, "Eighth Amendment Committee comes under tough scrutiny".

71 *Report of the Joint Committee on the Eighth Amendment of the Constitution*
(Houses of the Oireachtas, December 2017), Section 1.9.

72 Joint Committee on the Eighth Amendment of the Constitution, 11
October 2017, Houses of the Oireachtas website <https://www.oireachtas.
ie/en/debates/debate/joint_committee_on_the_eighth_amendment_of_the_
constitution/2017-10-11/3/> accessed 2 August 2018.

73 Joint Committee on Health and Children, 8 January 2013 <https://
www.oireachtas.ie/en/debates/debate/joint_committee_on_health_and_
children/2013-01-08/2/#s5> accessed 7 November 2018.

74 Barry Roche, "Mother might still be alive but for Eighth Amendment –
gynaecologist", *Irish Times*, 13 May 2018 <https://www.irishtimes.com/news/
ireland/irish-news/mother-might-still-be-alive-but-for-eighth-amendment-
gynaecologist-1.3493958> accessed 11 November 2018.

75 Joint Committee on the Eighth Amendment of the Constitution, 25
October 2017, Houses of the Oireachtas website <https://www.oireachtas.
ie/en/debates/debate/joint_committee_on_the_eighth_amendment_of_the_
constitution/2017-10-25/2/> accessed 11 November 2017.

76 Inquest into the death of Ms. Savita Halappanavar held before the coroner,
Dr. Ciaran MacLoughlin, on Wednesday, 10th April 2013 – day 3, JCEA
43RC(a), Coroner's Court, Galway <https://webarchive.oireachtas.ie/
parliament/media/committees/eighthamendmentoftheconstitution/jcea-

43rc(a)---coroner-inquest-into-death-of-ms.-savita-halappanavar.pdf>
accessed 15 July 2018; questions and answers 176–9.

77 Joint Committee on the Eighth Amendment of the Constitution,
25 October 2017 <https://www.oireachtas.ie/en/debates/
debate/joint_committee_on_the_eighth_amendment_of_the_
constitution/2017-10-25/5/; and Inquest into the death of Ms. Savita
Halappanavar, question 174.

78 Inquest into the death of Ms. Savita Halappanavar, question 177.

79 See also Joan McCarthy, "Reproductive Justice in Ireland: A Feminist
Analysis of the Neary and Halappanavar cases" in Mary Donnelly
and Claire Murray (eds), *Ethical and Legal Debates in Irish Healthcare:
Confronting Complexities* (Manchester: Manchester University Press, 2016),
pp.14–20.

80 Joint Committee on the Eighth Amendment of the Constitution, 18
October 2017.

81 Sabaratnam Arulkumaran *et al.*, *Final Report: Investigation of Incident
50278 from time of patient's self referral to hospital on the 21st of October 2012
to the patient's death on 28th of October, 2012*, Health Service Executive,
June 2013 <https://www.hse.ie/eng/services/news/nimtreport50278.pdf>
accessed 15 July 2018.

82 Joint Committee on the Eighth Amendment of the Constitution,
25 October 2017 <https://www.oireachtas.ie/en/debates/
debate/joint_committee_on_the_eighth_amendment_of_the_
constitution/2017-10-25/3/> accessed 30 July 2018.

83 Tom O'Malley, "Rape and Related Offences – A Legal Perspective",
Citizens' Assembly, 4 February 2017 <https://www.citizensassembly.ie/en/
Meetings/Tom-O-Malley-Paper.pdf> accessed 9 March 2017.

84 Joint Committee on the Eighth Amendment of the Constitution,
25 October 2017 <https://www.oireachtas.ie/en/debates/
debate/joint_committee_on_the_eighth_amendment_of_the_
constitution/2017-10-25/4/> accessed 1 August 2018.

85 Ibid.

86 Joint Committee on the Eighth Amendment of the Constitution,
13 December 2017, Houses of the Oireachtas website <http://
oireachtasdebates.oireachtas.ie/Debates%20Authoring/DebatesWebPack.
nsf/committeetakes/EAJ2017121300002?opendocument> accessed 16
December 2017.

87 *Report of the Joint Committee on the Eighth Amendment of the Constitution*,
sections 2.11–2.18.

88 Ibid., sections 2.20–2.23.

89 Ibid., sections 2.38–2.39.

90 Joint Committee on the Eighth Amendment of the Constitution,
29 November 2017 <https://www.oireachtas.ie/en/debates/

debate/joint_committee_on_the_eighth_amendment_of_the_
constitution/2017-11-29/3/> accessed 28 August 2018.

91 *Report of the Joint Committee on the Eighth Amendment of the Constitution*,
section 2.31.

92 The committee heard evidence from Eva Pajkrt, professor of obstetrics at the
Academic Medical Centre, University of Amsterdam; and from her colleague,
Sjef Gevers, formerly professor of health law at the same centre. Their
evidence to the committee sheds light on the major differences in outlook
between pro-life and pro-choice positions. Pajkrt informed the committee
that the Dutch system of healthcare was based on "patient autonomy and
what women want". Fine Gael TD Peter Fitzpatrick asked Pajkrt: if freedom
of choice resulted in no Down syndrome children being born, should society
accept the outcome? Was choice more important than the life of the unborn
with Down syndrome? Pajkrt's answer was unambiguous – the woman should
have the right to choose. After further discussion she revised her position – a
decision to terminate a pregnancy should be the choice of both the mother
and the father. Evidence of Professor Eva Pajkrt to the Joint Committee on
the Eighth Amendment of the Constitution, 23 November 2017 <https://
www.oireachtas.ie/en/debates/debate/joint_committee_on_the_eighth_
amendment_of_the_constitution/2017-11-23/2/> accessed 29 September
2018. Fitzpatrick then asked Gevers if, in the case of a pregnant woman, there
were two people to consider. Gevers responded that in the Netherlands, the
unborn was not, in a legal sense, thought to be a person. In Dutch law there
was increasing protection for unborn life as it developed in the womb. But
it was only after birth that the baby was considered a person and was given
the full rights of a person. Evidence of Professor Sjef Gevers to the Joint
Committee on the Eighth Amendment of the Constitution, 23 November
2017.

93 *Report of the Joint Committee on the Eighth Amendment of the Constitution*,
section 2.35.

94 Ibid., section 2.39.

95 Pro Life Campaign, "Today's abortion vote is appalling but public will have
final say on Eighth Amendment, says PLC", 13 December 2017 <http://
prolifecampaign.ie/main/portfolio/detail/14-12-17-todays-abortion-vote-
appalling-public-will-final-say-eighth-amendment-says-plc/> accessed 15
December 2017.

96 Ronan McGreevy, "Assembly selection defended: Chairwoman of
Citizens' Assembly says abortion outcome unaffected by audit", *Irish
Times*, 23 February 2018 <https://search-proquest-com.ucc.idm.oclc.org/
docview/2007254403/65364351C711406FPQ/47?accountid=14504>
accessed 25 February 2018.

97 Ronan McGreevy, "Committee 'couldn't find' any anti-abortion medical
experts to argue for Eighth", *Irish Times*, 20 February 2018 <https://www.

irishtimes.com/news/ireland/irish-news/committee-couldn-t-find-any-anti-abortion-medical-experts-to-argue-for-eighth-1.3397941> accessed 20 February 2018.

98 Thomas Ryan, letter to the editor, *Irish Times*, 23 February 2017 <https://www.irishtimes.com/opinion/letters/the-eighth-amendment-1.3402287> accessed 23 February 2018.

99 Thomas Ryan (see previous note) referred to a letter signed by 38 GPs and a number of other healthcare professionals opposing "the last legislative intervention" on the issue of abortion. See Dr Ann Barry *et al.*, letter to the editor, *Irish Times*, 29 May 2013 <https://search-proquest-com.ucc.idm.oclc.org/docview/1355766846/AAEAA021B9644D10PQ/118?accountid=14504> accessed 24 February 2018.

100 Dr Orla Halpenny, Doctors for Life, letter to the editor, *Irish Times*, 24 February 2018 <https://www.irishtimes.com/opinion/letters/the-eighth-amendment-1.3403495> accessed 24 February 2018.

101 Halpenny did not give the date of the invitation, but it is reasonable to assume that it was received before 13 December 2017 when the committee voted by a majority of 14 to 6 to recommend simple repeal of the Eighth Amendment.

CHAPTER TEN

---•---

The Repeal of the Eighth Amendment

2018

The Thirty-sixth Amendment and Draft Legislation

OPINION POLLS HAD CONSISTENTLY INDICATED THAT MORE citizens would vote to repeal the Eighth Amendment than to retain it. An opinion poll in early December 2017 found that 62 per cent would vote to repeal the Eighth Amendment so that the Oireachtas could legislate for greater access to abortion. Just how extensive people felt this access should be was not clear, although there were some indications. An Ipsos/MRBI poll in June 2017 found broad support for abortion on the grounds of fatal foetal abnormalities, rape, and when there was a threat to the health of the mother. Over 30 per cent of voters were unwavering supporters of repeal. About 20 per cent were staunchly defensive of the Eighth Amendment. The remainder of voters occupied the middle ground, although it was thought that most of them were leaning towards repeal. Winning the middle ground, therefore, would be decisive for winning the referendum.[1]

The government was under constant pressure to press ahead with the referendum. Movement for change came from the pro-choice Together for Yes (an umbrella group of about seventy organisations), opinion polls, the recommendations of the Citizens' Assembly and the Joint Committee on the Eighth Amendment, and most of the political opposition. It was no longer politically prudent to procrastinate! It remained to be seen what wording would be put before the people in arriving at a decision about Article 40.3.3. Should the government propose simple deletion of Article 40.3.3 or replacement with different wording? The Citizens' Assembly recommended that Article 40.3.3 should be replaced with a constitutional provision enabling the Oireachtas to legislate for terminations of pregnancy. The Joint Committee on the Eighth Amendment of the Constitution had recommended simple repeal of Article 40.3.3.

Legal opinion was split on what the courts were likely to decide if Article 40.3.3 was repealed without a replacement provision. If the people voted to delete Article 40.3.3 it would be clear that they wanted decisions about termination of pregnancy to be made by the Oireachtas and not decided by the Constitution. A second opinion held that implied rights of the unborn existed in the Constitution before the Eighth Amendment was passed in 1983 and that such rights would limit the scope for legislation. A third opinion held that simple deletion of Article 40.3.3 would prevent the Oireachtas from restricting abortion to very limited circumstances because maternal rights to privacy, autonomy and bodily integrity would take precedence over any rights of the unborn.[2] Government ministers were very much aware of the legal uncertainties and political risks arising from simple repeal.[3]

On 29 January 2018, the government, acting on the advice of the Attorney General, Séamus Woulfe, decided to ask the electorate to repeal Article 40.3.3 "in full" and to insert a new article to "expressly affirm that laws may be enacted by the Oireachtas providing for the regulation of termination of pregnancy".[4] Its Thirty-sixth Amendment of the Constitution Bill 2018 proposed to amend Article 40.3.3 to read as follows: "Provision may be made by law for the regulation of termination of pregnancy."[5] The government published its *Policy Paper: Regulation of Termination of Pregnancy* on 8 March, the day after the Supreme Court issued a ruling on the rights of the unborn external to Article 40.3.3.[6] The paper outlined 21 policy principles for the drafting of a general scheme of a Bill regulating the termination of pregnancy. This proposed legislation could only be enacted if the proposed amendment to the Constitution was passed and the Oireachtas approved of the legislation. Policy principles included "termination of pregnancy on the grounds of a foetal condition which is likely to lead to death before or shortly after birth"; and "termination of pregnancy up to 12 weeks of pregnancy without specific indication". Pregnant women who terminated, or attempted to terminate, their pregnancies would not be deemed guilty of an offence.[7]

The policy paper published by the government on 8 March required further examination, refinement and legal advice from the Office of the Attorney General. The outcome of this was the General Scheme of a Bill to Regulate Termination of Pregnancy (27 March 2018). Under Head 4 it would be legal to carry out a termination of pregnancy when two medical practitioners certify that there is:

> (a) a risk to the life of, or of serious harm to the health of, the pregnant woman, (b) the foetus has not reached viability, and (c) it is appropriate to carry out the termination of pregnancy in order to avert that risk.

Head 5 required certification from only one medical practitioner in emergency cases. Head 6 of the Bill provided for a termination of pregnancy when, in the "reasonable opinion" of two medical practitioners, there was "a condition affecting the foetus that is likely to lead to death of the foetus either before birth or shortly after birth". No gestational limits were specified. Head 7 of the Bill provided for termination of pregnancy within the first twelve weeks with the only restriction of a waiting period of seventy-two hours between certification and the procedure being carried out.[8]

An abortion regime as liberal as that in Britain would have been unacceptable to most of the Irish electorate. Defenders of the Eighth Amendment, very much aware of this, argued that the government's proposals were similar to Britain's 1967 Abortion Act. It was lawful to terminate a pregnancy in Britain if it had "not exceeded its twenty-fourth week" and "the continuance of the pregnancy would involve risk, greater than if the pregnancy were terminated, of injury to the physical or mental health of the pregnant woman".[9] This condition (Ground C) was invariably satisfied because continuing a pregnancy to term always presented a higher risk to maternal health than an abortion under clinical conditions. Those who opposed repeal of the Eighth Amendment pointed out that 97 per cent of abortions in Britain occurred on the basis of Ground C. However, it was reported that 92 per cent of terminations were carried out within thirteen weeks of pregnancy, and 81 per cent within ten weeks.[10]

Save the 8th saw very little difference between the General Scheme of a Bill to Regulate Termination of Pregnancy and Britain's Abortion Act. It claimed that "A Yes vote absolutely legalises abortion up to six months, or 'viability'" and "in some cases, where an unborn child is very seriously ill, it legalises abortion up to birth." The government's position was that the legislation would be restrictive, but this was contested on the basis that "serious risk" to health included mental health and 97 per cent of all abortions in the UK were carried out on mental health grounds.[11] The comparison of the proposed Irish legislation with the Abortion Act was highly questionable. The provision for abortion on request up to twelve weeks was in line with most European jurisdictions. Irish law would be more restrictive than most European jurisdictions when, as stated in the General Scheme of a Bill to Regulate Termination of Pregnancy, it would restrict reasons for termination of pregnancy to risk to life, risk of serious harm to health, and when the foetus suffered from an abnormality that was likely to cause death before birth or shortly after birth.[12]

Differences of opinion were expressed in the legal profession about the likely consequences of overturning the Eighth Amendment and the associated legislative proposals.[13] Senior figures included Senator Ivana Bacik, Professor William Binchy, Ronan Keane (a former chief justice), and Bryan McMahon (retired High Court judge). Keane took issue with McMahon and others who believed that repeal of the Eighth Amendment would eliminate all constitutional protection for the unborn. This idea, he believed, was "dangerously simplistic" and "misleading". The right to life of the unborn would be maintained, although it would be subject to legislation passed by the Oireachtas specifying under what conditions termination could take place. It would be open to the courts, "freed from the constraints imposed by the present wording of article 40.3.3" to rule that provisions enacted by the new Article 40.3.3 must strike an appropriate balance between the rights of the unborn and the mother – taking account of not only the mother's right to life but also her right to bodily integrity, health, privacy and personal autonomy.[14] It was essentially a rebalancing of rights in favour of the mother – not the obliteration of rights of the unborn. The constitutionality of any law could be challenged. How the courts might rule was not possible to predict "with certainty".[15] This lack of certainty gave rise to fears among those who were undecided or were slightly inclined towards repeal of the Eighth Amendment. This in turn played into the hands of No campaigners (i.e. those who advocated retaining the Eighth Amendment), who sought to win over those who were undecided or only slightly inclined towards Yes.

A Challenge to Democracy

On 6 March the Irish Catholic bishops issued a statement reiterating that the right to life was a fundamental right. It was not a right granted by the Constitution or by any law. All human beings had such a right – from conception onwards.[16] Article 40.3.3 didn't grant the right to life; it acknowledged the right to life – as indicated by the text. Human beings had rights over which the state had no authority. The Constitution confirmed the existence of such rights and gave them protection. The state had no moral right to withdraw such protection – even if a democratic parliamentary vote found to the contrary. Yet this "natural law" view of the Constitution was not quite so straightforward.[17] In some cases disagreements about the meaning and application of natural law arose, creating possibilities for natural law to be invoked in support of "diametrically opposed conclusions".[18] Furthermore, the Supreme Court had found that the Constitution was "the fundamental law of the State ... and at no stage recognised the provisions of the natural law as superior to the Constitution". Article 5 of the Constitution was quoted to bolster this finding. It declared that Ireland was "a sovereign, independent, democratic state".[19]

Some politicians were probably influenced by a Catholic, natural law interpretation of the Constitution. When a vote was taken in the Dáil (21 March) on the Thirty-Sixth Amendment of the Constitution Bill 2018 (Fifth Stage) the motion was declared carried by ninety-seven in favour to twenty-five against.[20] The majority of those who voted against the Bill were members of Fianna Fáil. The Bill was passed to the Seanad for consideration on 27–28 March and was passed by forty in favour and ten against. Most of those who voted against the Bill were members of Fianna Fáil.[21]

A secular view of the Constitution was that it was the people's document, despite the preamble which declared "In the Name of the Most Holy Trinity, from Whom is all authority and to Whom, as our final end, all actions both of men and States must be referred". How best to comply with "all our obligations to our Divine Lord, Jesus Christ" did not feature in debates about the Eighth Amendment. In twenty-first-century Ireland, the preamble seemed little more than a historical curiosity, reflecting pious aspirations out of place in a sovereign democratic republic. The people would decide their own laws, independent of any considerations of what the supreme deity might expect. Joe Humphreys, a journalist with the *Irish Times*, referred extensively to emeritus Professor

John Dillon of Trinity College Dublin to make the point that absolutism should be avoided. It was untenable to assert that the human embryo had an absolute right to life "independent of any human decision to grant it". A right deemed to be inalienable was, in reality, dependent on the people to affirm it and uphold it in law. Therefore, any rights relating to Irish embryos would be only those granted by the Irish people.[22] This secular outlook stood in stark contrast to the doctrines of the Roman Catholic Church.

Pro-life activists were sharply critical of politicians. Politicians had been manipulated and found very useful by the Pro-Life Amendment Campaign in 1983 when the Eighth Amendment was passed. They had served their purpose: now they needed to be restrained by the Constitution, which in turn needed to be interpreted in the light of immutable fundamental moral principles. A coalition of pro-life organisations claimed that the proposed amendment to the Constitution would give politicians "the power to introduce any legislation they want, no matter how liberal or extreme". Unborn babies would be deprived of all constitutional rights and the electorate would "never have a say on this matter again".[23] These statements, disseminated through their widely circulated pamphlet, *Your Guide to The Referendum – Information on the Government's Proposals*, were alarmist and misleading. There was an underlying assumption that politicians, given the opportunity, would loosen restrictions on the termination of pregnancy that exceeded the wishes of the people. But the historical record clearly indicated otherwise. Politicians were extremely reluctant to take the initiative and were led by public opinion on this matter. Always mindful of the next election, they were excessively cautious about broadening access to abortion beyond what they judged to be the minimum necessary. Demands for constitutional and legislative reforms were driven by civil society, not by politicians – most of whom would have avoided the issue given the opportunity. The obsession with untrustworthy politicians thinly masked a deeper fear. Many of those who advocated retention of the Eighth Amendment didn't trust the electorate to make the "right" choice. Democracy could no longer be relied upon to uphold traditional Catholic values.

"Don't Mention the Church"

On 28 March the government disclosed that the referendum to repeal the Eighth Amendment would be held on 25 May 2018. For several months concerns were expressed that the democratic process would be tainted, if not subverted, by a campaign of manipulation and misinformation waged through Google and social media accounts such as Facebook and Twitter – especially against the background of Brexit and the election of Donald Trump to the presidency of the USA. The issue of abortion extended beyond national frontiers and drew support from partisans on both sides.[24] Funding from abroad was a source of contention. Amnesty International (Ireland) and the Abortion Rights Campaign were ordered by the Standards in Public Office Commission (SIPO) to return donations they had received from George Soros's Open Society Foundation on the basis that the funding from a foreign source was for political purposes and therefore prohibitable by law.[25] No pro-life organisations were ordered by SIPO to return donations from abroad, although it seemed that they did receive foreign funding from sources such as the Pro-Life Action League in the USA.[26]

The internet and the World Wide Web transformed society and the way political elections and referendums were conducted, which indicated well in advance that the referendum campaign on abortion would be conducted in ways radically different from those employed in 1983 when the Eighth Amendment was passed. Reports circulated that Save the 8th had hired Kanto Systems, a London-based political consultancy firm with connections to the Brexit campaign. The Pro Life Campaign was reported to have hired the services of uCampaign, a conservative American firm that had created apps for Donald Trump, the National Rifle Association and Vote Leave in the UK.[27] The instruments of choice for the pro-life movement in Ireland were those applicable to social media rather than rosaries and crucifixes.

The abortion referendum received press coverage internationally. Columnists writing in *The Economist* (London) and the *New York Times* observed that revelations about the sexual abuse of children by priests and members of religious orders, the ruthless exploitation and incarceration of "fallen women" in Magdalene Laundries, involuntary adoptions, and the undocumented burials of numerous infants at "mother and baby" homes had eroded the Church's authority since 1983.[28] The essay in *The Economist* was headlined "Don't mention the Church." Catholic doctrine and the institutional Church were rarely mentioned in support of arguments against abortion. The religious affiliations of many pro-life activists were known, although pro-life organisations such as the Pro Life Campaign, Save the 8th, the Iona Institute and the Life Institute did not identify themselves in a denominational sense.[29]

The institutional Church did of course make its views known, although it was very much a voice in the background. On 6 January 2018 a pastoral letter from Archbishop Eamon Martin, Primate of All Ireland, urged all citizens committed to the common good to make their views known to their elected representatives.[30] This pastoral message would have been very potent in 1983. However, it exerted very limited influence in 2018 because the movement for change was coming, not from politicians, but from civil society. Politicians, therefore, didn't feel quite so intimidated by the prospect of "a belt of a crozier". They increasingly felt it necessary to re-examine their consciences, confronted as they were by a series of opinion polls indicating majority support for repealing the Eighth Amendment.

The bishops' pronouncements stood in stark contrast to the outlook of most Catholics. Contraception, divorce and same-sex marriage had all been legalised, contrary to principles of Catholic moral teaching. A rift had developed between bishops and most Catholics. Also, there was a poor relationship between many priests and their bishops. Frequently, priests realised through insights derived from pastoral experience that dogmatic statements from the hierarchy would have relatively little influence. On 4 May the Association of Catholic Priests (Ireland) (ACP) issued a statement calling for a more nuanced response to the issue of abortion. The ACP fully endorsed the teaching of the institutional Church that held that all human life was "sacred" from "beginning to end". Every "human person" had a fundamental right to life. Yet the complexity of life called for a more nuanced approach to pastoral work. Mindful that its members were unmarried and without children of their own, the ACP acknowledged that they were "not best placed to be in any way dogmatic" on the issue of whether or not to repeal the Eighth Amendment.

The ACP adopted a non-judgemental stance and its members would not tell anyone how they should vote. The association expressed concern that some Catholic priests were permitting their pulpits to be used by campaigners during Mass. This was inappropriate because Catholic opinion was deeply divided. Some Catholics would see the use of pulpits by campaigners as "an abuse of the Eucharist". In view of this, the ACP called for the practice to be discontinued for the remainder of the campaign.[31]

The ACP press release elicited a sarcastic response from Save the 8th. The pro-life organisation observed that the ACP "appears worried that Catholics may hear Catholic teaching reflected at Catholic masses".

Save the 8th was responding to invitations to "educate voters" about "the extremity of the Government's proposal". Nobody was compelled by Save the 8th, or by their Church, to listen to any speaker. If it was now seen as controversial to speak about the right to life in a Christian church, this would indicate that "hysteria" had "overtaken rational discourse".[32]

The ACP stated in its press release on 4 May that it would not participate further in the referendum debates. Relatively little was heard from members of the clergy. The Catholic bishops expressed their opinions through pastoral letters and homilies but were not very active.[33] Their rigid stance on abortion was faithfully advocated through the medium of the secular pro-life movement. This was especially evident when Bishop Alphonsus Cullinan (Waterford and Lismore) urged his priests to use documents issued by the Pro Life Campaign at Masses a few days before the referendum.[34] Cullinan was in a poor position, despite his episcopal status, to influence Catholics in his diocese. His credibility on moral issues had been damaged in late September 2017 when he expressed scepticism about the merit of vaccinating schoolgirls against human papillomavirus (HPV). Infection by HPV was one of the most common sexually transmitted diseases and in some cases caused cervical cancer. Cullinan had claimed that HPV vaccination was "only 70% safe" and speculated that it would "lull ... girls into a false sense of security", making it more likely that they would become promiscuous and at higher risk of infection.[35] This opinion had provoked widespread outrage. Paul Connors, National Director of Communications at the Health Service Executive, asserted that the bishop's comments were incompatible with the best scientific and medical evidence and put the health and lives of women at risk.[36] The ACP had called on Bishop Cullinan to withdraw his comments and requested that the Irish Catholic bishops disassociate themselves from his ill-informed opinions, observing that:

> Parents who may be convinced that he enjoys some competence in this area could follow his advice and unwittingly put their children at risk. Sadly, his comments also bring the Irish Catholic Church into further disrepute suggesting a nonchalance about women's health and an obsession with sexuality.[37]

On 2 October, Cullinan issued an apology through the website of the Irish Catholic Bishops' Conference, acknowledging that he had been misinformed about the HPV vaccination programme, and that HPV vaccines contributed "greatly" to reducing the frequency of cervical cancer.[38]

The background role of the bishops probably gave rise to some frustration and disillusionment among traditionally minded Catholics. A letter to the *Irish Times* complained about the lack of leadership and commitment from the hierarchy, although it acknowledged the publication of pastoral letters – "which most people ignore anyway".[39] These observations misunderstood the position of the hierarchy. The bishops, aware that their status in Irish society had been tarnished, probably calculated that robust engagement in debates would be counterproductive. Their greatest contribution to the debate was their unwavering reiteration of Catholic doctrine which held that human life was sacred from conception onwards. Pro-life activists embraced this concept, presenting it in secular rather than in theological terms. This in turn ruled out any prospect of compromise in dealing with the "hard cases" of rape, incest and "fatal" foetal abnormalities. The need to compromise was essential for winning over undecided voters, something the pro-life campaign seemed incapable of doing.

Hard Cases and Moral Dilemmas

In mid-February 2018 the Minister for Employment Affairs and Social Protection, Regina Doherty TD (Fine Gael), expressed concern that not enough was being done to explain the recommendations of the Joint Committee on the Eighth Amendment to the electorate. Failure to do so was likely to lead to a retention of the Eighth Amendment. There would then be no prospect of legislating for rape, fatal foetal abnormalities, and the illegal use of abortion pills without medical supervision. Access to abortion up to twelve weeks without the need to disclose a specific reason was regarded as a major problem for a large sector of the electorate. The public needed to be informed about the legal and medical reasons for this.[40]

Leading obstetricians spoke out in favour of repeal. At a press conference in Dublin, Professor Fergal Malone stated that about 2–3 per cent of the approximately 1,500 women who procured abortion pills from online sources each year would experience medical complications after taking the tablets. For example, in some cases, women were unaware that they had an ectopic pregnancy; patients delayed seeking help and sometimes presented with major bleeding into the abdomen from ruptured fallopian tubes. The Eighth Amendment was not so much preventing abortion as creating conditions that endangered the lives and health of women.[41] This was a moral issue that needed to be addressed.

A moral dilemma also arose in cases where women were liable to prosecution for inducing termination of pregnancy. Under the terms of the Protection of Life During Pregnancy Act 2013 (PLDPA) they could serve prison sentences up to fourteen years if found guilty. Some women would procure and use abortion pills regardless of the Eighth Amendment and the PLDPA. What course of action should be pursued in such cases? Defenders of the status quo seemed unable to answer this question.[42] Imposing prison sentences on women found guilty of illegally procuring an abortion was widely seen as indefensible, especially in cases where women had become pregnant due to rape. The logical response, apparently, was to amend the PLDPA, replacing the prison sentence with a token €1 fine. This amendment was proposed in a Private Members' Bill by Bríd Smith TD in the Dáil. It was voted down by government TDs based on advice from the Attorney General. The Minister for Health, Simon Harris, informed the Dáil that a duty was imposed on the state under Article 40.3.3 to defend "the right to life of the unborn". A €1 fine proposed in the Protection of Life During Pregnancy (Amendment) Bill 2017 was likely to elicit an "immediate successful legal challenge". It would be found unconstitutional on the basis that the punishment did not reflect the seriousness of the offence.[43]

Prison sentences were seen as unacceptable even by many pro-life activists! Was there another way to avoid sending women to prison? Section 22 of the PLDPA seemed to offer some hope of a resolution. It stated that a decision to prosecute could only be taken by or with the consent of the Director of Public Prosecutions. Dr Conor Hanly, lecturer in law at the National University of Ireland, Galway, pointed to this sub-section of the PLDPA as a solution to the problem. An important aspect of the DPP's discretion was a consideration of what best served the public interest. Hanly, who intended voting No, argued that prosecuting women in such circumstances did not serve the public interest.[44] A major problem with this argument is that the decision of the DPP not to prosecute could not be relied upon by all women who procured abortion pills. Unsafe use of illegally procured medication would continue. Consistently deciding not to prosecute would bring the law into disrepute and would be a failure to "defend and vindicate" the right to life of "the unborn". If the law was morally defensible and practicable it needed to be upheld; otherwise there was a need to amend or repeal it. Retaining Article 40.3.3 and compatible legislation under such circumstances was, arguably, very inimical to the public interest by failing to protect unborn human life, creating conditions that placed women's lives and health at risk, and bringing the law into disrepute.

The Pro Life Campaign argued that most jurisdictions, including those with liberal abortion laws, such as Britain, maintained sanctions against illegal abortions. Love Both observed that, although no woman had been prosecuted in Ireland for procuring an illegal abortion, it was still necessary to retain deterrents in law. However, the prosecution should be directed at the abortion provider and not at the woman who sought the abortion.[45] Senator Mullen had raised this point when the Thirty-sixth Amendment of the Constitution Bill was being debated in the Seanad. The purpose of the criminal law was "to deter, not always to punish, and ... the law may say it is a crime but people are treated with mercy and compassion."[46] Senator Michael McDowell, a barrister and former attorney general, challenged Mullen on this point on the basis that it would not be possible to decriminalise abortion if Article 40.3.3 was retained. Turning "a blind eye" to crime would not occur in every instance. A young woman had been prosecuted in Belfast for using abortion pills; why would it not happen in the Republic?[47] Defenders of the Eighth Amendment were unable to give a credible answer to this question.

Abortion and Disability

The issue of disability, especially relating to Down syndrome, was raised frequently by the pro-life campaign, sometimes with reference to eugenics and euthanasia to heighten fears about repeal of the Eighth Amendment.[48] When the government published its *Policy Paper: Regulation of Termination of Pregnancy* on 8 March it indicated that the intended legislation would not provide for termination of pregnancy in cases where a foetal condition was not likely to cause death before or shortly after birth.[49] This did little to assuage concerns about eugenics and euthanasia among some in the pro-life campaign. Bishop John Buckley (Cork and Ross) and Bishop Denis Nulty (Kildare and Leighlin) warned that repealing the Eighth Amendment could lead to the emergence of an "abortion culture", which would in turn prepare the way for the introduction of eugenics and euthanasia.[50] The association between euthanasia and the anticipated consequences of repealing the Eighth Amendment was not plausible. However, concerns about eugenics, although based on exaggerations and misunderstandings, could not be so easily dismissed.

On 23 January Fintan O'Toole, a columnist and literary editor for the *Irish Times*, anticipated that "the face of the campaign" for retaining the Eighth Amendment would be "a delightfully smiling kid with Down Syndrome". He was responding to a Love Both pamphlet with a photograph of a smiling child with Down syndrome (DS) and the caption "90% of babies diagnosed with Down Syndrome in Britain are aborted". He warned those campaigning for repeal that this was a powerful message which needed to be addressed. Repeal of the Eighth Amendment was thought to facilitate a eugenics programme where people with DS would be "engineered out of existence." This claim presented a major risk to the repeal campaign and needed to be challenged.

O'Toole observed that improved screening techniques and "relatively free access" to abortion services created the possibility of "essentially" eliminating DS.[51] Anti-abortion campaigners pointed to trends in Western European democracies, especially Iceland, Denmark and Britain. In its submission to the Citizens' Assembly, the Pro Life Campaign stated that, in Britain, 90 per cent of pregnant women who received a diagnosis of DS opted for abortion. In Denmark, there was "a goal" to eliminate DS by 2030. Iceland, it seemed, had already succeeded. Ireland was presented in a virtuous light with its "culture of equality and inclusion".[52] O'Toole argued that the presentation of statistical data was oversimplified and misleading. There was an underlying assumption that all Irish women who received diagnoses of DS would turn to abortion. The figure of 90 per cent for Britain was accurate but misleading; it did not include the 30–40 per cent of women who declined to be screened because they had already decided that they would maintain their pregnancy even if the test gave a positive result.[53] The emphasis on Iceland was excessive, considering its population of about 340,000, its low birth rate, and the few DS diagnoses per annum.

O'Toole made reference to Professor Eva Pajkrt's evidence to the Joint Committee on the Eighth Amendment of the Constitution to add further weight to his argument. In response to a question by Senator Rónán Mullen she informed the committee that the uptake of prenatal screening in the Netherlands was as low as 35 per cent. Many women believed that DS should not be screened for. In cases where there was a diagnosis of DS, usually among women who had requested screening, the termination rate was about 90 per cent. Prenatal screening did not drive down the birth rate of DS children to zero. In the Netherlands the frequency of DS births was stable at about 250 per annum. Healthcare services were based on patient autonomy and what women wished for.[54]

Mullen informed Professor Pajkrt that children in Ireland with DS were "more cherished than in many other countries". This echoed the Love Both pamphlet, which pointed to "a culture of equality and inclusion". These sentiments elicited a caustic response from O'Toole, who observed that it was all very well to speak about equality, inclusion, and cherishing DS children, but the state had fallen far short of providing much-needed services for DS. The Ireland that cherished DS children was the same Ireland where DS children had to wait two years for a wheelchair and three years for language therapy.[55]

Down Syndrome Ireland (which represented and supported about 3,500 members) did not look favourably on either side in the abortion debate when reference was made to DS to promote their cause. This was clearly indicated when the organisation's chief executive, Gary Owens, wrote to the *Irish Times* in response to media coverage, especially in relation to the Love Both pamphlet and O'Toole's article (although the latter was not specifically referenced). Owens was adamant that people with DS should not be referred to in arguments for or against abortion. Campaigners who did so were disrespectful to both children and adults with DS and to their families, which in turn caused much stress, especially to parents. The organisation's position in the referendum debate was one of neutrality. It was up to each person to make their own decision. Owens then asked "all political parties and any other interested groups to stop exploiting children and adults with DS to promote their campaign views".[56]

The opinions of people with disabilities, and their families, were probably as varied as those of the general population. Voluntary organisations representing their interests took different positions in the debate. Down Syndrome Ireland, as already observed, was resolutely neutral. Inclusion Ireland, an organisation for people with intellectual disabilities, joined the Together for Yes campaign.[57] Some parents with DS children, many of whom were already members of pro-life organisations, formed a new organisation, Disability Voices for Life, to campaign for retention of the Eighth Amendment.[58] Disability Voices for Life was closely associated with Save the 8th. The lack of support from voluntary organisations that worked to promote the welfare of people with disabilities tended to undermine the credibility of those who contended that repeal of the Eighth Amendment was somehow inimical to the best interests of those with disabilities and was disrespectful to both them and their families.[59] A diametrically opposite opinion viewed the Eighth Amendment as "a severe burden" on those with disabilities, most of whom were unemployed. They had low incomes and limited means of travel. Their wishes were frequently ignored in situations of crisis pregnancy. The risk of crisis pregnancy was higher than average for disabled people because of limited access to sex education, low awareness of appropriate contraceptive use, and vulnerability to abuse. Access to abortion services, in common with the rest of the population, would be an important step towards "disabled autonomy".[60]

The credibility of the pro-life campaign's claims about disabilities and abortion was called into question on 29 January when the "Statement from the Institute of Obstetricians and Gynaecologists" was published. The institute's purpose was to give the public "factual background information to inform the debate". Most of the controversy about disability and abortion was focused on DS (trisomy 21). Most women first received an appointment for antenatal care when they were between twelve and twenty weeks pregnant.[61] Non-invasive prenatal screening tests (NIPT, e.g. Panorama and Harmony) analysed free foetal DNA in the mother's bloodstream and could be carried out from as early as nine weeks but, because there was no testing facility in Ireland, the patient had to wait for a period usually not exceeding two weeks.[62] These tests were not diagnostic and required a further test to confirm or refute the diagnosis. Also, these tests were priced at more than €500 and were not funded by the state, which effectively restricted access for many women.[63] The institute concluded that:

> It is clear therefore that diagnosis of chromosomal abnormality, while technically possible, can rarely or realistically be achieved before twelve weeks. To suggest therefore that disability will be eliminated by enacting legislation in line with the recommendations of the Oireachtas committee is misleading.[64]

The information published by the institute was further disseminated by Dr Peter Boylan in an interview with the *Irish Times*.[65]

The government's policy paper (8 March) and its General Scheme of a Bill to Regulate Termination of Pregnancy (27 March 2018) did not permit legal termination of pregnancy in cases of severe abnormalities affecting the foetus that were not likely to lead to the death of the foetus, either before birth or shortly after birth. This, together with the fact that termination was permitted in all cases up to twelve weeks, made disability a non-issue in terms of the government's stated intentions. Pro-life campaigners saw it otherwise, expressing mistrust of politicians. It was anticipated that the restrictive legislation envisaged would quickly become more liberal, reflecting trends in other countries, especially Britain, Denmark and Iceland. Most such pregnancies would be terminated in the first few weeks when cheaper, reliable and faster tests for chromosomal abnormalities became widely accessible. It would be open to the government, freed of constitutional constraints if the referendum proposal was passed, to change legislation to address this issue, but this was untenable. The first twelve-week period with no restrictions (except the seventy-two-hour waiting period) was included in the General Scheme of the Bill to address issues relating to the illegal use of abortion pills and cases of rape.

Although Down Syndrome Ireland was not mentioned by name, Disability Voices for Life reacted against what it perceived as "a campaign to silence families" with a DS son or daughter. Caitríona Cronin claimed that:

> [I]n countries with legal abortion along the lines the government wishes to introduce, people like Joseph disappear at astonishing and cruel rates ... we want Joseph to grow up in a culture where people with disabilities are loved and valued and cherished. How can this happen when most babies with disabilities are being aborted – when they are no longer being born.[66]

This statement was misleading because it ignored the restrictions in the proposed legislation. Furthermore, there was the unfounded assumption that if no more DS babies were born this would somehow change attitudes towards those who were born, so that they were no longer loved, valued or cherished. The assumption that all women who received diagnoses of DS, or some other chromosomal anomaly, would choose to terminate their pregnancies was also contrary to research findings, as indicated by Eva Pajkrt's research relating to the Netherlands. The same point was applicable to Ireland – many pro-life campaigners could not have been unaware of this.[67] Women who were resolutely pro-life did not need the Eighth Amendment to make what was, for them, the right moral decision to continue their pregnancy.

The pro-life contention that prenatal diagnoses of Down syndrome would lead to very high percentages of terminations was supported by statistical data from Britain, Denmark and other jurisdictions. Yet there was a tendency by pro-life organisations to misrepresent the data, which in turn led to higher percentage figures for abortions. The frequently quoted 90 per cent abortion rate for DS in Britain was inaccurate because it should have been applied only to prenatal diagnoses.[68]

The General Scheme of a Bill to Regulate Termination of

Pregnancy and the "Statement from the Institute of Obstetricians and Gynaecologists" created difficulties for sustaining the idea of a government policy of eugenics. However, there was some basis for arguing that a relatively small number of abortions would occur following very early prenatal screening tests. On 10 May, following the publication of the government's *Policy Paper: Regulation of Termination of Pregnancy*, veteran pro-life campaigner Professor William Binchy and obstetrician Dr Trevor Hayes argued that abortions would be performed on grounds of disability, contrary to the opinions of Dr Peter Boylan and the Minister for Health, Simon Harris. The Institute of Obstetricians and Gynaecologists had acknowledged that it was possible to diagnose chromosomal abnormality within twelve weeks, but only in rare cases. Binchy and Hayes, speaking at a Love Both media conference in Dublin, argued that such cases might not be so rare, and they referred to Dr Peter McParland's evidence to the Citizens' Assembly on 7 January 2017.[69] McParland, director of foetal medicine at the National Maternity Hospital in Dublin, had informed the assembly that in the previous three years there had been a major improvement in prenatal diagnosis. It was possible to extract foetal DNA from maternal blood to diagnose common chromosomal anomalies, including Down, Edwards and Patau syndromes. This test was 99 per cent accurate and could be done as early as ten weeks into the pregnancy. McParland anticipated that there would be greater access to ultrasound scanning facilities, and that such facilities would be improved. Non-invasive testing would become less costly and more accessible.[70]

McParland observed that increasing numbers of women were choosing to travel abroad to terminate their pregnancies. This was corroborated by Dr Rhona Mahony when she was interviewed on RTÉ Radio One on 9 May. She stated that a screening test for Down syndrome, with 99 per cent accuracy, could be performed as early as nine weeks and that "most" women who were screened proceeded to have a diagnostic test.[71] This led to the question: Would women act on the results of the screening test alone, with its 99 per cent accuracy, when there was a limit of twelve weeks, as envisaged in the General Scheme of a Bill to Regulate Termination of Pregnancy? Binchy and Hayes thought not! Reference was made to Peter Boylan, who was quoted as saying that "women will wait the full diagnostic test with 100 per cent accuracy, which is usually available after 12 weeks gestation".[72] No source was given for the quotation, but reference to an interview of Boylan by TheJournal.ie indicates that the 99 per cent figure was an oversimplification and that he had been quoted out of context. The 99 per cent figure was not consistent from case to case and was influenced by variables such as the age of the mother. Also, some tests failed because samples did not contain sufficient quantities of foetal DNA and needed to be repeated, which was then very likely to delay results beyond the twelve-week limit in the proposed legislation.[73]

It is significant that Binchy and Hayes did not make reference to the statement issued by the Institute of Obstetricians and Gynaecologists on 29 January, which stated that screening test results were "rarely" available within the twelve-week period.[74] There was the likelihood, as envisaged by McParland, that the costs of screening tests would decrease and that such tests would become widely accessible sometime in the future. It was reasonable to speculate that the accuracy of screening tests would improve further. These developments would then facilitate higher abortion rates for pregnancies in the first twelve weeks of pregnancy in cases where chromosomal anomalies had been diagnosed. But there were no restrictions on abortion within the first twelve weeks. If it was legally permissible to terminate the life of a healthy foetus, there was no rational basis for prohibiting the termination of pregnancy in cases where chromosomal and other anomalies had been diagnosed.

Dr Hayes stated that he would "hate to see Irish society with no more babies with Down's Syndrome" because it "would defile the core identity we have of being Irish" – as if this was somehow a cultural choice or an essential feature of national identity.[75] DS is a spectrum of disorders "ranging from babies who won't survive the first trimester, babies with very serious heart defects, all kinds of other genetic anomalies, and babies that are quite well and relatively healthy".[76] Some parents would choose to terminate a pregnancy when there was a diagnosis of DS, preferring to try again and improve their prospects of having a healthy child, especially when special needs services were under-resourced. The referendum was essentially about granting the right to choose; it was not about enabling a state-sponsored scheme of eugenics. The association between abortion and disability, in the context of debates about the General Scheme of the Bill, lacked credibility and does not seem to have persuaded any significant sector of the electorate to swing decisively in favour of retaining the Eighth Amendment.

"Medical Myths" about the Eighth Amendment

On 6 April, in the *Irish Times*, Dr Eamon McGuinness challenged the opinion that the Eighth Amendment put women's lives at risk.

McGuinness was a former chairman of the Institute of Obstetricians and Gynaecologists (1993–1996) and served as a medical adviser to the Save the 8th campaign. He was therefore in a highly influential position. McGuinness's article was published under the provocative title "Medical myths about Eighth Amendment must be challenged." He was adamant that there was no constitutional restriction on his ability, or that of his colleagues, to save the lives of pregnant women when serious medical complications occurred. He pointed to the research findings of Maternal Death Enquiry (Ireland) to make the point that maternal deaths in the Republic were very rare. If doctors were obstructed by the Eighth Amendment from acting in the best interests of women, the outcome would be a significantly higher mortality rate.[77] Maternal Death Enquiry reports indicated that there was no significant statistical differences between Ireland and the UK in deaths per 100,000 maternities.[78] However, McGuinness's analysis did not consider the point that if abortion services in Britain were not accessible to women travelling from Ireland, the maternal mortality rate for Ireland would be much higher.[79]

McGuinness condemned what he regarded as "a campaign of fear and misinformation" about the Eighth Amendment in the context of providing timely and appropriate healthcare to pregnant women. Medical Council guidelines required doctors to provide treatment, even if this threatened the baby's life. McGuinness singled out a pro-repeal meeting in Kildare where it was claimed that a woman who had cancer while pregnant was unable to avail of chemotherapy in Ireland. He dismissed this as "simply false". McGuinness's assertion drew an angry response from Professor Louise Kenny, obstetrician and gynaecologist at Cork University Maternity Hospital. Kenny criticised the opinion that the Eighth Amendment didn't put women's lives at risk as disingenuous. She had treated Michelle Harte, who had had to travel to Britain for an abortion while terminally ill with cancer. A termination could have been performed in the first trimester of Ms Harte's pregnancy, but Professor Kenny was prevented from doing so by an absence of clear guidelines and uncertainty in relation to the legal interpretation of risk to the life of her patient. The assessment of the hospital ethics committee was that, in the absence of an "immediate risk" to Ms Harte's life, a termination should not be proceeded with. Delays and interruptions of treatment led to a rapid deterioration in her health and she died in November 2011.[80]

When McGuinness spoke at a Save the 8th press conference on 10 April he was questioned again about the adverse impact of the Eighth Amendment on healthcare services for pregnant women. An article by journalist Órla Ryan in TheJournal.ie indicates that he was out of touch with developments in his profession. He was still unaware of any maternal death due to the Eighth Amendment. When questioned about the case of Michelle Harte he replied that he did not wish to comment on it because he did not know the details of the case. He also declined to offer an opinion on the *P.P. v Health Service Executive* (2014) case because he could not remember it. McGuinness downplayed differences of opinion in the medical professions.[81] The Institute of Obstetricians and Gynaecologists had expressed support for the repeal of Article 40.3.3 on 10 January 2018.[82] McGuinness, who was still a member of the institute, declined to comment on its position. Many doctors, it seemed to him, had views similar to his. He was not aware of "a major disagreement" – "even among general practitioners".[83] This was evidently not true, as indicated by evidence submitted to the Citizens' Assembly by Doctors for Choice in February and March 2017. Additionally, a survey of nearly 400 GPs and hospital consultants the previous February indicated that 73 per cent were supportive of providing unrestricted access to abortion up to twelve weeks.[84] In early May more than 1,000 doctors signed a public declaration calling for the repeal of the Eighth Amendment.[85]

McGuinness had some influential allies in the medical profession. Dr John Monaghan, a consultant obstetrician and gynaecologist based in Portiuncula Hospital (Ballinasloe), was a member of the Medical Alliance for the 8th. At the launch of Save the 8th in March he stated that he had delivered between 4,000 and 5,000 babies during his career and Article 40.3.3 had never prevented him taking action to protect a woman's life. He believed that Peter Boylan should have stepped aside as chairman of the Institute of Obstetricians and Gynaecologists because of his active participation in the referendum debate. More significantly, he cast doubt on the level of support for repeal among the membership of the institute. He claimed that members did not get the opportunity to discuss the substantive issue of whether or not the Eighth Amendment should be repealed. Boylan had stated a few days previously that nineteen of the executive's approximately twenty-five members were at the meeting at which a decision was taken to support repeal.[86]

On 8 May, five obstetricians – Dr Peter Boylan, Dr Rhona Mahony, Dr Jennifer Donnelly (Rotunda Hospital, Dublin), Professor Mary Higgins and Dr Cliona Murphy – spoke out against the Eighth Amendment in a Together for Yes campaign video. Mahony stated, "we continue to play medical roulette with women's lives." Boylan maintained that the Eighth Amendment "makes it difficult for us to treat women with compassion and give them the proper care that they need." This provoked a reaction from Professor John Bonnar, Dr Eamon McGuinness, Dr Conor Carr, Dr James Clinch and Dr Michael O'Hare, all former chairmen of the Institute of Obstetricians and Gynaecologists. They singled out for censure the comments of Boylan and Mahony, who were then called upon to withdraw their statements on the basis that their claims were groundless. Bonnar and his colleagues each had about forty years' experience in obstetrics and gynaecology. Four of them had practised in the Republic of Ireland and had performed the necessary surgeries to save women's lives even when these operations resulted in termination of pregnancy. The Eighth Amendment was never a problem for them in carrying out ethically and medically indicated procedures.[87]

The generation gap between the first and second group of obstetricians and gynaecologists indicates that opinions about abortion in the medical profession had changed radically since 1983 – probably reflecting changes in public opinion generally. The Institute of Obstetricians and Gynaecologists informed the public that:

> Notwithstanding the provisions of the Protection of Life in Pregnancy Act, the existence of the Eighth Amendment poses major challenges for doctors when caring for pregnant women. Doctors have to decide how close to death a woman is in order to proceed with termination of pregnancy. The woman has no input into this decision other than to give her consent.[88]

This stance on the issue of abortion was a major problem for the pro-life movement. The institute was the national professional and training body for obstetrics and gynaecology in Ireland and was accredited by the Medical Council of Ireland. Seventeen members of the institute believed that it should adopt a neutral stance in keeping with the diversity of opinions of its members and that Peter Boylan should "temporarily stand aside" as chairman if he wished to continue participation in the referendum debate. Boylan refused, asserting that he was an advocate for the best interests of women in Ireland. Also, 81 per cent of members who responded to an internal survey expressed support for repeal.[89] Some of these, such as Rhona Mahony (master of the National Maternity Hospital), Fergal Malone (master of the Rotunda Hospital) and Peter Boylan, were in key positions of influence in the profession and their active participation in the referendum debates made a major impact on public opinion.[90]

Mental Health, Suicide, and Abortion

Section 9 of the PLDPA stated that it would be lawful to terminate a pregnancy if three medical practitioners (one obstetrician and two psychiatrists) jointly certified in good faith that there was a "real and substantial risk of loss of the woman's life by way of suicide" and that such a risk could only be averted by termination of pregnancy. Accessing termination of pregnancy through the PLDPA was less than straightforward. For example, a decision might be taken not to invoke the PLDPA and a young pregnant girl might instead be detained in a psychiatric unit under Section 25 of the Mental Health Act 2001. A psychiatrist could refuse to assess the girl or woman due to conscientious objection or a psychiatrist could assess her and refuse her. It might be necessary to see four or more medical practitioners. The process was so arduous that few people who were suicidal would persist in navigating their way through it.[91] Only seven terminations of pregnancy in response to the risk of suicide were carried out in the three-year period from 2014 to 2016.[92]

The argument that the risk of suicide would be unscrupulously used to liberalise access to abortion was clearly not sustainable in relation to the PLDPA. The PLDPA was so cumbersome that it was "effectively unworkable" for most women.[93] Despite this, the PLDPA was a step too far for some defenders of the Eighth Amendment. In the course of the Seanad debate on the Thirty-sixth Amendment of the Constitution Bill 2018, Senator Rónán Mullen claimed that there had been "some unjust deaths" due to the provision for termination on grounds of suicide risk in the PLDPA. Seven babies had died because of "a suicide ground that was never medically justifiable".[94] Consultant psychiatrist Professor Patricia Casey was, for similar reasons, sharply critical of the government's proposed legislation. Casey, a patron of the Iona Institute, had in January 2013 warned against "a floodgates phenomenon" in relation to a suicide risk clause in forthcoming legislation (the PLDPA) which had to take account of the Supreme Court ruling in the X Case judgment (1992).[95]

Her scepticism about mental health risks as grounds for abortion did not diminish in the following years. Speaking at a press conference organised by Save the 8th on 1 May 2018, she dismissed the idea of abortion as a solution to mental illness as "naive in the extreme". The government's General Scheme of a Bill to Regulate Termination of Pregnancy was "very vague in relation to psychiatric assessment".[96] The Bill referred to the "reasonable" opinions of medical professionals "formed in good faith".[97] Casey was not confident that medical professionals could be relied upon to exercise good judgement. A doctor – "specialty unspecified" – could perform an "immediate termination of pregnancy" if he or she was "of the reasonable opinion" that there was an "immediate risk of serious harm" to the mental health of the pregnant woman. Furthermore, such a termination of pregnancy would be lawful "up until birth".[98]

On 16 May Professor Casey and twenty-two other psychiatrists expressed concerns in an open letter about the proposed legislation on abortion. Demands for repeal of the Eighth Amendment were presented in the language of healthcare, but this, it was claimed, was misleading because in the "vast majority" of cases terminations would apply to healthy women and healthy babies. There were no restrictions in the first three months of pregnancy – the period in which about 90 per cent of abortions took place. A major defect in the legislation was that abortion could be permitted for health reasons. No distinction was drawn between physical and mental health in the General Scheme of a Bill to Regulate Termination of Pregnancy. Casey and her colleagues were especially concerned about the mental health aspect of the proposed legislation. They believed that the proposed legislation was very similar to the law regulating abortion in Britain. They referred to official statistics from Britain to make the point that 97 per cent of the almost 200,000 abortions per annum there were permitted on grounds of mental health issues. In support of this they referred to paragraph 2.38 of the *Report of the Joint Committee on the Eighth Amendment of the Constitution* (2017) which found that most of the abortions, relating to women travelling from Ireland, were really carried out for socio-economic reasons. Taking cognisance of the history of abortion in Britain, Casey and her colleagues were confident that Ireland would follow a very similar path and that most abortions after twelve weeks of pregnancy would be permitted on "spurious" mental health grounds.

A key assumption by Casey and her colleagues was that, after the twelve-week period, Irish law would "conform closely" to British law.[99] Their analysis failed to win over middle-ground voters. Furthermore, Casey and her fellow psychiatrists addressed only the mental health ground issue. Other important issues that featured prominently in public discourse, such as rape and fatal foetal anomalies, were ignored on the basis that abortions in Britain were performed "almost always for socio-economic reasons".[100] Many of these "socio-economic" reasons included being the victim of rape or domestic violence, and being homeless and living with children in temporary accommodation.

Statements issued by the Psychological Society of Ireland (PSI) contrasted sharply with those of Casey and her colleagues. In its press release of 11 May, the PSI emphasised the importance of "evidence-based facts" and expressed its intention to challenge the dissemination of "false facts". In doing so it referred to a range of peer-reviewed research publications, including two major reviews by the American Psychological Association and the Academy of Medical Royal Colleges (London). On the strength of these it claimed that: (1) abortion was not harmful to women's mental health; and (2) women who chose to have an abortion did so "because of the negative effects of continuing the pregnancy on their mental health and that of their existing children and significant others."[101]

The PSI press release did not exert any discernible influence on campaigners for a No vote. In the last few days of the referendum campaign they emphasised at every opportunity the supposed similarity between the General Scheme of a Bill to Regulate Termination of Pregnancy and abortion law in Britain. They argued that abortion would be legal up to six months on "vaguely defined mental-health grounds".[102] This stance probably alienated many potential retain voters and gave the repeal campaigners a considerable advantage. Questioning mental health as grounds for abortion implied that women could not be trusted – a point frequently made throughout the referendum campaign.

The medical and legal professions were divided on the issue of abortion. It is probable that the majority of members of both professions were in agreement with repealing the Eighth Amendment. Calls for repeal drew strong support from key sectors of the medical profession. Together for Yes elicited support from 1,642 doctors, of whom 1,532 were working in Ireland. These included 424 in general practice, 115 in obstetrics and gynaecology, and 107 in psychiatry.[103] Collectively, they played an important role in persuading a large sector of the electorate that there were sound medical reasons for repeal.

The Campaign

The Together for Yes organisation was formed in March 2018 when fifty-seven organisations came together to press for repeal of the Eighth Amendment. It represented a diverse cross-section of Irish society and it quickly grew to represent ninety-six organisations by 23 May.[104] Its two main opponents were Save the 8th and Love Both. Save the 8th was an umbrella organisation comprising Youth Defence and the Life Institute with some support from a number of local support groups. Love Both was the campaign name for the Pro Life Campaign – the successor organisation to the Pro-Life Amendment Campaign of 1981–1983.[105] These pro-life organisations pressed ahead with their campaign with greater speed than Together for Yes. Save the 8th lost no time in erecting posters nationwide. It anticipated that the public would be shocked by the statistics on its posters. This was justified on the basis that "the reality of abortion is shocking".[106] Photographs were not selected with accuracy in mind. Its first poster displayed a photograph of a newly born baby with the caption "IN ENGLAND I IN 5 BABIES ARE ABORTED. DON'T BRING THIS TO IRELAND: VOTE NO."The photograph was clearly at variance with the official statistics of England and Wales, which indicated that 90 per cent of abortions were performed at less than thirteen weeks' and 80 per cent at less than ten weeks' gestation.[107] The poster "IN BRITAIN, 90% OF BABIES WITH DOWN SYNDROME ARE ABORTED. DON'T LET THAT HAPPEN HERE" displayed a photograph of an infant at least several months old – not in the womb at a maximum of twelve weeks' gestation as stated in the proposed legislation for broad access to abortion.

Save the 8th posters were clearly intended to shock. Some posters displayed photographs of foetuses, although the medical terms "foetus" or "foetuses" were not used – despite the pro-life movement's professed respect for science in "demonstrating the humanity of the unborn".[108] All its posters used hard-hitting captions such as "A LICENCE TO KILL: VOTE NO TO ABORTION ON DEMAND"; "THIS IS ABORTION TO 6 MONTHS. IT'S IN THE LEGISLATION. VOTE NO"; "PREBORN BABIES WILL HAVE NO RIGHTS"; "REAL COMPASSION DOESN'T KILL: VOTE NO," and "IF KILLING AN UNBORN BABY AT SIX MONTHS BOTHERS YOU, THEN VOTE NO."[109] A Love Both poster showed an ultrasound image of a foetus with the caption: "I AM 9 WEEKS OLD: I CAN YAWN AND KICK: DON'T REPEAL ME: VOTE NO." Images of foetuses were usually displayed in isolation and without reference to their mothers. This provoked Dr Chris Fitzpatrick, consultant obstetrician-gynaecologist and a former master of the Coombe Hospital, to write in the *Irish Times*:

> [F]oetuses look down at me from posters high up on the lampposts. They are as big as new-born babies. They tell me that their hearts are beating. They tell me that they can kick and yawn. They ask me to protect them. Their words are meant to hit you where it hurts most – in your heart.[110]

The foetuses had no mothers, were advanced for their age and expressed adult thoughts. Their carefully chosen words were difficult to ignore. They knew "how to make you feel bad". As Fitzpatrick observed, the life of a mother with a crisis pregnancy was much too long and complicated to fit on a poster.[111]

Pro-life posters with misleading claims such as "abortion on demand" were probably counterproductive. Some pro-repeal posters were also subject to sustainable criticism, for example People Before Profit's "TRUST WOMEN: OUR BODIES OUR CHOICE: VOTE YES", which clearly ignored the issue of whether the unborn had any rights. The posters generally did not elicit a favourable response from the public, especially those with photographs of foetuses. Posters with graphic images of dead foetuses erected by the Irish Centre for Bio-ethical Reform (ICBR) outside Dublin's three maternity hospitals (Holles Street, the Coombe and the Rotunda) generated angry responses from the public. The ICBR (which had affiliates in several other countries) was unapologetic. Its mission was to educate the public about abortion. If photographs of aborted "babies" were "vile and disturbing" this was because abortion itself was "vile and disturbing".[112] There was clearly an awareness in the mainstream pro-life movement that the ICBR's initiatives were alienating potential No voters. John McGuirk, spokesman for Save the 8th, criticised the ICBR, pointing out that its actions were wrong and unhelpful. The ICBR was not affiliated with Save the 8th or with the other "major" pro-life organisations.[113]

Posters displayed near schools confronted parents with the onerous responsibility of explaining abortion to their children. A hard-line pro-life stance was unsympathetic towards parents in such difficult circumstances. Parents needed to be honest with their children. Children were cutting "straight through the choice ideology and demanding a straightforward explanation". If parents were experiencing difficulties in explaining abortion to their children, then it was probably because they knew it was wrong.[114] This failed to give due consideration to child psychology and the inability of children to understand complicated ethical issues. Young children needed to be shielded from discussions about abortion in the context of rape, mental health issues and foetal anomalies.[115]

In early May an online survey of parents found that the poster campaign had led to three-quarters of respondents having difficult conversations about abortion with their children. The strongest objections were expressed in relation to posters erected near schools, and with pictures.[116] The extent of public dissatisfaction with referendum posters was indicated in a Claire Byrne Live/Amárach Research poll that found that 74 per cent of 1,000 adults surveyed said that such posters should be banned.[117]

Social media was a crucially important element of both retain and repeal campaigns. In mid-April pro-life supporters found that their activities were restricted on Twitter; the company had taken measures to mitigate the risk that debates about the Eighth Amendment would be manipulated on its site.[118] In early May, Facebook decided it would no longer accept foreign advertisements relating to the Eighth Amendment. This may have been due to concerns that it would come under scrutiny about its role in influencing votes, as had occurred in the UK and the USA. Facebook's decision was welcomed by the repeal movement – they had concerns that a huge volume of advertisements in the last few weeks of the campaign could swing the vote towards retaining the Eighth Amendment.[119] Google's decision to ban all advertisements relating to the referendum inflicted another heavy blow on the pro-life movement, depriving it of an important platform. That this move favoured pro-choice supporters was evident from their enthusiastic approval.[120]

Both No and Yes sides of the referendum debate had to contend with difficult questions which were potentially lethal to their respective campaigns. The pro-life argument that abortion was not a solution for hard cases was well received by committed No voters but did not find much support from undecided voters – the critically important middle ground. In the early weeks of the debate the government's proposal to legalise abortion up to twelve weeks was difficult to accept for many voters. It seemed too extreme![121] Many politicians, such as the Tánaiste, Simon Coveney, who were in favour of repealing the Eighth Amendment, experienced difficulties in accepting this aspect of the accompanying legislative proposals. Even so, a key consideration for Coveney was the unsafe conditions in which abortion pills were being used.[122] Coveney's change of mind on the issue was probably indicative of evolving opinions among middle-ground voters. In the early weeks of the campaign, canvassers for Yes found that many voters were unwilling to accept abortion on request up to twelve weeks.

An *Irish Times*/MRBI opinion poll published on 20 April indicated that the Yes campaign was maintaining a strong lead over the No campaign. But the gap was narrowing. Forty-seven per cent were in favour of Yes; 28 per cent said that they would vote No. Twenty per cent were undecided – an increase of 5 per cent since January. Still, a critically important point was that support for retaining the Eighth Amendment had decreased by 1 per cent.[123] Together for Yes continued to place women's health at the centre of their campaign – a strategy acknowledged by John McGuirk as "very smart and effective". Medical professionals played a key role – especially obstetricians. Concerns about a lacklustre Yes campaign in late April were dissipated by the registration of 118,000 voters on the supplementary register by the closing date of 8 May.[124]

Opinion polls regularly commissioned by the *Irish Times* over the previous two years consistently indicated a clear majority in favour of repealing the Eighth Amendment. Therefore, the Yes campaign started from a very advantageous position. The No campaign needed to reach out to middle-ground and "soft" Yes voters. It failed to do so. The uncompromising stance and inability to advance persuasive proposals for "hard cases" appealed to committed defenders of the Eighth Amendment, but this fell far short of the majority it needed. The Yes campaign seemed less rigidly ideological, emphasising "care, compassion and change" more than "our bodies, our rights".[125]

An *Irish Times* opinion poll on 17 May indicated that 58 per cent of respondents supported repeal, with 42 per cent favouring retention. This prompted some supporters of a No vote to shift position, arguing that it was possible to reform the law for hard cases.[126] Both No and Yes campaigners knew that if public opinion was focused on permitting abortion for fatal foetal abnormalities, rape and incest, the Eighth Amendment would almost certainly be repealed. Shifting attention away from the hard cases by conceding on these, and redirecting attention towards the twelve weeks issue and "abortion on demand" was seen as a winning strategy.[127]

Dr Trevor Hayes, speaking at a Love Both conference on 22 May, asserted that the government had the opportunity to draft legislation for hard cases but had chosen not to do so. He believed that, if the Eighth Amendment was retained, the government would have to pass legislation for "exceptional cases".[128] On 23 May Archbishop Diarmuid Martin claimed that it was still possible to create a legislative framework to help doctors respond appropriately to complex medical cases.[129] Breda O'Brien, a columnist with the *Irish Times*, wrote: "I know it is possible to amend the Constitution and legislate for abortion in exceptionally traumatic cases like rape."[130] This was a clever idea in the sense that it appealed to people who were dissatisfied with the Eighth Amendment but had reservations about the government's proposed legislation. Yet it lacked credibility because the pro-life movement had not proposed an alternative constitutional amendment for consideration earlier during the referendum campaign.

The move towards compromise tended to create confusion and failed to gain consensus among No supporters.[131] It came too late in the campaign to have any prospect of success. Besides, it did not consider legal advice to the contrary. The Taoiseach, Leo Varadkar, dismissed it as a cynical tactic. He, and other supporters of repeal, referred to the advice of the two previous attorneys general[132] that any law passed to permit termination of pregnancy in cases of fatal foetal abnormality would be unconstitutional if the Eighth Amendment was retained.[133] Both Varadkar and Simon Harris argued that those who pressed for retaining the Eighth Amendment had had thirty to thirty-five years to propose alternative amendments to deal with hard cases and had failed to do so. Sinn Féin leader Mary Lou McDonald pointed out in the Dáil that pro-life campaigners had trenchantly opposed the passing of the PLDPA (the provisions of which were very restrictive on termination of pregnancy). There was no concession towards hard cases in 2013. *Irish Times* columnist Miriam Lord observed that predictions about the opening of "floodgates" were unfounded. The "absolutists" had "cried wolf once too often" and had undermined their own credibility.[134]

Voters who had been undecided swung decisively towards repeal to deliver a landslide victory for the Yes campaign. Ireland voted 66.4 per cent for repeal and 33.6 per cent for retain.[135] Many undecided voters had strong reservations about, or objections to, unrestricted abortion up to twelve weeks, but despite this they voted Yes because they saw the Eighth Amendment as deeply flawed in the context of addressing risks to women's health and safety.[136] Some commentators speculated that middle-ground voters might have been won over if a revised Article 40.3.3, to allow for abortion in hard cases, had been proposed early in the referendum campaign. However, John McGuirk argued that such a compromise would have split the movement. Many volunteers and donors would have withdrawn support.[137] Compromise might not have staved off defeat, although the margin between Yes and No would probably have been much smaller.

The referendum result led to a renewal of demands for changes to abortion law in Northern Ireland.[138] Thirty Irish and 143 British parliamentarians wrote to the British Prime Minister, Theresa May, calling for reform on the basis that abortion law in Northern Ireland breached Article 8 of the European Convention on Human Rights. They argued that abortion law was a human rights issue and not a "devolved matter".[139] Political conditions in Northern Ireland and Britain did not favour their initiative.

Sinn Féin and the Social Democratic and Labour Party (SDLP) had decided to no longer oppose the reform of Northern Ireland's restrictive abortion laws.[140] Still, the largest political party – the Democratic Unionist Party (DUP) – was resolutely a pro-life party and was adamant that it would not change its stance on abortion. It was in a strong position to block reform in the power-sharing system of Northern Ireland. Two majorities – Unionist and nationalist – were necessary for reforming the law. All the DUP needed to block reform was a little over 25 per cent of the vote.[141] Also, the Northern Ireland Assembly (the devolved legislature) was in a state of suspension after collapsing in January 2017 due to policy disagreements between the leadership of the DUP and Sinn Féin. Extending abortion rights to Northern Ireland found support from both Conservative and Labour MPs, but the prime minister's office insisted that abortion was a devolved matter. The DUP's ten MPs held the balance of power in Westminster, keeping May's Tory government in power. But the DUP lost its veto in July 2019 when two Labour Party MPs in Westminster tabled amendments to the government's Northern Ireland Bill on abortion and same-sex marriage. The amendments won cross-party support and the amendments were passed by large majorities. On 22 October 2019, abortion was decriminalised and same-sex marriage was to become legal in Northern Ireland from January 2020.[142]

The Catholic bishops were dismayed at the referendum result south of the border.[143] Archbishop Eamon Martin expressed sadness that Ireland had "obliterated the right to life of all unborn children". He had been challenged by personal stories in the course of the referendum campaign and came to realise how little he knew about the problems that women had to struggle with. Even so, he warned, abortion was not the solution for tragic and desperate cases.[144] In a radio interview with RTÉ's Sean O'Rourke, Bishop Kevin Doran stated that those Catholics who had voted Yes, "knowing and intending that abortion would be the outcome", had committed a sin and should consider going to confession.[145] Bishop Alphonsus Cullinan agreed with Doran that Catholics who had voted Yes should go to confession. A clear majority of Catholics in his diocese disagreed with him: almost 70 per cent of voters in Waterford voted Yes to repealing the Eighth Amendment.[146]

Members of the Oireachtas were not inclined towards repentance and were mindful of the democratic imperative to implement the will of the people. The Thirty-sixth Amendment of the Constitution Act 2018 was enacted by the Oireachtas on 18 September after delays caused by three unsuccessful challenges to the validity of the referendum. The new Article 40.3.3 read: "Provision may be made by law for the regulation of termination of pregnancy."[147] The Eighth Amendment had been repealed! But the PLDPA remained in place as the operative law until new legislation was passed. The government pressed ahead with legislation, as it had indicated it would during the referendum campaign. Simon Harris was determined to adhere closely to what the electorate had voted for in the General Scheme of a Bill to Regulate Termination of Pregnancy.[148] The large electoral majority in favour of Yes made it difficult for TDs and senators who had supported retention of the Eighth Amendment to sustain their opposition. Many of them felt it was their democratic duty to vote for the proposed legislation.[149] Simon Harris promised that the government would move quickly to legislate for abortion services.[150] The Health (Regulation of Termination of Pregnancy) Bill 2018 was debated in the Oireachtas from 27 September to 13 December and was passed by a large majority in both houses. The key provisions of the General Scheme of a Bill to Regulate Termination of Pregnancy were retained in the Bill.[151] The Bill was signed into law by President Michael D. Higgins on 20 December 2018. The new law governing terminations of pregnancy took effect on 1 January 2019 (although several hospitals committed to providing abortion services were not ready to do so).[152]

Abortion is not a settled issue in Ireland – or elsewhere. The Health (Regulation of Termination of Pregnancy) Act 2018 is not immutable. Some pro-choice supporters will press for loosening restrictions on abortion. The pro-life movement will campaign for the repeal of the Thirty-sixth Amendment and the subsequent legislation. It is likely to be a very long campaign![153] Those who are most conservative will press for the restoration of a pro-life clause in the Constitution, similar to the Eighth Amendment but even more restrictive in that it will rule out suicide as a basis for termination of pregnancy. They will also insist that human life deserves full human rights protection in law from conception. This is likely to cause deep divisions in the movement. Strict adherence to these concepts imposed a rigid ideology on the pro-life campaign in 2018 that proved fatal to its objective of retaining the Eighth Amendment.[154]

Endnotes

—•—

1   Pat Leahy, "Opinion polls suggest middle ground will be decisive", *Irish Times*, 14 December 2017.

2   Brian Murray, "Legal Consequences of Retention, Repeal, or Amendment of Article 40.3.3 of the Constitution", Citizens' Assembly, 4 March 2017 <https://www.citizensassembly.ie/en/Meetings/Brian-Murray-s-Paper.pdf> accessed 11 March 2017.

3   Noel Whelan, "Simple repeal of Eighth Amendment carries risks", *Irish Times*, 19 January 2018 <https://search-proquest-com.ucc.idm.oclc.org/docview/1988763759/47009D2C03FA4A7EPQ/86?accountid=14504> accessed 19 January 2018.

4   Séamus Woulfe, "Information note on legal advice received on options for a Referendum on Article 40.3.3 of the Constitution" <https://static.rasset.ie/documents/news/2018/01/ag-advice-summary.pdf> accessed 31 January 2018.

5   Thirty-sixth Amendment of the Constitution Bill 2018, 7 March 2018 <https://data.oireachtas.ie/ie/oireachtas/bill/2018/29/eng/initiated/b2918.pdf> accessed 24 October 2018.

6   There was some uncertainty about the right to life of the unborn arising from an immigration case. A High Court judgment in the case of *I.RM. and ors v The Minister for Justice and Equality and Ors* (2016) found that the unborn had constitutional rights other than provided in Article 40.3.3. The High Court also found that the unborn is a child under Article 42A and was protected by the provisions of that article. *M v The Minister for Justice & Ors* (2018 IESC 14) Supreme Court of Ireland, 7 March 2018, section 2.3 <http://www.supremecourt.ie/Judgments.nsf/1b0757edc371032e802572ea0061450e/af9213ad1cf44a3c80258249002acd3d?OpenDocument> accessed 7 March 2018. The state submitted that the unborn has no constitutionally protected rights beyond the right to life in Article 40.3.3 and therefore could not have invoked on its behalf any other constitutional rights (section 7.15). The Supreme Court judgment on 7 March 2018 found that the Minister for Justice (and therefore the state) was "not obliged to treat the unborn as having constitutional rights other than the rights contained in Article 40.3.3". It also found that "the most plausible view of the pre Eighth Amendment law was that there was uncertainty in relation to the constitutional position of the unborn which the Eighth Amendment was designed to remove"

(section 13.3). Nevertheless, the state was "entitled to take account of the respect which is due to human life" as an "aspect of the common good" when legislating (section 10.63). The Supreme Court judgment removed uncertainty about the constitutional status of the unborn, clearing the path for the government to press ahead with a referendum on Article 40.3.3 before the end of May.

7   Appendix 2, *Policy Paper: Regulation of Termination of Pregnancy*, approved and published by the government on 8 March 2018 <http://health.gov.ie/wp-content/uploads/2018/03/Policy-paper-approved-by-Goverment-8-March-2018.pdf> accessed 7 May 2018.

8   General Scheme of a Bill to Regulate Termination of Pregnancy, 27 March 2018 <http://health.gov.ie/wp-content/uploads/2018/03/General-Scheme-for-Publication.pdf accessed 8 May 2018).

9   Section 1, Abortion Act 1967, United Kingdom of Great Britain and Northern Ireland <https://www.legislation.gov.uk/ukpga/1967/87/section/1> accessed 10 May 2018.

10 Sarah Bardon, "The claim: Ireland could introduce an abortion law similar to Britain's", *Irish Times*, 23 May 2018, p. 7.

11 Save the 8th, "Abortion Until 6 Months", April 2018 <https://www.save8.ie/did-you-know-this-is-abortion-up-to-6-months/> accessed 10 May 2018.

12 Mairead Enright *et al.*, letter to the editor, *Irish Times*, 9 April 2018 <https://search-proquest-com.ucc.idm.oclc.org/docview/2022902932/E7A4FE80CC2E4595PQ/89?accountid=14504> accessed 9 April 2018. This letter was signed by several Irish and British professors and lecturers in law, including Senator Ivana Bacik and Professor Fiona de Londras. For further points about how the Irish Bill would be more restrictive than the UK's Abortion Act 1967, see Sally Sheldon *et al.*, letter to the editor, *Irish Times*, 23 April 2018 <https://search-proquest-com.ucc.idm.oclc.org/docview/2028721567/2480E698EBBF447CPQ/82?accountid=14504> accessed 23 April 2018. Professor Sheldon's letter was co-authored by several university lecturers (all UK) and one solicitor.

13 For differences of opinion in the legal profession see, for example, Mairead Enright *et al.* (op. cit.) and Séamas Ó Tuathail *et al.*, letter to the editor, *Irish Times*, 23 April 2018 <https://search-proquest-com.ucc.idm.oclc.org/docview/2028721567/2480E698EBBF447CPQ/82?accountid=14504> accessed 23 April 2018.

14 Ronan Keane, "Repeal does not mean the unborn have no right to life", *Irish Times*, 16 May 2018 <https://search-proquest-com.ucc.idm.oclc.org/docview/2038990392/51D67B8B79584ABCPQ/87?accountid=14504> accessed 16 May 2018.

15 Ronan Keane, letter to the editor, *Irish Times*, 21 May 2018 <https://www.irishtimes.com/opinion/letters/referendum-on-the-eighth-amendment-1.3501920> accessed 21 May 2018.

16 Irish Catholic Bishops' Conference, "Our Common Humanity", 6 March 2018 <https://www.catholicbishops.ie/2018/03/06/our-common-humanity-statement-on-the-second-day-of-the-spring-2018-general-meeting-of-the-irish-catholic-bishops-conference/> accessed 28 May 2018.

17 The concept of natural law in a legal and constitutional context is discussed in *M v The Minister for Justice & Ors* (2018 IESC 14), Supreme Court of Ireland, 7 March 2018, sections 10.11, 10.17, 10.28 and 10.44–47.

18 Ibid., paragraph 10.46.

19 Ibid., paragraph 10.46. See also Keane, "Repeal does not mean the unborn have no right to life".

20 Vote on Thirty-sixth Amendment of the Constitution Bill 2018: Fifth Stage, Dáil Éireann, 21 March 2018 <https://www.oireachtas.ie/en/debates/vote/dail/32/2018-03-21/27/> accessed 21 September 2018.

21 Thirty-sixth Amendment of the Constitution Bill 2018, Seanad Éireann, 28 March 2018 <https://www.oireachtas.ie/en/debates/vote/seanad/25/2018-03-28/2/?highlight%5B0%5D=thirty&highlight%5B1%5D=sixth&highlight%5B2%5D=amendment> accessed 22 September 2018.

22 Joe Humphreys, "Is there a right to life? You might not like the answer", *Irish Times*, 24 April 2018 <https://search-proquest-com.ucc.idm.oclc.org/docview/2029223301/7164D45CCCAF4233PQ/65?accountid=14504> accessed 24 April 2018.

23 *Your Guide to The Referendum – Information on the Government's Proposals*, May 2018. Publishers and sponsors included Family & Life, Life Institute, www.save8.ie, www.protectthe8th.ie, and Coalition Against Abortion on Demand. The booklet was reported to look like an official government publication and was circulated to 200,000 households. Pat Leahy, "Save the Eighth group defends booklet design", *Irish Times*, 16 May 2018.

24 Hugh Linehan, "Will Eighth Amendment referendum campaign be manipulated online?" *Irish Times*, 20 November 2017 <https://search-proquest-com.ucc.idm.oclc.org/docview/1965941130/2777F748E12B4619PQ/42?accountid=14504> accessed 20 November 2017.

25 Amnesty International successfully challenged the Standards in Public Office Commission's order in the High Court. Aodhan O Faolain, "Sipo's order that Amnesty should return €137,000 grant is quashed after High Court appeal", TheJournal.ie, 31 July 2018 <https://www.thejournal.ie/sipo-amnesty-decision-4156736-Jul2018/> accessed 15 December 2018.

26 Ed O'Loughlin, "As Irish abortion vote nears, fears of foreign influence rise", *New York Times*, 26 March 2018 <https://search-proquest-com.ucc.idm.oclc.org/docview/2019741852/70F07B3255C44BFBPQ/2?accountid=14504> accessed 20 April 2018.

27 *Economist*, "Don't mention the Church", vol. 426, no. 9084 (24 March 2018) <https://search-proquest-com.ucc.idm.oclc.org/

docview/2017355779/9F9C8952DC8F4C11PQ/10?accountid=14504>
accessed 20 April 2018.

28 Ibid.; and O'Loughlin, "As Irish abortion vote nears, fears of foreign
    influence rise".

29 *Economist*, op. cit.

30 Archbishop Eamon Martin, "Pastoral Message for the new year 2018
    from Archbishop Eamon Martin: 'To Serve Human Life is to Serve
    God' (Pope Francis)", Irish Catholic Bishops' Conference <https://www.
    catholicbishops.ie/2018/01/06/pastoral-message-for-the-new-year-2018-
    from-archbishop-eamon-martin-to-serve-human-life-is-to-serve-god-
    pope-francis/> accessed 8 January 2018.

31 Association of Catholic Priests, "ACP Statement about the upcoming
    referendum on the Eighth Amendment", 4 May 2018 <https://www.
    associationofcatholicpriests.ie/2018/05/acp-statement-on-the-upcoming-
    referendum-on-the-eight-amendment/> accessed 7 May 2017.

32 "Save the 8th Statement On Pro-Life Speakers at Catholic Masses", 5 May
    2018 <https://www.save8.ie/save-the-8th-statement-on-pro-life-speakers-
    at-catholic-masses/> accessed 8 May 2018.

33 For some statements by individual bishops and archbishops
    see Barry Roche, "Bishop says culture of abortion would
    be 'horrendous'", *Irish Times*, 8 May 2018 <https://search-
    proquest-com.ucc.idm.oclc.org/docview/2035453235/
    ABC7884B2DEA435EPQ/38?accountid=14504> accessed 8 May 2018;
    and Patsy McGarry, "Pope's message on fake news welcomed", *Irish
    Times*, 14 May 2018 <https://search-proquest-com.ucc.idm.oclc.org/
    docview/2038137921/7B7D35945F184915PQ/54?accountid=14504>
    accessed 14 May 2018; "Bishop says wildlife will be protected
    better: Bishop said if the amendment is repealed the unborn baby
    will be left with no protection", *Irish Times*, 21 May 2018 <https://
    search-proquest-com.ucc.idm.oclc.org/docview/2041434788/
    A66B53F0A07F4786PQ/22?accountid=14504> accessed 21 May 2018.

34 Fiachra Ó Cionnaith, "Call to use no vote as starting point", *Irish
    Examiner*, 23 May 2018, p. 6.

35 Paul Cullen, "Catholic bishop claims cervical cancer vaccine 'only 70%
    safe'", *Irish Times*, 27 September 2017 <https://www.irishtimes.com/
    news/health/catholic-bishop-claims-cervical-cancer-vaccine-only-70-
    safe-1.3235705> accessed 30 September 2017.

36 Rónán Duffy, "FactCheck: Is the Bishop of Waterford right to say the
    HPV vaccine is '70% safe'?", TheJournal.ie <http://www.thejournal.ie/hov-
    bishop-factcheck-3620053-Sep2017/> accessed 30 September 2017.

37 "Statement from the Association of Catholic Priests Responding to
    Comments made on the HPV vaccine", 1 October 2017 <http://www.
    associationofcatholicpriests.ie/2017/10/statement-from-the-association-of-

catholic-priests-acp%e2%80%88-responding-to-comments-made-on-the-hpv-vaccine/> accessed 12 October 2017.

38 Irish Catholic Bishops' Conference, "Statement by Bishop Alphonsus Cullinan on HPV vaccines", 2 October 2017 <http://www.catholicbishops. ie/2017/10/02/statement-by-bishop-alphonsus-cullinan-on-hpv-vaccines/> accessed 7 October 2017.

39 Noel Kennedy, letter to the editor, *Irish Times*, 14 May 2018.

40 Ronan McGreevy, "Committee 'couldn't find' any anti-abortion medical experts to argue for Eighth", *Irish Times*, 20 February 2018 <https://www. irishtimes.com/news/ireland/irish-news/committee-couldn-t-find-any-anti-abortion-medical-experts-to-argue-for-eighth-1.3397941> accessed 20 February 2018.

41 Evelyn Ring, "Eighth 'has led to dangerous abortions'", *Irish Examiner*, 22 May 2018, p. 6.

42 Áine Carroll, "Anti-abortion campaigners dodging the issue: what to do with unwanted pregnancies if Eighth is repealed", *Irish Times*, 18 April 2018 <https://search-proquest-com.ucc.idm.oclc.org/ docview/2026045109/806D78EAAF3849D5PQ/85?accountid=14504> accessed 20 April 2018.

43 Protection of Life During Pregnancy (Amendment) Bill 2017: Second Stage [Private Members], Dáil Debates, 7 March 2017 <https://www. oireachtas.ie/en/debates/debate/dail/2017-03-07/30/> accessed 18 October 2018; and Fintan O'Toole, "Eighth demands punishment for women", *Irish Times*, 1 May 2018 <https://search-proquest-com.ucc.idm.oclc.org/ docview/2032559721/EBB4E07422794B5FPQ/63?accountid=14504> accessed 1 May 2018.

44 Dr Conor Hanly, letter to the editor, *Irish Times*, 18 May 2018 <https://search-proquest-com.ucc.idm.oclc.org/docview/2040319173/ C545F39D6F2D4E0FPQ/105?accountid=14504> accessed 18 May 2018.

45 "Should abortion be decriminalised?", Love Both <https://loveboth.ie/ should-abortion-be-decriminalised/> accessed 24 May 2018.

46 Thirty-sixth Amendment of the Constitution Bill 2018: Second Stage, Seanad Éireann Debates, 27 March 2018 <https://www.oireachtas.ie/en/ debates/debate/seanad/2018-03-27/12/> accessed 21 October 2018.

47 Thirty-sixth Amendment of the Constitution Bill 2018: Committee Stage, Seanad Debates, 28 March 2018.

48 David Quinn, "Repeal vote is a rubber stamp for eugenics", *Sunday Times*, 10 December 2017, p. 13; and RTÉ, "Catholic bishop warns about arguments for abortion", RTÉ News, 27 January 2018 <https://www.rte.ie/news/ ireland/2018/0127/936344-catholic-bishop-warns-about-arguments-for-abortion/> accessed 27 January 2018.

49 Policy 5, Appendix 2: *Policy Paper: Regulation of Termination of Pregnancy* (8 March 2018), allowed for termination of pregnancy in cases where there was

a foetal condition which was "likely to lead to death before or shortly after birth".

50 Barry Roche, "Repealing Eighth 'could lead to euthanasia and eugenics'", *Irish Times*, 16 April 2018.

51 Fintan O'Toole, "Down syndrome will be central issue in abortion referendum", *Irish Times*, 23 January 2018 <https://search-proquest-com.ucc.idm.oclc.org/docview/1992712965/1F34273BEAC942C6PQ/58?accountid=14504> accessed 16 February 2018.

52 Pro Life Campaign, "The Eighth Amendment – A Life-Saving Beacon of Hope", presented to the Citizens' Assembly, 3 March 2017 <https://www.citizensassembly.ie/en/Meetings/Pro-Life-Campaign-s-Paper.pdf> accessed 30 September 2018.

53 O'Toole did not give the sources for his 30–40 percentage range. The estimated percentage for England and Wales in 2013, based on available data, was 19%, but the "true percentage" was thought to be much greater because there was no data on 43% of women who had received a postnatal diagnosis. Joan K. Morris and Anna Springett, *The National Down Syndrome Cytogenetic Register for England and Wales: 2013 Annual Report*, December 2014, p. 7 <http://www.binocar.org/content/annrep2013_FINAL.pdf> accessed 6 October 2018.

54 Evidence of Professor Eva Pajkrt to the Joint Committee on the Eighth Amendment of the Constitution, 23 November 2017 <https://www.oireachtas.ie/en/debates/debate/joint_committee_on_the_eighth_amendment_of_the_constitution/2017-11-23/2/> accessed 29 September 2018.

55 O'Toole, "Down syndrome will be central issue".

56 Gary Owens, letter to the editor, *Irish Times*, 25 January 2018 <https://www.irishtimes.com/opinion/letters/eighth-amendment-and-disability-1.3367321> accessed 25 January 2018.

57 Jack Quann, "Disability group Inclusion Ireland to join campaign to repeal Eighth Amendment", 13 April 2018, Newstalk.com <https://www.newstalk.com/Disability-group-Inclusion-Ireland-to-join-campaign-to-repeal-Eighth-Amendment> accessed 8 October 2018.

58 Patsy McGarry, "Child with Down Syndrome to feature in anti-abortion billboard campaign", *Irish Times*, 29 January 2018 <https://www.irishtimes.com/news/social-affairs/religion-and-beliefs/child-with-down-syndrome-to-feature-in-anti-abortion-billboard-campaign-1.3372867> accessed 31 January 2018.

59 Anne Trainer, Disability Voices for Life, stated that: "babies with a disability are aborted in disproportionate numbers, with 90% being aborted in Britain. This reality is absolutely heart-breaking and the reality is that abortion discriminates against babies diagnosed with a disability. This is the real

disrespect to both children and adults with Down Syndrome and their families." Save the 8th, Disability Voices for Life <https://www.save8.ie/abortion-disability/disability-voices-for-life/> accessed 9 May 2018.

60 Stuart Neilson, letter to the editor, *Irish Times*, 14 May 2018.

61 The combined results of ultrasound scans (11 to slightly less than 14 weeks) and measurements of maternal blood proteins (10–13 weeks) provided a basis for calculating risks of chromosomal abnormalities. These were screening tests – not diagnostic tests.

62 The usual waiting period was given as 10 to 14 days by Dr Peter Boylan (chairman of the Institute of Obstetricians and Gynaecologists), and Dr Cliona Murphy (chairwoman-elect). Letter to the editor, *Irish Times*, 4 April 2018.

63 Fianna Fáil TD Mary Butler gave an estimate of 10–15% for pregnant women who underwent non-invasive prenatal testing for chromosomal anomalies. Stephen O'Brien, "Pro-life TDs seek disability clause in abortion bill", *Sunday Times*, 3 June 2018, p. 1.

64 "Statement from the Institute of Obstetricians and Gynaecologists", 29 January 2018 <https://www.rcpi.ie/news/releases/statement-from-the-institute-of-obstetricians-and-gynaecologists-2/> accessed 29 January 2018.

65 Sarah Bardon, "Focusing on Down syndrome misguided, says Boylan", *Irish Times*, 29 January 2018 <https://search-proquest-com.ucc.idm.oclc.org/docview/1991848056/F8BF870E10D24106PQ/10?accountid=14504> accessed 29 January 2018.

66 Save the 8th, Disability Voices for Life, op. cit. See also McGarry, "Child with Down Syndrome to feature in anti-abortion billboard campaign."

67 For example, members and supporters of Disability Voices for Life closely associated with Save the 8th.

68 See for example Aoife Barry, "FactCheck: Are 90% of babies with Down syndrome in Britain aborted?" TheJournal.ie, 4 February 2018 <http://www.thejournal.ie/factcheck-babies-abortion-3823611-Feb2018/> accessed 6 October 2018. In England and Wales (accounting for the vast majority of the population in Britain), 65% of diagnoses for Down syndrome were made prenatally in 2013. See Morris and Springett, *The National Down Syndrome Cytogenetic Register for England and Wales: 2013 Annual Report*, p. 1.

69 Love Both, "Three mothers that faced pressure to terminate their pregnancies", 10 May 2018 <https://loveboth.ie/three-mothers-pressure-abortion/> accessed 5 October 2018; and Patsy McGarry, "Love Both challenges Minister on claim about abortion on disability grounds", *Irish Times*, 11 May 2018 <https://search-proquest-com.ucc.idm.oclc.org/docview/2036892082/96F336D60BE14F28PQ/46?accountid=14504> accessed 11 May 2018.

70 Peter McParland, "Antenatal Diagnosis and Management of Fetal Abnormalities", Paper presented to the Citizens' Assembly <https://www.

citizensassembly.ie/en/Meetings/Dr-Peter-McParland-Paper.pdf> accessed 5 October 2018.

71 RTÉ Radio 1, "Dr Mahony about abortion of babies with Down Syndrome", transcript of interview of Dr Rhona Mahony by Claire Byrne, *News at 1*, 9 May 2018, Love Both website <https://loveboth.ie/rhona-mahony-down-syndrome-test/> accessed 5 October 2018.

72 Love Both, "Three mothers that faced pressure to terminate their pregnancies", 10 May 2018; and McGarry, "Love Both challenges Minister".

73 YouTube interview of Dr Peter Boylan accessed through "Q&A: The Answers to your Questions about the Eighth Amendment", TheJournal.ie, 16 May 2018 <http://www.thejournal.ie/eighth-amendment-ref-q-a-3999597-May2018/> accessed 10 October 2018.

74 "Statement from the Institute of Obstetricians and Gynaecologists", 29 January 2018.

75 Love Both, "Three mothers that faced pressure", 10 May 2018; and McGarry, "Love Both challenges Minister".

76 RTÉ Radio 1, "Dr Mahony about abortion of babies with Down Syndrome", 9 May 2018, transcript, Love Both website.

77 Eamon McGuinness, "Medical myths about Eighth Amendment must be challenged", *Irish Times*, 6 April 2018 <https://www.irishtimes.com/opinion/medical-myths-about-eighth-amendment-must-be-challenged-1.3451748> accessed 6 April 2018.

78 Maternal Death Enquiry Ireland, *Data Brief No. 1* (December 2015) <https://www.ucc.ie/en/media/research/maternaldeathenquiryireland/MDEIrelandDataBriefNo1December2015.pdf> accessed 4 November 2017; and *Data Brief No. 2* (December 2016) <https://www.ucc.ie/en/media/research/maternaldeathenquiryireland/MDEIrelandDatabriefNo2December2016.pdf> accessed 4 November 2017; M.F. O'Hare, E. Manning, P. Corcoran, and R.A. Greene, *Confidential Maternal Death Enquiry in Ireland: Report for 2013–2015* (Cork: December 2017) <https://www.ucc.ie/en/media/research/maternaldeathenquiryireland/Confidential-Maternal-Death-Enquiry-Report-2013---2015--Web.pdf> accessed 29 October 2018.

79 This point was made by Professor Sabaratnam Arulkumaran, who was president-elect of the International Federation of Obstetrics and Gynaecology when he gave evidence to the Joint Committee on the Eighth Amendment of the Constitution. Joint Committee on the Eighth Amendment of the Constitution, 18 October 2017, Houses of the Oireachtas website <https://www.oireachtas.ie/en/debates/debate/joint_committee_on_the_eighth_amendment_of_the_constitution/2017-10-18/3/> accessed 20 October 2017.

80 Áine McMahon, "Eighth Amendment has caused death of cancer patients, says obstetrician", *Irish Times*, 9 April 2018 <https://

search-proquest-com.ucc.idm.oclc.org/docview/2022902451/
E7A4FE80CC2E4595PQ/9?accountid=14504> accessed 9 April 2018.

81 Órla Ryan, "Pro-life doctor says no woman has died because of the Eighth
Amendment", TheJournal.ie, 10 April 2018 <https://www.thejournal.ie/
eamon-mcguinness-eighth-amendment-3949918-Apr2018/> accessed 29
October 2018.

82 Statement from the Institute of Obstetricians and Gynaecologists, 10
January 2018 <https://www.rcpi.ie/news/releases/statement-from-the-
institute-of-obstetricians-and-gynaecologists/> accessed 30 October 2018.

83 Ryan, op. cit.

84 "75% of doctors support 12-week access to abortion", *Irish Examiner*,
8 February 2018 <https://search-proquest-com.ucc.idm.oclc.org/
docview/1999156799/7C848271DA424DFFPQ/1?accountid=14504>
accessed 16 May 2018.

85 Sorcha Pollak, "More than 1,000 doctors call for Yes vote", *Irish
Times*, 14 May 2018 <https://search-proquest-com.ucc.idm.oclc.org/
docview/2038137870/7B7D35945F184915PQ/53?accountid=14504>
accessed14 May 2018.

86 Elaine Edwards, "Doctors agree plan in event of repeal", *Irish Times*, 14
April 2018, p. 4.

87 John Bonnar *et al.*, letter to the editor, *Irish Times*, 11
May 2018 <https://search-proquest-com.ucc.idm.oclc.org/
docview/2036892729/96F336D60BE14F28PQ/110?accountid=14504>
accessed 11 May 2018. See also Greg Daly, "Top Obstetricians condemn
medical scaremongering around Eighth", *Irish Catholic*, 10 May 2018
<https://www.irishcatholic.com/top-obstetricians-condemn-medical-
scaremongering-around-eighth/> accessed 1 November 2018. This letter
was also published on the Save the 8th website.

88 Institute of Obstetricians and Gynaecologists, "Repeal of the Eighth
Amendment: Information for the public" <https://www.rcpi.ie/faculties/
obstetricians-and-gynaecologists/repeal-the-eighth-amendment-info-
for-the-public/> accessed 15 May 2018. The institute's website stated
that it had nearly 200 members. Boylan informed the *Irish Times* that
SurveyMonkey forms had been sent out to all members requesting their
opinions about the referendum and the associated proposals for reform.
Seventy-nine or eighty members responded. Of these, 81% supported
repeal. Dr Trevor Hayes said that the institute was more divided on the
issue than the survey indicated, arguing that there was "a tight time frame"
to respond to the survey and that fewer than half of the members had
responded.

89 Harry McGee, "Boylan stands over claim majority of
institute's members support repeal", *Irish Times*, 16 May
2018 <https://search-proquest-com.ucc.idm.oclc.org/

docview/2038985449/51D67B8B79584ABCPQ/60?accountid=14504>
accessed 16 May 2018.

90 Ring, "Eighth 'has led to dangerous abortions'"; Fiachra Ó Cionnaith
and Eoin English, "Professor: Savita would be alive today if not for 8th",
Irish Examiner, 22 May, p. 6; and Elaine Edwards, "Halappanavar inquiry
chairman calls for repeal", *Irish Times*, 23 May, p. 7.

91 Kitty Holland, "Accessing abortion is a 'lottery' under Irish rules –
psychiatrist", *Irish Times*, 12 June 2017 <http://www.irishtimes.com/
news/social-affairs/accessing-abortion-is-a-lottery-under-irish-rules-
psychiatrist-1.3116997> accessed 16 June 2017.

92 Ciarán D'Arcy, "What is the situation with abortion in Ireland?", *Irish
Times*, 17 December 2017 <https://search-proquest-com.ucc.idm.oclc.org/
docview/1977074550/98232BC1419B4E49PQ/18?accountid=14504>
accessed 17 December 2017.

93 Kitty Holland, "Protection of Life During Pregnancy Act is 'unworkable'",
Irish Times, 13 June 2017.

94 Thirty-sixth Amendment of the Constitution Bill 2018: Second Stage,
Seanad Éireann Debates, 27 March 2018.

95 Joint Committee on Health and Children, 8 January 2013 <https://
www.oireachtas.ie/en/debates/debate/joint_committee_on_health_and_
children/2013-01-08/2/#s5> accessed 7 November 2018; and Lloyd Mudiwa,
"Barbed exchange between medics", *Irish Medical Times*, 18 January 2013
<https://www.imt.ie/news/barbed-exchanges-between-medics-18-01-2013/>
accessed 6 November 2018.

96 Patsy McGarry, "Psychiatrist says to suggest abortion a solution to mental
illness 'naive in the extreme'", *Irish Times*, 1 May 2018 <https://www.
irishtimes.com/news/social-affairs/psychiatrist-says-to-suggest-abortion-
a-solution-to-mental-illness-naive-in-the-extreme-1.3480660> accessed 4
November 2018.

97 General Scheme of a Bill to Regulate Termination of Pregnancy, Heads 4, 5,
7 and 11.

98 McGarry, "Psychiatrist says to suggest abortion a solution".

99 Save the 8th press conference, "Statement from Psychiatrists", 16 May 2018
<https://www.save8.ie/statement-from-psychiatrists/> accessed 30 October
2018.

100 Ibid.

101 Psychological Society of Ireland: "Psychological Society of Ireland releases
fact-based position on abortion and mental health, and supports repeal of
the Eighth Amendment" <https://www.psychologicalsociety.ie/> accessed
12 May 2018; and "5 Facts on The Eighth Amendment and Mental Health"
<https://www.psychologicalsociety.ie/> accessed 12 May 2018.

102 Cora Sherlock, "Say no to abortion on demand", *Irish Times*, 24 May 2018,
p. 4; Elaine Loughlin and Fiachra Ó Cionnaith, "No canvassers 'ridiculing

mental health': Harris", *Irish Examiner*, 22 May 2018, p. 1; and Pat Leahy, "Referendum campaign", *Irish Times*, 24 May 2018, p. 2.

103 Together for Yes website, "As doctors we make difficult decisions every day: 1,642 of us are agreed on this one" <http://www.togetherforyes.ie/doctors/> accessed 13 November 2018.

104 Together for Yes <https://www.togetherforyes.ie/about-us/campaign-platform-members/> accessed 10 December 2018.

105 Luke Field, "The Abortion Referendum of 2018 and a Timeline of Abortion Politics in Ireland to Date", *Irish Political Studies*, vol. 33, issue 4 (2018), p. 620.

106 Save the 8th, "Our Posters" <https://www.save8.ie/posters/> accessed 23 May 2015.

107 Department of Health and Social Care (UK), *Abortion Statistics, England and Wales: 2017*, June 2018 <https://assets.publishing.service.gov.uk/government/uploads/system/uploads/attachment_data/file/714183/2017_Abortion_Statistics_Commentary.pdf> accessed 10 December 2018.

108 Sherlock, op. cit. Cora Sherlock was spokeswoman for Love Both.

109 Save the 8th, "Our Posters".

110 Chris Fitzpatrick, "Life doesn't fit on anti-abortion posters", *Irish Times*, 23 April 2018 <https://search-proquest-com.ucc.idm.oclc.org/docview/2028721464/FFAF0465A7F14380PQ/80?accountid=14504> accessed 23 April 2018.

111 Ibid.

112 Billy O'Riordan, "Anti-abortion group seeks to defend graphic imagery on posters", *Irish Examiner*, 30 May 2018 <https://www.irishexaminer.com/breakingnews/views/analysis/anti-abortion-group-seeks-to-defend-graphic-imagery-on-posters-845795.html> accessed 14 December 2018.

113 "Save the 8th: Graphic posters 'wrong and unhelpful'", *Irish Examiner*, 1 May 2018 <https://www.irishexaminer.com/breakingnews/ireland/save-the-8th-graphic-posters-wrong-and-unhelpful-840262.html> accessed 9 December 2018; Patsy McGarry, "Anti-abortion group targets hospitals", *Irish Times*, 2 May 2018 <https://search-proquest-com.ucc.idm.oclc.org/docview/2033122916/FF2DB3D6F5C2462FPQ/41?accountid=14504> accessed 3 May 2018.

114 Samuel Shepard, letter to the editor, *Irish Times*, 18 April 2018 <https://search-proquest-com.ucc.idm.oclc.org/docview/2026043471/C2CACD20807E46ACPQ/89?accountid=14504> accessed 19 April 2018.

115 See Katie Harrington, letter to the editor, *Irish Times*, 19 April 2018 <https://search-proquest-com.ucc.idm.oclc.org/docview/2026745727/6B206A0CEA394406PQ/108?accountid=14504> accessed 19 September 2018.

116 Catherine Shanahan, "Parents angered by referendum posters", *Irish Examiner*, 7 May 2018 <https://www.irishexaminer.com/ireland/parents-

angered-by-referendum-posters-470336.html> accessed 11 December 2018.

117 Gráinne Ní Aodha, "Most Irish people think referendum posters should be banned", TheJournal.ie, 26 May 2018 <https://www.thejournal.ie/referendum-posters-ban-4034334-May2018/> accessed 11 December 2018.

118 Peter Murtagh, "Twitter rejects restriction accusation from Irish anti-abortion campaigners", *Irish Times*, 14 April 2018, p. 4.

119 Pat Leahy, "Social media group's move reflects repeal nerves", *Irish Times*, 9 May 2018 <https://search-proquest-com.ucc.idm.oclc.org/docview/2035909708/F760F3456B25418CPQ/65?accountid=14504> accessed 9 May 2018.

120 Pat Leahy, "Google ban is unprecedented, so why did they do it?", *Irish Times*, 10 May 2018 <https://search-proquest-com.ucc.idm.oclc.org/docview/2036541119/F245D3E7582421CPQ/44?accountid=14504> accessed 10 May 2018.

121 Harry McGee, "How the tide turned against the Eighth", *Irish Times*, 28 May 2018 <https://search-proquest-com.ucc.idm.oclc.org/docview/2044968134/C9B12D887BEA42ABPQ/15?accountid=14504> accessed 28 May 2018.

122 Simon Coveney, "Here's how my thinking shifted on the Eighth Amendment", Independent.ie, 26 March 2018 <https://www.independent.ie/irish-news/simon-coveney-heres-how-my-thinking-shifted-on-the-eighth-amendment-36743798.html> accessed 18 December 2018.

123 Some of those interviewed said that they would not vote or declined to answer. Pat Leahy, "Repeal side well ahead despite dip in support", *Irish Times*, 20 April 2018 <https://search-proquest-com.ucc.idm.oclc.org/docview/2027380697/16E3869566784158PQ/5?accountid=14504> 20 April 2018.

124 McGee, "How the tide turned against the Eighth".

125 Pat Leahy, "Yes campaign's outreach to middle ground delivered the landslide", *Irish Times*, 28 May 2018 <https://search-proquest-com.ucc.idm.oclc.org/docview/2044967711/C9B12D887BEA42ABPQ/12?accountid=14504> accessed 28 May 2018.

126 McGee, "How the tide turned against the Eighth".

127 Fiach Kelly, "Retain campaign makes bid to shift narrative", *Irish Times*, 23 May, p. 6.

128 Elaine Loughlin, "Cross-party event cut short as heckler targets Harris", *Irish Examiner*, 23 May 2018, p. 6; Pat Leahy and Sarah Bardon, "Varadkar rejects idea from No side of laws for 'hard cases'", *Irish Times*, 23 May 2018, p. 1.

129 Archbishop Diarmuid Martin, "The Defence of Human Life", 23 May 2018, Archdiocese of Dublin <http://www.dublindiocese.ie/choose-life-2018/> accessed 28 May 2018.

130 Breda O'Brien, "If you vote for choice you are facilitating abortions", *Irish Times*, 24 May 2018, p. 16.

131 McGee, "How the tide turned against the Eighth".

132 The two attorneys general were John Rogers SC and Michael McDowell SC. Fiach Kelly, "Amendment limiting abortion to rape cases 'unworkable', say former AGs", *Irish Times*, 16 May 2018 <https://search-proquest-com.ucc.idm.oclc.org/docview/2038990025/51D67B8B79584ABCPQ/59?accountid=14504> accessed 16 May 2018.

133 Leahy and Bardon, op. cit.

134 Miriam Lord, "Stony silence as absolutist bluff called", *Irish Times*, 23 May 2018, p. 5.

135 Stephen O'Brien, "Varadkar hails quiet revolution", *Sunday Times*, 27 May 2018, p. 1.

136 Jody Corcoran, "Abortion landslide down to reluctant, not silent, Yes", *Sunday Independent*, 3 June 2018, p. 3.

137 Stephen O'Brien, "How the 'No' Campaign fell apart", *Sunday Times*, 3 June 2018, p. 17.

138 Fionola Meredith, "Abortion referendum aftermath: Is Northern Ireland next?", *Irish Times*, 9 June 2018 <https://www.irishtimes.com/news/social-affairs/abortion-referendum-aftermath-is-northern-ireland-next-1.3522667> accessed 23 June 2018.

139 Tim Shipman and Caroline Wheeler, "Northern Irish flock to Britain weekly for abortions: Abortion law reform demanded [Ulster Region]", *Sunday Times* (London), 22 July 2018 <https://search-proquest-com.ucc.idm.oclc.org/docview/2072972929/8AD109881E574741PQ/40?accountid=14504> accessed 26 July 2018; and Lord Steel *et al.*, letter to the editor, *Sunday Times* (London), 22 July 2018 <https://search-proquest-com.ucc.idm.oclc.org/docview/2072971781/F261FB2E77464D02PQ/1?accountid=14504> accessed 26 July 2018.

140 Martin Fletcher, "Focus of abortion reform now moves north of border", *Sunday Times*, 27 May 2018, p. 2.

141 Newton Emerson, "The DUP flexes religious muscle while terminating moves towards liberalism", *Sunday Times*, 27 May 2018, p. 16.

142 Gerry Moriarty and Freya McClements, "Abortion decriminalised in NI despite unionist opposition", *Irish Times*, 22 October 2019 <https://search-proquest-com.ucc.idm.oclc.org/docview/2307239589/B1F6A6273B634695PQ/1?accountid=14504> accessed 22 October 2019; Rory Carroll, "Northern Ireland to legalise abortion and same-sex marriage", *Guardian*, 22 October 2019 <https://www.theguardian.com/uk-news/2019/oct/21/northern-ireland-set-to-legalise-abortion-and-same-sex-marriage> accessed 22 October 2019.

143 Patsy McGarry, "Ireland 'obliterated' right to life of the unborn, says Catholic primate", *Irish Times*, 28 May 2018.

144 Joe Little, "Archbishop says he is deeply saddened over referendum result", RTÉ News, 28 May 2018 <https://www.rte.ie/news/2018/0527/966293-

diarmuid-martin/> accessed 28 May 2018.

145 Gráinne Ní Aodha, "Bishop says Catholics who voted Yes have sinned and should go to confession", TheJournal.ie, 28 May 2018 <http://www.thejournal.ie/bishop-catholics-who-voted-yes-sinned-4039904-May2018/> accessed 28 May 2018.

146 Ryan Nugent, "Catholics who voted Yes must repent to be worthy of communion: bishop", Independent.ie, 2 June 2018 <https://www.independent.ie/irish-news/politics/catholics-who-voted-yes-must-repent-to-be-worthy-of-communion-bishop-36970575.html> accessed 3 June 2018.

147 Thirty-sixth Amendment of the Constitution Act 2018, 18 September 2018 <https://data.oireachtas.ie/ie/oireachtas/act/2018/C36/mul/enacted/36th-amdt-of-the-constitution-act-2018.pdf> accessed 24 October 2018.

148 Ailbhe Conneely, "Harris seeks availability of second doctor in abortion cases", RTÉ News, 29 November 2018 <https://www.rte.ie/news/politics/2018/1128/1013989-abortion-dail/> accessed 1 January 2019.

149 Pat Leahy, "Many anti-repeal TDs will back legislation", *Irish Times*, 28 May 2018 <https://search-proquest-com.ucc.idm.oclc.org/docview/2044967023/74D30A4F40924292PQ/8?accountid=14504> accessed 31 December 2018.

150 Pat Leahy and Sarah Bardon, "Harris pledges swift action on abortion laws", *Irish Times*, 28 May 2018 <https://search-proquest-com.ucc.idm.oclc.org/docview/2044967575/74D30A4F40924292PQ/1?accountid=14504> accessed 31 December 2018.

151 Health (Regulation of Termination of Pregnancy) Bill 2018 <https://data.oireachtas.ie/ie/oireachtas/bill/2018/105/eng/ver_b/b105b18d.pdf> accessed 1 January 2019.

152 RTÉ News, "Abortion services to be provided in Ireland from today", 1 January 2019 <https://www.rte.ie/news/ireland/2019/0101/1019777-abortion-services-ireland/> accessed 1 January 2019.

153 See David Quinn, "Unborn have no voice, so how could they win?" *Sunday Times*, 27 May 2018, p. 15.

154 There was a lesson to be learned from history if pro-life campaigners had looked back to the referendum in 2002 when it was proposed to reverse the Supreme Court X Case judgment concerning suicide. Referendum Commission, "Protection of Human Life in Pregnancy: Referendum on the Twenty-Fifth Amendment of the Constitution (Protection of Human Life in Pregnancy) Bill 2001" <https://www.refcom.ie/previous-referendums/protection-of-human-life/> accessed 2 January 2019. The proposed constitutional amendment and its associated Protection of Human Life in Pregnancy Bill 2001 was defeated by a very narrow margin: 50.42% voted No and 49.58% voted Yes. The most extreme wing of the pro-life movement contributed to the defeat because they urged a No vote on the basis that the amendment did not offer sufficient protection for the unborn. Legal

protection would only apply from implantation in the womb – not from conception. It is ironic that the Irish Catholic bishops, given their propensity for absolutist pronouncements, expressed a more nuanced view. They saw the proposal as "limited" and "imperfect" but believed that Catholics were free in conscience to vote Yes. Louise Fuller, *Irish Catholicism since 1950: The Undoing of a Culture* (Dublin: Gill and Macmillan, 2002), p. 249. This in turn relates to two related points raised in the Introduction: (1) sometimes it is necessary to tolerate a lesser evil to avoid a greater evil; and (2) not all acts considered immoral should be punishable by civil law. For the first point see Pope John Paul II, *Evangelium Vitae* (25 March 1995), paragraph 73. An invocation of these moral concepts offers the necessary flexibility to the pro-life campaign to navigate a reasonable path towards optimising respect and legal protection for unborn human life.

---— • ———

Conclusion

In 1994 sociologists Christopher T. Whelan and Michael P. Hornsby-Smith observed that what was so noticeable about Irish society was "not so much secularisation as the emergence of the 'new Catholic'". Characteristics that distinguished "new Catholics" from traditionalist Catholics included a liberal outlook on sexual issues and an attitude that questioned the hierarchy's assertion of absolute authority on questions relating to personal morality. Eternal damnation was no longer quite so feared and there was much less emphasis on sin. A more optimistic outlook prevailed as sin and hell were pushed towards the outer margins of religious thinking.[1] A process of transformation within Irish Catholicism, against a background of profound social and cultural changes, had been in progress since the 1960s and influenced many Catholics to be more independent-minded.[2] By the late 1990s pronouncements by the bishops exerted relatively little influence on the opinions of lay Catholics. The fallout from a stream of clerical scandals in the 1990s further eroded clerical power in the Church.[3] Internationally, the exclusively male leadership of the Church, and its lack of solidarity with women's rights, may be seen as another major contributing factor to the decline of ecclesiastical influence.[4] In Ireland this is especially true in relation to such issues as contraception, abortion and *in vitro* fertilisation.[5]

Chrystel Hug expressed it rather forcefully in 1999 when she wrote that "Irish Catholics have reclaimed the right to think for themselves" on issues of sexual morality. The "moral majority" – comprising militant pro-life supporters, anti-divorce activists, ultra-Catholic lay organisations, and traditionalists – were no longer the majority. An "ethical dissensus" more in keeping with the ideals of a pluralist liberal democracy had emerged.[6] A small minority of Catholics disagreed with the doctrines of their Church to the point of leaving the Church. Others abstained from the sacraments and stopped going to church. Many struggled to reach a practical accommodation, merging conflicting secular and religious values in response to their individual circumstances and personal needs. In matters of assisted human reproduction this has led to moral ambivalence.[7]

The power vacuum created by the decline of clerical power within the Church was quickly filled by the emergence of a "more fundamentalist Catholic lay movement" that was staunchly supportive of the Eighth Amendment, which in turn created difficulties for the resolution of bioethical issues. Orla McDonnell and Jill Allison pointed to the anti-abortion clause as "the most enduring aspect of Catholic conservative political control over social values both within the health field and more broadly in terms of national identity".[8] The sharp decline of conservative Catholicism was nowhere more conspicuously evident than in the outcome of the referendums in 2015 (marriage equality) and 2018 (abortion).

The bishops, despite their huge loss of influence, do not see themselves as being without a voice on moral issues in the public arena. Their declared mission is to preach the gospel. Abdicating all responsibility to the laity is not seen as an option. This raises questions about their role in public life and, more important, the role of religion in liberal democracies. In a liberal democracy the freedom to practise one's religion is broadly accepted. This means that no religion is favoured over another, and no religion is discriminated against. Tolerance for religion is upheld provided that human rights are respected and that religious organisations are not subversive of democracy. The institutional Church expressed support for democracy and religious freedom but opposed a number of liberal reforms. The bishops appealed to Catholic consciences – to influence public opinion as much as possible – in the knowledge that politicians would be far more concerned to reflect public opinion than to change it.[9] Irish politicians were generally averse to risk-taking on highly contentious biomedical issues. The dominant political tendency was to procrastinate through the mechanism of government-appointed commissions, Oireachtas committees and protracted consultations. When pressed to legislate, members of the Oireachtas did so only minimally, and under cover of substantial shifts in public opinion, commissions of enquiry, and legal imperatives emanating from judgments of the Supreme Court and the European Court of Human Rights. The ingrained political instinct for survival in general elections served the interests of traditionalist Catholicism well – until 2015, when the marriage equality referendum was passed.

Catholicism will continue to exert significant influence over public discourse and the legislative process, contrary to the wishes of those who seek to exclude it from the public arena. It can be argued that the exclusion of religious influence is a violation of religious freedom and is not tenable in a pluralist democracy. Even so, as emphasised by Patrick Hannon (professor emeritus of moral theology), the style and content of what the Church has to say must be appropriate to contemporary culture if it is to carry weight in public debate.[10] But secularists are very likely to question the value of any religious opinion concerning matters of public policy. Assertions of moral authority based on divine revelation are not amenable to rational discourse, are outside the domain of scientific investigation, and tend towards premature conclusions rather than contributing to constructive debates. All these are obstacles to credibility. Cardinal Cahal B. Daly seemed to take account of this issue in his introduction to *The Bishops and the Law on Public Morality* (2006). Although he reiterated that Catholic moral doctrine was based "ultimately on the authority of divine revelation", he maintained that data sourced from research in the social sciences, and, more generally, the insights derived from human reasoning, were additional sources of moral truths. Therefore, rational debate about morality and law was not exclusively in the hands of the secularists.[11] Donal Murray, retired bishop of Limerick, expressed the point more forcefully (with reference to abortion), that an opinion, consistent with the church's position, can be reached on the basis of human rights and without reference to religious beliefs. Therefore, public policy should be decided on the basis of human rights because the Church does not wish to impose its religious views on non-Catholics.[12] However, condemning abortion on the basis of human rights is far from straightforward. It raises the question: What are "human rights"? Does any organisation have primacy in terms of moral credibility in addressing issues relating to human rights? Human rights treaty-monitoring committees of the UN and Amnesty International – as discussed earlier – have reached conclusions very different from those of the Catholic Church in the context of the abortion issue in Ireland.[13] This casts serious doubt on the credibility of traditionalist and institutional opinions in the Catholic Church about abortion and related issues (especially contraception).[14]

Archbishop Diarmuid Martin of Dublin observed that, although religious faith should never be imposed on non-believers, the values that are derived from faith do have a legitimate role in public life. He believed that, despite the failures of Church institutions, and of individual Christians, the overall impact of Christian faith and practice had given rise to the "fundamental good principles" that inspired the best traits of Irish society. Faith was not a private matter for each person. Martin was speaking about the role of Catholic faith in pluralistic societies against the background of debates about the Protection of Life During Pregnancy Bill in the Dáil. Supporting the pro-life movement was intrinsically linked to searching for the deepest meaning of life.[15]

Archbishop Martin and other thoughtful Catholics insist that there is no conflict between faith and reason. Nevertheless, sustaining harmony between faith and reason is not without major difficulties. Doctrinal teachings are so inflexible that reasoning in the service of faith is highly biased towards predetermined conclusions, thus compromising the integrity of the reasoning process. In other words, when a conclusion is fixed, research and rational debate are moulded to sustain it. This has created a formidable obstacle to progress in bioethical matters, which in turn has eroded confidence in the teaching authority of the Church. The vast majority of Roman Catholics do not think that the papacy's assertion of a moral distinction between natural and artificial means of contraception is reasonable. They are not likely to change their opinions on this issue. The Church's assertion that "the human being is to be respected and treated as a person from the moment of conception"[16] is implausible. This moral prescription is especially restrictive on the reproductive freedom of couples and on human embryonic stem cell research. It detracts from the credibility of the Church's teaching against abortion. Advocates of Catholic morality will frequently press for legislation that reflects their religious beliefs, although they generally tend to argue on the basis of human rights rather than referring to theological concepts. For example, belief in the presence of immortal souls in human embryos and foetuses is unlikely to sway public opinion to retain or enact anti-abortion legislation.[17]

Shifts in public opinion about what is or is not immoral will influence changes in state law. The institutional Church will find it extremely difficult to adapt to such changes. The teaching authority has painted itself into a corner, damaging its credibility and greatly diminishing its influence. There seems to be little room for manoeuvre. It would be difficult for the teaching authority to change its stance without a major loss of credibility, considering that pronouncements from the Vatican were made so authoritatively. And yet it will continue to lose credibility by reiterating moral concepts that have been widely rejected by both Catholics and non-Catholics.

From an orthodox Catholic perspective, it can be argued that the Church cannot simply change its teaching to adapt itself to trends in contemporary culture. The teaching authority of the Church – "the bishops in communion with ... the Bishop of Rome" – asserts that it is the sole authentic interpreter of the "sacred deposit" of the faith (the *depositum fidei*). All divinely revealed truths are derived from this source. The teaching authority cannot change the Word of God – it can only teach what it has received.[18] Dogmas are revealed truths and must be believed.[19] Furthermore, "loyal submission of the will and intellect must be given" by Catholics, even when the pope is not speaking *ex cathedra* (i.e. infallibly).[20]

The heavy demands of Rome impose an excessive burden of loyalty on Irish Catholics, who are, as already observed, less amenable to dictation from the hierarchy. Many of them will see conflict between faith and reason in some papal pronouncements. Moral ambivalence aside, is there a way out of their dilemma? Is there, for example, some scope for revisions of doctrine in matters of birth control and assisted human reproduction? In theory – yes! Church documents such as *Mysterium Ecclesiae* (1973) acknowledge that there is a difference between a dogmatic truth and the interpretation and understanding of a dogmatic truth. Advances in knowledge and understanding can facilitate changes in Church teaching.[21]

Sources for the inspiration of doctrine indicate possibilities for change. Maynooth theologian Pádraig Corkery pointed to three such sources in his *Bioethics and the Catholic Moral Tradition* (2010): "the Christian Scriptures, the ongoing living tradition of a believing community" and "natural law".[22] Although scripture provided a basis for moral theology it did not give clear answers to many contemporary moral issues that arose in healthcare and assisted human reproduction. Catholic "tradition" was "dynamic and ongoing" – not "static and complete". The concept of natural law was based on the idea that God endowed human beings with rational faculties to discern the difference between right and wrong without recourse to divine revelation. This all seemed very well – but theologians held different opinions about what it was and how it was to be applied to various moral issues.[23]

The fluidity of the underlying sources of Catholic doctrine, then, seems to offer opportunities for a reinterpretation of some Church dogmas together with prospects for revising a number of controversial non-dogmatic teachings, such as the ordination of married and women priests. However, when recent Church history is considered, there is little reason for confidence that such developments will occur. The centralisation of power in Rome presents a formidable obstacle to changes in doctrine that would enhance the prospect of greater harmony between the Church and contemporary culture in Ireland. If the Irish Catholic bishops, for example, contemplated changing their stance on birth control or assisted human reproduction they would be most unlikely to do so in the absence of major revisions in moral theology authorised by Rome. Therefore, Irish Catholicism will probably be characterised by a broad spectrum of Catholic faith and practice ranging from the traditionalists, ever loyal to Rome and probably in a small minority, to à la carte Catholics who will be more receptive and adaptable to the currents of cultural change that will sometimes be incompatible with the authoritative teachings of the Church. The hierarchy, aware of such ambivalence, and mindful of its own diminished influence, will probably place much less emphasis on doctrines that attract relatively little assent within the Church. As observed earlier, very little is now said about hell, but it remains an article of faith. The ambivalence of religious faith will be facilitated by softer ecclesiastical pronouncements because the "faithful" are now far less inclined to obey directives from their clergy "with docility".[24] David Quinn, writing in the *Irish Catholic*, observed that Pope Francis, two years into his pontificate, had "aroused fear among traditionalists and hope among many liberals" that he intended to revise some of the Church's moral teachings, especially in relation to marriage and sexual morality. The "generally soft tone" of what he said, and the occasional lack of clarity, gave rise to such fears and hopes. Even so, Quinn saw the pope as essentially conservative or traditionalist. Although some concessions might be made, such as divorced and remarried Catholics being allowed to receive Communion, no radical changes would be made to the Church's teaching about abortion, contraception or marriage.[25] A softer, less judgemental, and somewhat ambiguous presentation of doctrine will probably help many Catholics to reconcile their own personal needs with the teachings of their Church that might otherwise prove unsustainable.[26]

Pope Francis reiterated the importance of upholding the doctrines of the Church, although not in a way that was harshly judgemental and exclusionary towards those living in "irregular" situations such as divorcees and homosexuals.[27] His pastoral style is to some extent evident amongst the Irish Catholic bishops. When Kevin Doran, bishop of Elphin, declared in early March 2015 that gay parents of children were, somehow, not really parents, he provoked a storm of criticism. He subsequently apologised for the inappropriate choice of words that had caused so much offence. Archbishop Diarmuid Martin, mildly critical of Doran's *faux pas*, did not express disagreement on a doctrinal basis.[28] The credibility of preaching the gospel depended very much on the sensitivity of the language used. The archbishop believed that Church teaching inspired joy and was not about "negative rules and regulations". It was about love, truth and freedom. It was about feeling special in a vast universe. That brought to mind the words of Pope Benedict: "We are not some casual and meaningless product of evolution. Each of us is the result of a thought of God. Each of us is willed, each of us is loved, each of us is necessary."[29] The great appeal of the Catholic faith, for Martin, was that it elevated humans to cosmic significance. No matter how tough and cruel life was on earth, the prospect of a blissful afterlife for good Christians would make it all worthwhile. God was not a relentless and harsh judge. Yet Martin was very much aware that all was not sweetness and light. He was critical of those Catholics who had marginalised their faith in their day-to-day lives, going so far as to label them "Nicodemus Catholics ... living in a sort of *de facto* atheism".[30]

The choices that Irish Catholics make in their personal lives, and as voters in general elections and referendums, will frequently not be compatible with Catholic doctrine. Their decisions and lifestyle choices will emerge from the complex interplay between religious faith, rational choices and personal needs. They are by far the largest sector of the population in the Republic of Ireland and they will continue for many more years to play a central and unpredictable role in the ever-changing relationships between morality, law and social life.[31]

Endnotes

———•———

1   Michael P. Hornsby-Smith and Christopher T. Whelan, "Religious and Moral Values" in Christopher T. Whelan (ed.) *Values and Social Change in Ireland* (Dublin: Gill and Macmillan, 1994), p. 44.

2   This was not a smooth linear progression from conservative to liberal. The passing of the Health (Family Planning) Act 1979 was followed by what historian Brian Girvin termed "conservative retrenchment". Liberal influence on the issues of abortion, divorce and homosexuality was ineffective throughout the 1980s. See Brian Girvin, "An Irish Solution to an Irish Problem: Catholicism, contraception and change, 1922–1979", *Contemporary European History*, vol. 27, no. 1 (2018), pp. 1–22.

3   Louise Fuller, *Irish Catholicism since 1950: The Undoing of a Culture* (Dublin: Gill and Macmillan, 2002), p. 251 *et seq.* For a sociological study of Roman Catholics retaining their faith in contemporary Ireland – "outside or in addition to the institutional Church", see Gladys Ganiel, *Transforming Post-Catholic Ireland: Religious Practice in Late Modernity* (Oxford: Oxford University Press, 2016). Quotation from p. 5.

4   See Peter Steinfels, "Bishops and Abortion Law: Learning from the American experience", *Doctrine and Life*, vol. 63, no. 7 (September 2013), p. 16.

5   For the institutional Church's lack of concern about women's welfare on the issue of *in vitro* fertilisation, see Susan Ryan-Sheridan, *Women and the New Reproductive Technologies in Ireland* (Cork: Cork University Press, 1994), pp. 38–40. For the issues of contraception and abortion, see Sandra McAvoy, "The Catholic Church and Fertility Control in Ireland: The Making of a Dystopian Regime" in Aideen Quilty, Sinéad Kennedy and Catherine Conlon (eds), *The Abortion Papers Ireland* Volume 2 (Cork: Attic Press, 2015), pp. 47–62.

6   Chrystel Hug, *The Politics of Sexual Morality in Ireland* (London: Macmillan Press, 1999), pp. 241–2.

7   See Jill Allison, *Motherhood and Infertility in Ireland: Understanding the Presence of Absence* (Cork: Cork University Press, 2013), pp. 98–103, 186.

8   Orla McDonnell and Jill Allison, "From Biopolitics to Bioethics: Church, state, medicine and assisted reproductive technology in Ireland", *Sociology of Health and Illness*, vol. 28, no. 6 (2006), pp. 819, 832–3.

9   See Hug, op. cit., pp. 100–1. Direct episcopal influence on the legislature is,

and will be, minimal, in stark contrast to the early decades of independent Ireland when some leading Irish politicians were very explicit in docile obedience to hierarchical judgements. J.H. Whyte, *Church and State in Modern Ireland 1923–1979* (Dublin: Gill and Macmillan, 1984 (2nd edn)), pp. 36, 48, 231–5.

10 Patrick Hannon, *Church, State, Morality and Law* (Dublin: Gill and Macmillan, 1992), p. 7.

11 Cardinal Cahal B. Daly, Introduction, *The Bishops and the Law on Public Morality*, July 2005 <http://www.armagharchdiocese.org/2008/05/01/july-the-bishops-and-the-law-on-public-morality/> accessed 2 November 2014.

12 Donal Murray, "Some Thoughts on the Abortion Debate", *Doctrine and Life*, vol. 63 (February 2013), pp. 12–13. For the same point see also the evidence of Bishop Christopher Jones (Diocese of Elphin) to the Joint Committee on Health and Children, 10 January 2013 <https://www.oireachtas.ie/en/debates/debate/joint_committee_on_health_and_children/2013-01-10/2/#s3> accessed 9 November 2018. Bishop Jones attended as a representative of the Irish Catholic Bishops' Conference.

13 See Chapter 7; and Amnesty International, *She is Not a Criminal: The Impact of Ireland's Abortion Law* (London: 2015).

14 The Catholic hierarchy's reiteration of *Humanae Vitae* especially undermines its credibility. Bishop Kevin Doran (chairman of the Committee of Bioethics of the Irish Catholic Bishops' Conference) called for the principles of the encyclical to be expounded in "a fresh way" at a conference organised by the Nazareth Family Institute. In the course of his lecture he denied that contraception had "liberated" women by enabling them to control their fertility. He claimed that "the fact that they are less likely to become pregnant also takes away from women one of the principal motives or freedoms for saying no to unwanted sex." He linked "the contraceptive mentality" with the "surprisingly high number" of people who were supportive of same-sex marriage. He made no reference to any research in the social sciences supportive of his implausible claims. Minister for Health Simon Harris responded through social media, saying that increasing access to contraception would continue to be a feature of public health policy. Colin Gleeson, "Minister responds to bishop on birth control", *Irish Times*, 6 August 2018 <https://search-proquest-com.ucc.idm.oclc.org/docview/2083431635/9FA2DDAD17434F2DPQ/30?accountid=14504> accessed 7 August 2018.

15 "Homily of Archbishop Diarmuid Martin at Mass in Church of Saint Dominick, Dublin, 6 July 2013" <http://www.catholicbishops.ie/2013/07/06/homily-archbishop-diarmuid-martin-mass-church-saint-dominick-dublin/> accessed 14 December 2013.

16 Congregation for the Doctrine of the Faith, *Instruction Dignitas Personae on Certain Bioethical Questions* (8 September 2008), paragraph 4 <http://www.

vatican.va/roman_curia/congregations/cfaith/documents/rc_con_cfaith_
doc_20081208_dignitas-personae_en.html> accessed 24 December 2011.

17 Professor Robert P. George observed that belief in ensoulment and
immortality is not generally the basis of state laws against homicide.
"Infanticide and Madness", *Journal of Medical Ethics*, vol. 39, no. 5 (May
2013), p. 300.

18 *Catechism of the Catholic Church* (Dublin, Veritas, 1995), paragraphs 84–6.

19 Sacred Congregation for the Doctrine of the Faith, *Declaration in Defence
of the Catholic Doctrine on the Church Against Some Present-Day Errors
(Mysterium ecclesiae*, 24 June 1973), in Austin Flannery (general ed.), *Vatican
Council II: More Postconciliar Documents* (Collegeville, Minn.: Liturgical Press,
1982 (1st edn)), p. 433.

20 *Dogmatic Constitution of the Church* (*Lumen Gentium*, 21 November 1964),
paragraph 25 in Austin Flannery (general ed.), *Vatican Council II: The
Conciliar and Post Conciliar Documents* (Dublin: Dominican Publications,
1992 (new revised edn)), p. 379.

21 Sacred Congregation for the Doctrine of the Faith, *Declaration in Defence of
the Catholic Doctrine*, pp. 433–5. See also the Synod of Bishops, *On Dangerous
Opinions and on Atheism* (*Ratione habita*, 28 October 1967), p. 663; both in
Flannery, op. cit. (1982).

22 Pádraig Corkery, *Bioethics and the Catholic Moral Tradition* (Dublin: Veritas,
2010), p. 11.

23 Ibid., pp. 11–35; quotations from p. 29.

24 Quotation from *Catechism of the Catholic Church*, paragraph 87.

25 David Quinn, "Less doctrinal emphasis does not equate to radical change",
Irish Catholic, 12 March 2015.

26 For critical analyses of Pope Francis's soft pastoral approach, especially
in relation to sexual morality and bioethics, see Mark J. Cherry, "Pope
Francis, Weak Theology, and the Subtle Transformation of Roman Catholic
Bioethics", *Christian Bioethics*, vol. 21, no. 1 (2015), pp. 84–8; and Christopher
Tollefsen, "The Future of Roman Catholic Bioethics", *Journal of Medicine and
Philosophy*, vol. 43 (2018), pp. 667–85.

27 Pope Francis's conciliatory attitude towards disaffected Catholics was clearly
evident in his lengthy apostolic exhortation *Amoris Laetitia* (19 March 2016)
<http://www.catholicbishops.ie/wp-content/uploads/2016/04/Amoris-
Laetitia.pdf> accessed 9 April 2016. He was critical of the obsession, in the
Church, with contraception, abortion and gay marriage. Antonio Spadaro SJ,
"A Big Heart Open to God: An interview with Pope Francis", *America: The
Jesuit Review*, 30 September 2013; and Colum Lynch, "Can Pope Francis
Get the Catholic Church's Mind Off of Sex?", *Foreign Policy*, 11 May 2015
<https://foreignpolicy.com/2015/05/11/can-pope-francis-get-the-catholic-
churchs-mind-off-of-sex/> accessed 1 May 2019.

28 Patsy McGarry, "Bishop of Elphin expresses regret over comments about

gay parents", *Irish Times*, 16 March 2015 <http://www.irishtimes.com/news/social-affairs/religion-and-beliefs/bishop-of-elphin-expresses-regret-over-comments-about-gay-parents-1.2140902?mode=print&ot=example.AjaxPageLayout.ot> accessed 16 March 2015.

29 "Homily of Archbishop Diarmuid Martin at Mass in Church of Saint Dominick, Dublin, 6 July 2013."

30 Homily notes of Diarmuid Martin, Archbishop of Dublin, "Ordination of Dominican Deacons", at St Saviour's Priory, Dominick Street, 15 March 2015 <http://dublindiocese.ie/2015/03/15/ordination-of-dominican-deacons/> accessed 17 March 2015.

31 Religious beliefs inevitably influence constitutional reform and legislative changes. This occurs mainly when individual politicians vote in conformity with a religiously informed conscience and when churches and their members lobby politicians for changes to the law. See L. Skene and M. Parker, "The Role of the Church in Developing the Law", *Journal of Medical Ethics*, vol. 28 (2002), pp. 215–18.

APPENDIX

———————•———————

Seeking Moral Boundaries: Abortion and

Infanticide

DEBATES ABOUT ABORTION ARE INEVITABLY INCONCLUSIVE. THIS should not be surprising, given that whatever foundational principles are proposed are unlikely to command consensus. Also, many relevant terms, such as "personhood" and "a life worth living", are highly subjective. All this gives rise to a broad spectrum of opinion, ranging from the belief that human life is sacred from conception onwards, to the polar opposite that abortion on request is morally permissible without any gestational time limits. Some philosophers even argue that infanticide is morally permissible! A comprehensive survey of the vast volume of philosophical literature on the subject is not possible here, but it is worthwhile to give some attention to a highly controversial essay by philosophers Alberto Giubilini and Francesca Minerva. Their essay "After-birth Abortion: Why should the baby live?" was first published online on 23 February 2012 and later appeared in the *Journal of Medical Ethics* (May 2013). Their thesis, and the responses to it, facilitates a limited exploration of some important points relating to immortal souls, personhood, and moral hazards relating to "slippery slopes".

Giubilini and Minerva argued that abortion should be permissible, but unlike many supporters of freedom to choose, they went one step further. They believed that it was ethically permissible to kill a neonate (newborn baby) – including those without disability – in all circumstances where it was acceptable to kill a foetus. They choose to use the self-contradictory expression "after-birth abortion" rather than "infanticide" to emphasise that a neonate in this context was comparable to a foetus and not to a child. Both a foetus and a neonate are human beings and potential persons, but neither is a person with a moral right to life. A person was defined as "an individual who is capable of attributing to her own existence some (at least) basic value such that being deprived of this existence represents a loss to her". Being human was not in itself a sufficient reason for a right to life. It was not immoral to terminate the life of a potential person because the person did not actually exist. It was not possible to harm a person who did not exist. The interests of actual persons outweighed the "alleged right" of "merely potential people to become actual ones". The authors went so far as to claim that "the alleged interest of potential people to become actual ones ... amounts to zero." Once a person existed, that person had a right to opportunities for a life worth living. But when did a subject become a person or cease being a person? Giubilini and Minerva could not give precise answers to these questions. It was therefore unclear what limit would be imposed for the termination of an infant's life if it was sought for non-medical reasons. The authors could only offer an answer in a general sense. Personhood depended on the level of neurological development, which was subject to assessment by neurologists and psychologists.[1]

The main arguments expressed by Giubilini and Minerva were not original. Proposals for the moral equivalence of abortion and infanticide had been made by Michael Tooley as far back as 1972.[2] In later years, infanticide was proposed for acceptance by other philosophers, such as Peter Singer (Princeton University) and Helga Kuhse. Giubilini and Minerva's paper provoked much debate among moral philosophers, but unlike Tooley's thesis, the reaction extended far beyond the boundaries of academic discourse. Many journal articles were now published online and with so many pro-life websites it was relatively easy to provoke opposition to opinions expressed in academic journals. The authors were subjected to virulent commentary, even to the point of receiving death threats. This indicated the potency of the abortion issue to provoke extreme emotional responses.

There was some disquiet in the pro-choice camp. The essay by Giubilini and Minerva almost certainly confirmed the worst fears of pro-life lobbies. Undermining the rights of unborn human life would in turn threaten vulnerable members of society. A dividing line needed to be established to protect those who deserved a right to life, from those who did not. For those who were extremely liberal on abortion that dividing line was birth.[3] Those who were resolutely pro-life, and who wished to avoid "slippery slope" arguments, argued that human life should be protected from conception onwards.

The belief that a pre-implantation embryo should be accorded the same status as a person was difficult to sustain. It raised the question: What property of the embryo justifies such a status? The official Roman Catholic response is that an embryo has a spiritual/immortal soul that does not perish when the body dies, although the Church does not say dogmatically and precisely at what stage of embryonic development the immortal soul (not "produced" by the parents) is "immediately created by God".[4] Terminating the life of an embryo could thus be seen as murder. Such an opinion is groundless in a legal context. Robert P. George, professor of law (Harvard and Princeton) observed, in relation to this issue, that laws against homicide are not grounded on a belief in immortal souls.[5] Philosophically, it can be challenged on the basis that there is no evidence for the existence of immortal souls. Professor Michael J. Selgelid (director of the Monash Bioethics Centre, Melbourne) observed that if evidence is claimed on the basis of sacred texts, further questions arise about what should, and should not, be seen as good standards of evidence.[6] From a religious point of view, it could be argued that the presence of an immortal soul in humans is evident in the human mind. This idea is philosophically very weak. It is a god-of-the-gaps type of argument, relying on the spiritual or divine to fill in the many questions about human psychology that still – and may for ever – remain unanswered. Michael Tooley, professor of philosophy at the University of Colorado, argued that the idea of an "immaterial" rational mind can be accepted as a scientific hypothesis and refuted on a scientific basis. The gradual emergence of mental capacities as children grow towards adulthood, the gradual decline of mental capacities in old age, and the adverse effects of head injuries, psychotropic drugs and disease (such as Alzheimer's disease) all point to the mind as physical matter. Specialised functions in the brain associated with language, spatial perception, motor skills, memories, etc., are located in different areas of the brain and if these areas are damaged there is a corresponding loss of functionality. This is what one would expect from a mind dependent on complex neuronal circuitry.[7]

The extreme anti-abortion stance, that personhood is present from conception, marginalises the biomedical sciences. If personhood is accepted from conception onwards there is little scope for science to contribute to ethical discourses about unborn human life. Philosophy is also marginalised and offers little more than an endorsement of conformist theological abstractions. C.A.J. Coady (University of Melbourne) argued that, even within theology, there are difficulties in reconciling the "tiny person" hypothesis with St Thomas Aquinas's understanding of human personhood. Coady pointed to an inconsistency among "strong" anti-abortionists arising from their reactions to the deaths of embryos and foetuses by natural causes. Funeral rites were generally not held in response to spontaneous abortions. Nor were IVF embryos baptised before death or before being "allowed to die". Coady argued that the physical structures associated with sensation and thought should be present before moral significance is granted to the human individual. This level of development, it seems, occurs near the end of the second trimester.[8]

Selgelid observed that a "highly plausible" way of viewing unborn human life is: (1) little if any moral status should apply to early-stage embryos; and (2) newborn babies should be entitled to the same rights as older children and adults. Embryonic and foetal development could then be seen as a process giving rise to a gradual accumulation of rights equal to those of children and adults.[9] The moral status attributed to a foetus is not seen as absolute and is commonly regarded as lower than that of an individual whose level of mental development has generated a range of traits and capacities such as self-awareness, the formation of social relationships and emotional experiences. Medical research does not to date reliably and accurately indicate to what extent these "morally valuable capacities" have developed.[10] Besides, it may be argued that some mental capacities are significant in a moral context only when a "certain threshold" has been acquired.[11] Some philosophers have argued that the emergence of consciousness, thought to occur near the end of the second trimester, is an important contributor to moral status – to the extent that there is now "someone" rather than "something" present. This coincides with viability, which also elevates the moral status of the foetus.[12]

Viability is based on the opinion that when it is possible for a foetus to survive termination of pregnancy it should be regarded as an independent human being and has a right to life. This was the basis of the US Supreme Court's judgment in the landmark case *Roe v Wade*. The convergence of two important contributors to moral status – viability and consciousness – seem to present a strong case against abortion except in exceptional circumstances, such as an elevated risk to the mother's life. This opinion can be critiqued on a number of points.

The viability of a foetus is dependent on the available medical technology and has been reduced from twenty-eight weeks down to about twenty-three weeks. In 1992 (*Planned Parenthood v Casey*) the US Supreme Court replaced the trimester framework with viability as the point where the state could protect the foetus except in cases where the pregnancy was a threat to the health or life of the mother.[13] The merit of viability is that it prohibits the killing of a foetus which, if relocated outside the mother's body, would be a premature infant. However, viability is not straightforward. For example, the viability of individual foetuses can vary considerably, depending on access to medical technology. Furthermore, viability is likely to change over time with further advances in medical technology.[14] It might even be possible with future technological advances to proceed with problematic pregnancies *ex utero* using artificial wombs. In cases of women with no womb, or a womb incapable of sustaining a pregnancy, it may be possible to generate children through IVF and artificial gestation. This would undermine the concept of viability in the context of abortion.

Some philosophers point to the emergence of consciousness or self-consciousness as features that elevate the foetus's right to life.[15] In a theoretical sense this presents a strong argument against abortion except in exceptional circumstances. Although theoretically neat, it has little to offer in practice. Consciousness and self-consciousness are internal subjective phenomena and are not objectively measurable. Although it is thought that a foetus becomes aware of its environment before birth, it is not known when this occurs. Philosophers Paul S. Penner and Richard T. Hull argued that abortions should not be performed after twenty-three weeks "except under special circumstances". Biomedical research indicates that a foetus begins to store and process receptor data in its cerebral cortex well before birth, possibly as early as twenty-three weeks. This data has served as the foundation of what would become a unique person. Therefore, it was critically important not to kill "a person in the making".[16] There is much yet to be discovered about foetal brain development. Even so, higher levels of neurological development give rise to increasing difficulties when seeking to justify late-term abortions.

Where, then, does one draw the line? Some liberal supporters of the right to choose point to birth. Some may see birth as theoretically arbitrary, but, mindful of other moral considerations, may choose it because they believe a line must be drawn somewhere. It is sometimes argued that birth itself does not generate any major development in psychological capacities. It is plausibly assumed that mental development correlates with brain development and that, with some degree of individual variation, mental development correlates with age.[17] Birth is seen as a mere change of location without any significant change in intrinsic properties. Therefore, there is no significant change in the moral status of the neonate. There is some scientific merit in this specific point, considering that a well-developed late-term foetus of thirty-eight weeks is more developed than a premature baby after twenty-four weeks of pregnancy. Jeff McMahan (Rutgers University) and Julian Savulescu (Oxford Uehiro Centre for Practical Ethics) observed that there is a period of approximately four months during which an individual could be a foetus or an infant, depending on whether or not birth has occurred.[18] Neil Levy (University of Melbourne) made the point that if it is accepted that mental development determines moral significance, a foetus may in some cases have greater moral status than a neonate. The distinction, then, between a foetus and an infant seemed to be blurred when considering abortion and infanticide. Birth, apparently, was not a good boundary for those who wished to avoid the uncertainties of slippery slope arguments and the unintended consequences of crossing over an assumed moral line. But this could be used as an argument against abortion rather than bolstering the case for infanticide. Besides, it fails to take account of the broader moral context by focusing only on the intrinsic properties of the foetus.

Many philosophers challenged the idea that birth is an insignificant event when considering infanticide.[19] Savulescu, in response to Giubilini and Minerva, pointed to an obvious difference between infanticide and abortion. In the case of infanticide a baby is killed when she or he could otherwise be cared for by people other than the mother.[20] Justin Oakley (Monash University) argued that the woman's right to bodily autonomy is not applicable to cases of infanticide because the baby is no longer within her body. Justifications for terminating the life of a foetus are not straightforwardly applicable to newly born infants.[21] Bertha Alvarez Manninen (Arizona State University) argued that location does matter, despite no significant change in the "nature" of the foetus/neonate (i.e. in a moral context). Late-term abortion is justified on the basis that a woman's right to bodily autonomy is greater than the right to life of the foetus (although Manninen conceded that the primacy of maternal bodily autonomy is not without its difficulties). The woman had a right to an abortion because she had a right to withdraw sustenance from the foetus. She did not have the right to kill the foetus *per se*, although the act of terminating a pregnancy before viability would have the same outcome. If the foetus survived, the mother had no right to kill it. Therefore, there was a clear distinction between the status of a foetus and a neonate. Manninen accepted the validity of Giubilini and Minerva's point about the lack of significant cognitive differences between a late-term foetus and a neonate, but this tended to persuade her against late-term abortions rather than influencing her to support infanticide.[22]

Lindsey Porter (University of Sheffield) pointed to the importance of moral context. During pregnancy there is a unique relationship between the mother and the foetus. Even if it is accepted that the foetus has a right to life this does not rule out abortion because the woman's right to choose not to sustain that life is seen as greater. Therefore, a right to life is not seen as decisive! The circumstances for infanticide are very different because the physical integrity of the mother is no longer an issue. There are other carer relationships to consider, especially concerning the father. The moral context is never the same for abortion and infanticide.[23]

Infanticide is almost certainly seen as immoral in most cultures.[24] It is antagonistic to deeply embedded moral intuitions. Some philosophers point to the role of emotions and intuitions as critically important for the formation of moral norms. Andrew McGee (Queensland University of Technology) argued that there is "something primal" about protecting our offspring. An obvious objection is that moral discourse should be rational to the point of excluding emotions and instincts. McGee's counterargument is that caring for our children is a core part of our nature and needs to be taken into consideration. Emotions are an important part of our nature. The intense pain and grief following the loss of a child is evidence of this. Maternal and paternal instincts, and our emotional nature in general, are "background conditions" which serve as the foundation for moral norms. Emotions and interpersonal relationships cannot be ignored when considering the meaning and value of human life. McGee was aware of the possibility that emotions can confuse moral debate. However, he believed that, in relation to some issues, a consideration of emotions was essential because "they help reveal rather than conceal the moral status of the entity towards which those emotions are directed."[25]

Jacqueline A. Laing (London Metropolitan University) speculated about the adverse consequences for society if attitudes of care and protection for the unborn and the young were eroded by the widespread practice of abortion and infanticide. This might lead to a lack of respect for future generations, undermine the caring ethic of medical professionals, diminish the trust of patients towards the medical profession, and drive down birth rates. Laing envisaged a dystopia where attitudes of care and protection would be undermined. Vulnerable adults would be at risk in a healthcare system excessively driven by considerations of driving down costs. The "slippery slope" would lead to paediatric euthanasia, to euthanasia of the terminally ill, and euthanasia of those who were depressed and lonely.[26]

Laing was not writing in response only to the article by Giubilini and Minerva. She was also critical of the highly controversial Groningen Protocol. In the Netherlands, neonatal euthanasia is legal in very limited circumstances. The conditions include: incurable and intense suffering (e.g. the severest type of epidermolysis bullosa – a lethal skin disease), certainty of diagnosis and prognosis, and informed consent from both parents. In some cases, neonatal euthanasia is chosen in preference to second trimester abortion because, for some conditions, diagnosis and prognosis are more easily established after birth. Also, more time is available for medical specialists to discuss alternative treatments with parents, including palliative care. In some cases, the distinction between euthanasia and palliative care can be blurred. Research by A.A. Eduard Verhagen (University Medical Centre, Groningen) indicated that predictions about a downward slide on the "slippery slope," arising from access to neonatal euthanasia, did not occur in the Netherlands.[27]

Giubilini and Minerva provoked much criticism from their fellow philosophers. C.A.J. Coady believed that death might be "preferable" to life in cases of very severe congenital abnormalities. However, he was critical of advocates of infanticide who viewed healthy babies as "simply disposable".[28] Oakley believed that a decision about infanticide should not be influenced mainly by a consideration of parental burdens but instead by whether or not a medical diagnosis and prognosis pointed to a future of intense and relentless suffering for the child.[29] This was a very different ethical stance from that of Giubilini and Minerva, who argued that it was morally permissible to terminate the lives of healthy neonates – even in cases where the child could be handed over for adoption. This elicited very little support from philosophers.

Giubilini and Minerva pointed to mental development as a determinant of personhood. Personhood entailed some degree of rationality and self-awareness. Charles Camosy (Fordham University) argued that considerations of rationality and self-awareness could give rise to some absurd conclusions. For example, he assumed that it was not very controversial to observe that: "a pig, though having a significant moral value, is not a person with a (legal) right to life." Pigs were mentally "sophisticated" to the point where they could even be taught to play video games. A one-year-old human infant could not be taught to play a video game.[30] At what point would an infant's rationality and self-awareness be greater than that of a pig? At what point could a human infant be considered a person? Giubilini and Minerva had not specified a limit for cases where non-medical reasons were given for infanticide. They left it to neurologists and psychologists to make a judgement. It seemed to Camosy that Giubilini and Minerva had been somewhat evasive in not pursuing their argument to its logical conclusion. Infanticide might be permitted up to the third year of life, depending on how rationality and self-awareness were defined.[31]

Manninen believed that women had a right to choose abortion because every person had a right to decide whether or not their body was to sustain the life of another human being. Infanticide was an entirely different matter. If rationality was necessary for personhood, then it seemed that infanticide might be permissible up to "the late toddler stages". How was rationality to be assessed, given that its acquisition, and frequently its loss, is gradual rather than instantaneous? Many mentally impaired individuals would be vulnerable if rationality were the criterion for a right to life. Manninen believed that consensus would never be achieved on the issue of personhood and that pro-choice advocates should cease to argue their case on this basis. Those who argued for the right to abortion were losing public support by denying that human foetuses had little if any moral status. They were confirming the worst fears of those who might be won over by linking infanticide to abortion. Infanticide was discrediting pro-choice. For Manninen, the argument based on the primacy of bodily autonomy was sufficient, avoiding the complexities and pitfalls of foetal moral status and personhood.[32] The criterion of personhood for a right to life is generally seen as too demanding.[33]

In the context of Irish public debate, it is almost certainly the case that most people see the argument from personhood as setting the bar too high when considering the right to life of the foetus. Neither does public opinion in Ireland support the idea that human life is sacred from conception. To what extent it grants legal protection to human embryos and foetuses remains to be seen. The outcome of the 2018 referendum on abortion and the enactment of the Health (Regulation of Termination of Pregnancy) Act 2018 confirms the fluidity of public opinion on bioethical issues.

Endnotes

———————•———————

1   Alberto Giubilini and Francesca Minerva, "After-birth Abortion: Why should the baby live?", *Journal of Medical Ethics*, vol. 39, no. 5 (May 2013), pp. 261–3. The authors pointed out that the rights of actual people did not always outweigh the rights of future generations. Consideration had to be given to the welfare of future generations. This was a different issue from the one relating to the "alleged interest" of individual foetuses and newborns.

2   Helga Kuhse, "Some Comments on the Paper 'After-birth Abortion: Why should the baby live?'", *Journal of Medical Ethics*, vol. 39, no. 5 (May 2013), p. 323. For differences between Michael Tooley's infanticide thesis and Giubilini and Minerva's argument, see Lindsey Porter, "Abortion, Infanticide and Moral Context", *Journal of Medical Ethics*, vol. 39, no. 5 (May 2013), p. 351.

3   See Kuhse, op. cit., p. 324.

4   See *Catechism of the Catholic Church* (Dublin: Veritas, 1995), paragraphs 363–7. According to Massimo Reichlin, St Thomas Aquinas believed that God creates and infuses the spiritual soul into a well-developed human body. There is a gender difference – 40 days for males and 90 days for females. Massimo Reichlin, "The Argument from Potential: A reappraisal", *Bioethics*, vol. 11, no. 1 (1997), p. 16.

5   Robert P. George, "Infanticide and Madness", *Journal of Medical Ethics*, vol. 39, no. 5 (May 2013), p. 300.

6   Michael J. Selgelid, "Moral Uncertainty and the Moral Status of Early Human Life", *Journal of Medical Ethics*, vol. 39, no. 5 (May 2013), p. 324.

7   Michael Tooley, "Philosophy, Critical Thinking and 'After-birth Abortion: Why should the baby live?'", *Journal of Medical Ethics*, vol. 39, no. 5 (May 2013), p. 270–1.

8   C.A.J. Coady, "The Common Premise for Uncommon Conclusions", *Journal of Medical Ethics*, vol. 39, no. 5 (May 2013), p. 285.

9   Selgelid, op. cit., p. 324.

10 Justin Oakley, "'After-birth Abortion' and Arguments from Potential", *Journal of Medical Ethics*, vol. 39, no. 5 (May 2013), p. 324.

11 Neil Levy, "The Moral Significance of Being Born", *Journal of Medical Ethics*, vol. 39, no. 5 (May 2013), p. 327.

12 Jeff McMahan, "Infanticide and Moral Consistency", *Journal of Medical Ethics*, vol. 39, no. 5 (May 2013), p. 274.

13 Ibid.

14 Paul S. Penner and Richard T. Hull, "The Beginning of Individual Personhood", *Journal of Medicine and Philosophy*, vol. 33 (2008), p. 177.

15 Consciousness may be defined as "the phenomenon of immediately experiencing the physical world". Self-consciousness is "the phenomenon of immediately experiencing one's own consciousness and, therefore, of one's place in the physical world". Ibid., p. 175.

16 Ibid., pp. 176–82; quotations from p. 181.

17 Levy, op. cit., p. 326.

18 McMahan, op. cit., p. 274; and Julian Savulescu, "Abortion, Infanticide and Allowing Babies to Die, 40 Years On", *Journal of Medical Ethics*, vol. 39, no. 5 (May 2013), p. 258.

19 For example, Regina A. Rini, "Of Course the Baby Should Live: Against 'after-birth abortion'", *Journal of Medical Ethics*, vol. 39, no. 5 (May 2013), pp. 353–6.

20 Savulescu, op. cit, p. 258.

21 Oakley, op. cit., p. 325.

22 Bertha Alvarez Manninen, "Yes, the Baby Should Live: A pro-choice response to Giubilini and Minerva", *Journal of Medical Ethics*, vol. 39, no. 5 (May 2013), pp. 334–5.

23 Porter, "Abortion, infanticide and moral context", pp. 350–2.

24 See McMahan, op. cit., p. 274.

25 Andrew McGee, "The Moral Status of Babies", *Journal of Medical Ethics*, vol. 39, no. 5 (May 2013), p. 346.

26 Jacqueline A. Laing, "Infanticide: A reply to Giubilini and Minerva", *Journal of Medical Ethics*, vol. 39, no. 5 (May 2013), pp. 336–40. See also Leslie Francis and Anita Silvers, "Infanticide, Moral Status and Moral Reasons: The importance of context", *Journal of Medical Ethics*, vol. 39, no. 5 (May 2013), p. 290.

27 A.A. Eduard Verhagen, "The Groningen Protocol for Newborn Euthanasia; Which way did the slippery slope tilt?", *Journal of Medical Ethics*, vol. 39, no. 5 (May 2013), pp. 293–5.

28 Coady, "The Common Premise for Uncommon Conclusions", p. 288.

29 Oakley, "'After-birth abortion' and arguments from potential", p. 325.

30 Charles Camosy, "Concern for Our Vulnerable Prenatal and Neonatal Children: A brief reply to Giubilini and Minerva", *Journal of Medical Ethics*, vol. 39, no. 5 (May 2013), p. 297; in reference to the People for the Ethical Treatment of Animals (PETA) website, accessed 1 March 2012.

31 Camosy, op. cit., p. 297.

32 Manninen, "Yes, the Baby Should Live", pp. 333–4.

33 See, for example, Rini, "Of Course the Baby Should Live", pp. 353–6; and Ciara Staunton, "A Moral Gap? Examining Ireland's failure to regulate embryonic stem cell research" in Mary Donnelly and Claire Murray (eds), *Ethical and Legal Debates in Irish Healthcare: Confronting Complexities* (Manchester: Manchester University Press, 2016), p. 153.

BIBLIOGRAPHY

———•———

Primary Sources

Official Publications

Abortion Act 1967, United Kingdom of Great Britain and Northern Ireland <https://www.legislation.gov.uk/ukpga/1967/87/section/1> accessed 10 May 2018.

Arulkumaran, Sabaratnam *et al.*, *Final Report: Investigation of Incident 50278 from time of patient's self referral to hospital on the 21st of October 2012 to the patient's death on 28th of October, 2012*, Health Service Executive, June 2013 <https://www.hse.ie/eng/services/news/nimtreport50278.pdf> accessed 15 July 2018.

Barrington, Eileen, "Article 40.3.3 of the Constitution and Fatal Foetal Abnormalities", Citizens' Assembly, 7 January 2017 <https://www.citizensassembly.ie/en/Meetings/Eileen-Barrington-Paper.pdf> accessed 9 January 2017.

Central Statistics Office, *Census 2011, Profile 7: Religion, Ethnicity and Irish Travellers* (Dublin: Stationery Office, October 2012) <http://www.cso.ie/en/media/csoie/census/documents/census2011profile7/Profile,7,Education,Ethnicity,and,Irish,Traveller,entire,doc.pdf> accessed 20 March 2015.

— *Census 2016 Summary Results – Part 1*, Chapter 8, p. 72 <http://www.cso.ie/en/media/csoie/releasespublications/documents/population/2017/Chapter_8_Religion.pdf> accessed 13 April 2017.

Citizens' Assembly, *First Report and Recommendations of the Citizens' Assembly: The Eighth Amendment of the Constitution*, 29 June 2017 <https://www.citizensassembly.ie/en/The-Eighth-Amendment-of-the-Constitution/Final-Report-on-the-Eighth-Amendment-of-the-Constitution/Final-Report-incl-Appendix-A-D.pdf> accessed 27 January 2018.

Citizens Information Board, "Surrogacy" <http://www.citizensinformation.ie/en/birth_family_relationships/adoption_and_fostering/surrogacy.html> accessed 9 November 2013.

— "Children and Family Relationships Act 2015", *Relate*, vol. 42, issue 5

(May 2015) <http://www.citizensinformationboard.ie/publications/relate/
relate_2015_05.pdf> accessed 8 September 2015.

Clark, Judge Maureen Harding, *The Lourdes Hospital Inquiry: An Inquiry into
peripartum hysterectomy at Our Lady of Lourdes Hospital, Drogheda* (Dublin:
Government Publications, January 2006) http://health.gov.ie/wp-content/
uploads/2014/05/lourdes.pdf> accessed 7 February 2018.

— *The Surgical Symphysiotomy Ex Gratia Payment Scheme*, 19 October 2016
<http://health.gov.ie/wp-content/uploads/2016/11/The-Surgical-
Symphysiotomy-Ex-Gratia-Payment-Scheme-Report.pdf> accessed 8
February 2018.

Commission on Assisted Human Reproduction, *Report of the Commission on
Assisted Human Reproduction* (Dublin: Stationery Office, 2005).

Criminal Law Amendment Act 1885 <http://www.irishstatutebook.ie/eli/1885/
act/69/enacted/en/print> accessed 4 June 2019.

Criminal Law (Suicide) Act 1993 <http://www.irishstatutebook.ie/eli/1993/
act/11/enacted/en/print> accessed 15 April 2016.

Dáil Éireann Parliamentary Debates.

Denham, Susan, Nial Fennelly, Hugh Geoghegan, Adrian Hardiman and John
Murray, Supreme Court of Ireland judgment delivered on 15 December 2009,
Neutral Citation [2009] IESC 82, Supreme Court Record No. 469/06 &
59/07, accessed from the Supreme Court of Ireland website, 19 December
2009.

Department of Health, General Scheme of the Assisted Human Reproduction
Bill 2017 <https://health.gov.ie/wp-content/uploads/2017/10/AHR-general-
scheme-with-cover.pdf> accessed 4 January 2019.

— General Scheme of a Bill to Regulate Termination of Pregnancy, 27 March
2018 <http://health.gov.ie/wp-content/uploads/2018/03/General-Scheme-
for-Publication.pdf> accessed 8 May 2018.

— "Government approves the drafting of the Assisted Human Reproduction
Bill", 3 October 2017 <https://health.gov.ie/blog/press-release/government-
approves-the-drafting-of-the-assisted-human-reproduction-bill/> accessed
24 January 2019.

— "Government decision on ABC Expert Group option", 18 December 2012
<http://www.dohc.ie/press/releases/2012/20121218.html> accessed 25
January 2014.

— "Govt to legislate for Assisted Human Reproduction & Associated Research",
press release, 25 February, 2015 <http://health.gov.ie/blog/press-release/govt-
to-legislate-for-assisted-human-reproduction-associated-research/> accessed
12 January 2016.

— *Notifications in Accordance with Section 20 of The Protection of Life During
Pregnancy Act 2013*, June 2015 <http://health.gov.ie/wp-content/
uploads/2015/06/annual-report-2014-Protection-of-Life-During-
Pregnancy1.pdf> accessed 1 July 2015.

— *Statement from the Department of Health regarding the Governance arrangements in relation to the new National Maternity Hospital*, 18 April 2017 <http://health.gov.ie/blog/press-release/statement-from-the-department-of-health-regarding-the-governance-arrangements-in-relation-to-the-new-national-maternity-hospital/> accessed 6 February 2017.

Department of Health and Social Care (UK), *Abortion Statistics, England and Wales: 2017*, June 2018 <https://assets.publishing.service.gov.uk/government/uploads/system/uploads/attachment_data/file/714183/2017_Abortion_Statistics_Commentary.pdf> accessed 10 December 2018.

Department of Health and Social Security (UK), *Report of the Committee of Inquiry into Human Fertilisation and Embryology* (London: HMSO, 1984).

Department of Justice and Equality, "Children and Family Relationships Bill 2013: Briefing Note", 5 November 2013 <http://www.justice.ie/en/JELR/Children%20and%20Family%20Relationships%20Bill%202013%20141113.pdf/Files/Children%20and%20Family%20Relationships%20Bill%202013%20141113.pdf> accessed 11 January 2014.

— "Minister Fitzgerald publishes General Scheme of the Children and Family Relationships Bill", press release, 25 September 2014 <http://www.justice.ie/en/JELR/Pages/PR14000257> accessed 27 September 2014.

Department of Social Protection, "Statement in Relation to High Court judgment in the case of MR, DR, OR and CR v An tÁrd Chlaraitheoir [Registrar General], Ireland and the Attorney General," 6 June 2013 <https://www.welfare.ie/en/pressoffice/pdf/pr060613a.pdf> accessed 8 January 2014.

Doctors for Choice Ireland, "Doctors for Choice Position Paper for Citizens' Assembly, 23 February 2017", presented to the Citizens' Assembly, session 1 on 5 March 2017 <https://www.citizensassembly.ie/en/Meetings/Doctors-for-Choice-s-Paper.pdf> accessed 7 March 2017.

— PowerPoint presentation, Citizens' Assembly, 5 March 2017 <https://www.citizensassembly.ie/en/Meetings/Doctors-for-Choice-Powerpoint.pdf> accessed 7 March 2017.

Doctors for Life Ireland, "Presentation on the Eighth Amendment to the Citizens' Assembly 2017", 5 March 2017 <https://www.citizensassembly.ie/en/Meetings/Doctors-for-Life-Paper.pdf> accessed 7 March 2017.

European Commission, "Research, funding: Seventh Framework Programme nears fruition", research news and events web page <http://ec.europa.eu/research/biosociety/news_events/news_seventh_framework_programme_fruition_en.htm> accessed 6 March 2007.

European Court of Human Rights, *D v Ireland* (application number 26499/02).

— "Grand Chamber Judgment: Evans v. The United Kingdom", press release issued by the Registrar, 10 April 2007.

— Grand Chamber judgment, *Case of A, B and C v. Ireland*, 16 December 2010.

European Court of Human Rights, Council of Europe, *European Convention on Human Rights* <http://www.echr.coe.int/Documents/Convention_ENG.pdf> accessed 5 March 2016.

Every Life Counts, paper presented to the Citizens' Assembly, 5 March 2017 <https://www.citizensassembly.ie/en/Meetings/Every-Life-Counts-Paper.pdf> accessed 25 March 2017.

Farsides, Bobbie, "The moral status of the human fetus: a pro-choice approach", Citizens' Assembly, 7 January 2017 <https://www.citizensassembly.ie/en/Meetings/Professor-Bobbie-Farsides-Paper.pdf> accessed 5 March 2017.

Fleming v Ireland & Ors, Neutral Citation [2013] IESC 19, Supreme Court Record Number 019/2013, judgment of C.J. Denham <http://www.supremecourt.ie/Judgments.nsf/60f9f366f10958d1802572ba003d3f45/94ff4efe25ba9b-4280257b5c003eea73?OpenDocument&Highlight=0,Fleming> accessed 9 June 2015.

Fleming v Ireland and Ors, High Court Judgment, [2013] IEHC 2, 1 January 2013, judgment of P. Kearns <http://www.courts.ie/Judgments.nsf/597645521f07a-c9a80256ef30048ca52/911cb02a6531c7a380257aef0037c379?OpenDocument> accessed 16 April 2016.

Government of Ireland, General Scheme of the Protection of Life during Pregnancy Bill 2013, 30 April 2013, Interpretation, pp. 4-5 <http://www.merrionstreet.ie/wp-content/uploads/2013/04/Protection-of-Life-During-Pregnancy-Bill-PLP-30.04.13-10.30.pdf> accessed 19 January 2014.

— *Policy Paper: Regulation of Termination of Pregnancy* (Appendix 2), approved and published by the government on 8 March 2018 <http://health.gov.ie/wp-content/uploads/2018/03/Policy-paper-approved-by-Goverment-8-March-2018.pdf> accessed 7 May 2018.

Harney, Mary, "Statement by Mary Harney TD, Minister for Health and Children, on the R v R: High Court Frozen Embryos Case", 15 November 2006 <http://www.dohc.ie/press/releases/2006/20061115.html> accessed 10 March 2007.

Hayes, Nóirín, Opening Statement to the Joint Committee on Health, 19 December 2018 <https://data.oireachtas.ie/ie/oireachtas/committee/dail/32/joint_committee_on_health/submissions/2018/2018-12-19_opening-statement-professor-noirin-hayes-school-of-education-tcd_en.pdf> accessed 5 February 2019.

Health Information and Quality Authority, "Patient Safety Investigation Report published by Health Information and Quality Authority", press release, 9 October 2013 <http://www.hiqa.ie/press-release/2013-10-09-patient-safety-investigation-report-published-health-information-and-qualit> accessed 1 November 2013.

Health (Regulation of Termination of Pregnancy) Bill 2018 <https://data.oireachtas.ie/ie/oireachtas/bill/2018/105/eng/ver_b/b105b18d.pdf> accessed 1 January 2019.

Health Service Executive, *National Standards for Bereavement Care following*

Pregnancy Loss, 10 August 2016 <http://www.hse.ie/eng/services/news/media/pressrel/%20NationalStandardsBereavementCare%20.html> accessed 20 August 2016.

— *National Standards for Bereavement Care Following Pregnancy Loss and Perinatal Death*, Version 1.15 (10 August 2015) <http://www.hse.ie/eng/about/Who/acute/bereavementcare/standardsBereavementCarePregnancyLoss.pdf> accessed 20 August 2016.

"Information note on legal advice received on options for a Referendum on Article 40.3.3 of the Constitution," https://static.rasset.ie/documents/news/2018/01/ag-advice-summary.pdf> accessed 31 January 2018.

Inquest into the death of Ms. Savita Halappanavar held before the coroner, Dr. Ciaran MacLoughlin, on Wednesday, 10th April 2013 – day 3, JCEA 43RC(a), Coroner's Court, Galway <https://webarchive.oireachtas.ie/parliament/media/committees/eighthamendmentoftheconstitution/jcea-43rc(a)---coroner-inquest-into-death-of-ms.-savita-halappanavar.pdf> accessed 15 July 2018.

Irish Council for Bioethics, *Ethical, Scientific, and Legal Issues Concerning Stem Cell Research: Opinion*. Dublin: 2008.

— *Public Attitudes Towards Bioethics: Irish Council for Bioethics Research September 2005* <http://www.bioethics.ie/publications/index.html> accessed 5 March 2007.

— *Stem Cell Information Leaflet*, March 2007.

Joint Committee on Health, proceedings on the General Scheme of the Assisted Human Reproduction Bill 2017, 17 January–19 December 2018, Houses of the Oireachtas website.

— proceedings, 17 January 2018, 28 February 2018, and 19 December 2018, Houses of the Oireachtas website.

— *Report on Pre-Legislative Scrutiny of the General Scheme of the Assisted Human Reproduction Bill*, 10 July 2019 <https://data.oireachtas.ie/ie/oireachtas/committee/dail/32/joint_committee_on_health/submissions/2019/2019-07-10_submissions-report-on-pre-legislative-scrutiny-of-the-general-scheme-of-the-assisted-human-reproduction-bill_en.pdf> accessed 30 July 2019.

Joint Committee on Health and Children, 29 JHC 1, no. 60, 21 July 2005 (Dublin: Stationery Office).

— 29 JHC 1, no. 61, 15 September 2005 (Dublin: Stationery Office).

— 29 JHC 1, no. 95, 4 July 2006 (Dublin: Stationery Office).

— 29 JHC 1, no. 111, 12 December 2006 (Dublin: Stationery Office).

— proceedings, 8 January 2013 <https://www.oireachtas.ie/en/debates/debate/joint_committee_on_health_and_children/2013-01-08/2/#s5> accessed 7 November 2018).

— proceedings, 10 January 2013 <https://www.oireachtas.ie/en/debates/debate/joint_committee_on_health_and_children/2013-01-10/2/#s3> accessed 9 November 2018).

Joint Oireachtas Committee on the Eighth Amendment, press release, 12
   July 2017 <https://webarchive.oireachtas.ie/parliament/mediazone/
   pressreleases/2017/name-43149-en.html> accessed 2 July 201.
— proceedings, September–December 2017, Houses of the Oireachtas website.
M v The Minister for Justice & Ors (2018 IESC 14), Supreme Court of
   Ireland, 7 March 2018, section 2.3 <http://www.supremecourt.
   ie/Judgments.nsf/1b0757edc371032e802572ea0061450e/
   af9213ad1cf44a3c80258249002acd3d?OpenDocument> accessed 7 March
   2018.
M.R. & Anor v An tArd Chlaraitheoir & Ors, Neutral Citation [2013]
   IEHC 91, High Court Record Number 2011 46 M, 5 March
   2013, judgment by Mr Justice Henry Abbott <http://www.
   courts.ie/Judgments.nsf/597645521f07ac9a80256ef30048ca52/
   e3f0dc917872554c80257b250052dab3?OpenDocument> accessed from the
   Court Services website 9 November 2013 and 8 February 2014.
*M.R. and D.R. (suing by their father and next friend O.R.) & ors v An t-Ard-
   Chláraitheoir & ors*, Supreme Court judgment, J. Clarke, C.J. Denham, J.
   Hardiman, J. MacMenamin, J. Murray, Donal J. O'Donnell, 7 November
   2014, Neutral Citation [2014] IESC 60, Appeal No. 263/2013.
M.R. v T.R. & Ors, judgment of Mr Justice McGovern delivered on the 15th day
   of November 2006, Citation Number [2006] IEHC 359 <http://www.bailii.
   org/ie/cases/IEHC/2006/H359.html> accessed 22 December 2009.
Madden, Deirdre, Opening Statement to the Joint Committee on Health on
   the General Scheme of the Assisted Human Reproduction Bill 2017, 17
   December 2018 <https://data.oireachtas.ie/ie/oireachtas/committee/dail/32/
   joint_committee_on_health/submissions/2018/2018-12-19_opening-
   statement-professor-deirdre-madden-school-of-law-ucc_en.pdf> accessed 5
   February 2019.
McCaffrey, M.J., letter to the Joint Oireachtas Committee on the Eighth
   Amendment, dated 7 November 2017 <https://webarchive.oireachtas.ie/
   parliament/media/committees/eighthamendmentoftheconstitution/JCEA-
   55RC---Response-from-Dr.-Marty-McCaffrey.pdf> accessed 2 July 2018.
McParland, Peter, "Antenatal Diagnosis and Management of Fetal
   Abnormalities", Citizens' Assembly, 7 January 2017 <https://www.
   citizensassembly.ie/en/Meetings/Dr-Peter-McParland-Paper.pdf> accessed 9
   September 2017.
Morris, Joan K., and Anna Springett, *The National Down Syndrome Cytogenetic
   Register for England and Wales: 2013 Annual Report*, December 2014 <http://
   www.binocar.org/content/annrep2013_FINAL.pdf> accessed 6 October
   2018.
Mullen, Rónán, Jim Walsh and John Hanafin, Stem-Cell Research (Protection of
   Human Embryos) Bill 2008: Explanatory Memorandum (Dublin: Stationery
   Office, 20 November 2008.

Murphy, Judge Yvonne, *Independent Review of Issues relating to Symphysiotomy*, 11 March 2014 <http://health.gov.ie/wp-content/uploads/2014/07/Scanned-Murphy-report-redacted-version1.pdf> accessed 8 February 2018.

Murray, Brian, "Legal Consequences of Retention, Repeal, or Amendment of Article 40.3.3 of the Constitution", Citizens' Assembly, 4 March 2017 <https://www.citizensassembly.ie/en/Meetings/Brian-Murray-s-Paper.pdf> accessed 11 March 2017.

National Collaborating Centre for Mental Health, *Induced Abortion and Mental Health* (London: December 2011) <https://www.aomrc.org.uk/wp-content/uploads/2016/05/Induced_Abortion_Mental_Health_1211.pdf> accessed 5 November 2018.

O'Dowd, John, "The Unborn, within and beyond the Eighth Amendment", paper read to the Citizens' Assembly, 4 March 2017 <https://www.citizensassembly.ie/en/Meetings/John-O-Dowd-Paper.pdf> accessed 11 March 2017.

Offences Against the Person Act 1861 <http://www.irishstatutebook.ie/eli/1861/act/100/enacted/en/print> accessed 4 June 2019.

Office of the Attorney General, Children and Family Relationships Act 2015 <http://www.irishstatutebook.ie/eli/2015/act/9/enacted/en/pdf> accessed 28 August 2015.

O'Friel, Emma, Opening Statement to the Joint Committee on Health, 19 December 2018 <https://data.oireachtas.ie/ie/oireachtas/committee/dail/32/joint_committee_on_health/submissions/2018/2018-12-19_opening-statement-emma-o-friel_en.pdf> accessed 5 February 2019.

Olika vägar till föräldraskap, Stockholm 2016 <http://www.sou.gov.se/wp-content/uploads/2016/02/SOU-2016_11_webb.pdf> accessed 23 January 2019.

P.P. v Health Service Executive, Neutral Citation [2014]IEHC 622, High Court Record Number 2014 10792 P, 26 December 2014, judgment by Mr Justice P. Kearns, pp. 1–9 <http://www.courts.ie/Judgments.nsf/09859e7a3f34669680256ef3004a27de/fb8a5c76857e08ce80257dcb003fd4e6?OpenDocument> accessed 13 January 2015.

Pro Life Campaign, "The Eighth Amendment – A Life-Saving Beacon of Hope: Submission to the Citizens' Assembly", 16 December 2016 <https://www.citizensassembly.ie/en/Submissions/Submissions-Received/> accessed 14 March 2017.

Protection of Life During Pregnancy Act 2013 <http://www.oireachtas.ie/documents/bills28/acts/2013/a3513.pdf> accessed 19 January 2014.

Protection of Life in Pregnancy (Amendment) (Fatal Foetal Abnormalities) Bill 2013, no. 115 of 2013, proposed to the Dáil by Deputy Clare Daly, 21 November 2013.

Protection of Life in Pregnancy (Amendment) (Fatal Foetal Abnormalities) (No.

2) Bill 2013, sponsored by Mick Wallace TD, 28 November 2013 <https://www.oireachtas.ie/documents/bills28/bills/2013/12213/b12213d.pdf> accessed 10 September 2016.

Referendum Commission, *Marriage Referendum and Age of Presidential Candidates Referendum* <http://refcom2015.ie/marriage/> accessed 16 May 2015.

Report of the Expert Group on the Judgment in A, B and C v Ireland, November 2012 <http://www.dohc.ie/publications/pdf/Judgment_ABC.pdf?direct=1

Report of the Joint Committee on the Eighth Amendment to the Constitution (Houses of the Oireachtas, December 2017) <http://www.oireachtas.ie/parliament/media/committees/eighthamendmentoftheconstitution/Report-of-the-Joint-Committee-on-the-Eighth-Amendment-web-version.pdf> accessed 22 December 2017.

Rose, Joanna, Opening Statement to the Joint Committee on Health, 19 December 2018 <https://data.oireachtas.ie/ie/oireachtas/committee/dail/32/joint_committee_on_health/submissions/2018/2018-12-19_opening-statement-dr-joanna-rose_en.pdf> accessed 5 February 2019.

Seanad Éireann Parliamentary Debates.

Sedgh, Gilda (Guttmacher Institute), "Key Facts on Abortion Worldwide", Citizens' Assembly, 4 February 2017 <https://www.citizensassembly.ie/en/Meetings/Gilda-Sedgh-Paper.pdf> accessed 6 March 2017.

Shatter, Alan, Minister for Justice and Equality, and Minister for Defence, "Minister Shatter publishes General Scheme of Children and Family Relationships Bill for consultation", press release, 30 January 2014 <http://www.merrionstreet.ie/index.php/2014/01/minister-shatter-publishes-general-scheme-of-children-and-family-relationships-bill-for-consultation/?cat=12> accessed 2 February 2014.

Thirty-sixth Amendment of the Constitution Act 2018, 18 September 2018 <https://data.oireachtas.ie/ie/oireachtas/act/2018/C36/mul/enacted/36th-amdt-of-the-constitution-act-2018.pdf> accessed 24 October 2018.

Thirty-sixth Amendment of the Constitution Bill 2018, 7 March 2018 <https://data.oireachtas.ie/ie/oireachtas/bill/2018/29/eng/initiated/b2918.pdf> accessed 24 October 2018.

United Nations Committee against Torture, "Consideration of reports submitted by State parties under article 19 of the Convention" (17 June 2011) <http://tbinternet.ohchr.org/_layouts/treatybodyexternal/Download.aspx?symbolno=CAT/C/IRL/CO/1&Lang=E> accessed 21 May 2016.

United Nations Committee on Economic, Social and Cultural Rights, "Concluding observations on the third periodic report on Ireland", 8 July 2015 <http://tbinternet.ohchr.org/_layouts/treatybodyexternal/Download.aspx?symbolno=E%2fC.12%2fIRL%2fCO%2f3&Lang=en> accessed 21 May 2016.

United Nations Committee on the Rights of the Child, "Concluding observations on the combined third and fourth periodic reports of Ireland", 1 March 2016

<http://tbinternet.ohchr.org/_layouts/treatybodyexternal/Download.aspx?sym
bolno=CRC%2fC%2fIRL%2fCO%2f3-4&Lang=en> accessed 21 May 2016.
United Nations General Assembly, Convention on the Rights of the Child
(ratified 20 November 1989) <https://www.ohchr.org/en/professionalinterest/
pages/crc.aspx> accessed 10 February 2019.
— Declaration of the Rights of the Child (20 November 1959) <http://www.
unicef.org/malaysia/1959-Declaration-of-the-Rights-of-the-Child.pdf>
accessed 6 June 2016.
— Universal Declaration of Human Rights (10 December 1948) <http://www.
ohchr.org/EN/UDHR/Documents/UDHR_Translations/eng.pdf> accessed
6 June 2016.
United Nations Human Rights Committee, "Concluding observations
on the fourth periodic report of Ireland", 19 August 2014 <http://
tbinternet.ohchr.org/_layouts/treatybodyexternal/Download.
aspx?symbolno=CCPR%2fC%2fIRL%2fCO%2f4&Lang=en> accessed 21
May 2016.
— "Views adopted by the Committee under article 5(4) of the Optional Protocol,
concerning communication No. 2324/2013", 9 June 2016 <http://tbinternet.
ohchr.org/_layouts/treatybodyexternal/Download.aspx?symbolno=CCPR/
C/116/D/2324/2013&Lang=en> accessed 10 June 2016.
Youth Defence, paper presented to the Citizens' Assembly, 5 March 2017
<https://www.citizensassembly.ie/en/Meetings/Youth-Defence-s-Paper.pdf>
accessed 23 March 2017.

Books, Articles, Press Releases and Website Documents

American Psychological Association, "Mental Health and Abortion: Overview",
<http://www.apa.org/pi/women/programs/abortion/index.aspx> accessed 2
May 2018.
— *Report of the APA Task Force on Mental Health and Abortion*, 2008 <http://www.
apa.org/pi/women/programs/abortion/mental-health.pdf> accessed 2 May
2018.
Amnesty International, *She is Not a Criminal: The Impact of Ireland's Abortion Law*
(London: 2015).
Archbishops and Bishops of Ireland, *Human Life is Sacred: Pastoral Letter
of the Archbishops and Bishops of Ireland to the clergy, religious and faithful*
(Archbishops and Bishops of Ireland: May 1975).
Association of Catholic Priests (Ireland), "The National Maternity Hospital",
10 May 2017 <https://www.associationofcatholicpriests.ie/2017/05/the-
national-maternity-hospital/> accessed 27 May 2017.
— "Statement from the Association of Catholic Priests Responding to
Comments made on the HPV vaccine", 1 October 2017 <http://www.
associationofcatholicpriests.ie/2017/10/statement-from-the-association-of-

catholic-priests-acp%e2%80%88-responding-to-comments-made-on-the-hpv-vaccine/> accessed 12 October 2017).

— "ACP Statement about the upcoming referendum on the Eighth Amendment", 4 May 2018 <https://www.associationofcatholicpriests.ie/2018/05/acp-statement-on-the-upcoming-referendum-on-the-eight-amendment/> accessed 7 May 2017).

Benedict XVI, Pope, "Address of His Holiness Pope Benedict XVI to participants of the symposium on the theme: 'Stem cells: What future for therapy? Scientific aspects and bioethical problems'", *Cell Proliferation* 41, issue s1 (February 2008), pp. 4–6.

Bishops' Commission for Doctrine of the Irish Episcopal Conference, *In Vitro Fertilisation: Statement of Bishops' Commission for Doctrine of the Irish Episcopal Conference. The Furrow* 37, no. 3 (March 1986), pp. 197-200.

Bishops' Committee for Bioethics, *Assisted Human Reproduction: Facts and Ethical Issues* <http://www.catholiccommunications.ie/pastlet/ahr.html> accessed 1 November 2004; revised version of booklet published under the same title (Dublin: Veritas, 2000).

Brennan, Bishop Denis, "Homily of Bishop Brennan, Ferns Diocese at Knock Shrine, Sunday 7 July 2013", (press release on 8 July 2013) <http://www.catholicbishops.ie/2013/07/08/homily-bishop-brennan-ferns-diocese-knock-shrine-sunday-7-july-2013/> accessed 14 December 2013).

Burke, Cardinal Raymond (interview), "To decriminalise abortion is a contradiction of the most fundamental principle of the legal system", *Catholic Voice*, 24 April 2014 <http://www.catholicvoice.ie/index.php/6-to-decriminalise-abortion-is-a-contradiction-of-the-most-fundamental-principle-of-the-legal-system?showall=&start=1> accessed 20 December 2015.

Catechism of the Catholic Church (Dublin: Veritas, 1995).

Catholic Communications Office, "Winter 2012 General Meeting of the Irish Catholic Bishops' Conference", 5 December 2012 <http://www.catholicbishops.ie/2012/12/05/initial-response-report-expert-group/> accessed 14 December 2013.

— "Statement by the four Archbishops of Ireland in response to the decision today by the Government to legislate for abortion", 18 December 2012 <http://www.catholicbishops.ie/2012/12/18/statement-archbishops-ireland-response-decision-today-government-legislate-abortion/> accessed 25 January 2014.

— "Statement by Bishop John Buckley, Bishop of Cork and Ross in response to the decision by the Government to legislate for abortion", 19 December 2012 <http://www.catholicbishops.ie/2012/12/19/statement-bishop-john-buckley-bishop-cork-ross-response-decision-government-legislate-abortion/> accessed 25 January 2014.

— "Spring 2013 General Meeting of the Irish Bishops' Conference, 6 March

2013" <http://www.catholicbishops.ie/2013/03/06/spring-2013-general-meeting-irish-bishops-conference/> accessed 14 December 2013.

— "Preliminary response by the Catholic Bishops of Ireland to Protection of Life during Pregnancy Bill 2013", 3 May 2013 <http://www.catholicbishops.ie/2013/05/03/preliminary-response-catholic-bishops-ireland-protection-life-pregnancy-bill-2013/> accessed 19 January 2013.

— "Bishop John Buckley's Homily for Mass celebrating the fiftieth anniversary of the Church of the Holy Family, Caheragh, West Cork", 30 June 2013 <http://www.catholicbishops.ie/2013/06/30/bishop-john-buckleys-homily-mass-celebrating-fiftieth-anniversary-church-holy-family-caheragh-west-cork/> accessed 14 December 2013.

— "Cardinal Seán Brady raises legal and Constitutional concerns about the Protection of Life During Pregnancy Bill 2013", 1 July 2013 <http://www.catholicbishops.ie/2013/07/01/cardinal-sean-brady-raises-legal-constitutional-concerns-protection-life-pregnancy-bill-2013/> accessed 14 December 2013.

— "Homily of Archbishop Diarmuid Martin at Mass in Church of Saint Dominick, Dublin, 6 July 2013", <http://www.catholicbishops.ie/2013/07/06/homily-archbishop-diarmuid-martin-mass-church-saint-dominick-dublin/> accessed 14 December 2013.

— "Homily of His Excellency Archbishop Charles J Brown – Apostolic Nuncio in Ireland at Mass for Saint Oliver Plunkett", 7 July 2013 <http://www.catholicbishops.ie/2013/07/07/homily-excellency-archbishop-charles-brown-apostolic-nuncio-ireland-mass-saint-oliver-plunkett/> accessed 14 December 2013.

— "Homily of Bishop Noel Treanor at Saul Mountain, Downpatrick, Diocese of Down and Connor", 7 July 2013 <http://www.catholicbishops.ie/2013/07/07/homily-bishop-noel-treanor-saul-mountain-downpatrick-diocese-connor/> accessed 14 December 2013.

— "Bishops' briefing note on the Protection of Life During Pregnancy Bill 2013", 8 July 2013 <http://www.catholicbishops.ie/2013/07/08/bishops-briefing-note-protection-life-pregnancy-bill-2013/> accessed 14 December 2013).

— "Homily notes of Bishop Brendan Leahy for Vigil for Life – Saint John's Cathedral, Limerick", 9 July 2013 <http://www.catholicbishops.ie/2013/07/09/homily-notes-bishop-brendan-leahy-vigil-life-saint-johns-cathedral-limerick/> accessed 14 December 2013.

Catholic Communications Office press releases:

"Catholic Bishops' Winter Meeting", 10 December 2003 <http://www.catholiccommunications.ie/Pressrel/10-december-2003.html (accessed 12 October 2004).

"Comments of Archbishop Diarmuid Martin on the Report of the Commission on Assisted Human Reproduction", 12 May 2005 <http://www.catholiccommunications.ie/Pressrel/12-may-2005.html> accessed 20 May 2005.

"Irish Bishops' Conference, June General Meeting 2005", 16 June 2005 <http://www.catholiccommunications.ie/Pressrel/16-june-2005.html> accessed 28 June 2005.

"Bishops express concern in advance of EU Parliament vote on funding of research on human embryos", 14 June 2006 <http://www.catholiccommunications.ie/Pressrel/14-june-2006.html> accessed 15 June 2006.

"Statement of Archbishop Diarmuid Martin", 15 November 2006 <http://www.catholiccommunications.ie/Pressrel/15-november-2006.html> accessed 21 November 2006.

"Homily of Bishop Brennan, Ferns Diocese at Knock Shrine, Sunday 7 July 2013", 8 July 2013 <http://www.catholicbishops.ie/2013/07/08/homily-bishop-brennan-ferns-diocese-knock-shrine-sunday-7-july-2013/> accessed 14 December 2013.

Catholic Communications Office "Choose Life" newsletters:

Issue 1, 22 May 2013 <http://www.catholicbishops.ie/2013/05/22/choose-life-2013-newsletter-parishes/> accessed 26 January 2014.

Issue 2, 29 May 2013 <http://www.catholicbishops.ie/2013/05/29/choose-life-2013-newsletter-issue-2/> accessed 26 January 2014.

Issue 3, 6 June 2013 <http://www.catholicbishops.ie/2013/06/06/choose-life-2013-newsletter-issue-3/> accessed 26 January 2013.

Issue 4, 12 June 2013 <http://www.catholicbishops.ie/2013/06/12/choose-life-newsletter-issue-4/> accessed 26 January 2014.

Issue 5, 20 June 2013 <http://www.catholicbishops.ie/2013/06/20/issue-5-choose-life-2013-newsletter/> accessed 26 January 2014.

Issue 6, "A time for clarity and truth", 26 June 2013 <http://www.catholicbishops.ie/2013/06/26/choose-life-newsletter-issue-6-time-clarity-truth/> accessed 26 January 2014.

Issue 7, 3 July 2013 <http://www.catholicbishops.ie/2013/07/03/choose-life-newsletter-issue-7/> accessed 26 January 2014.

Issue 8, 11 July 2013 <http://www.catholicbishops.ie/2013/07/11/issue-8-choose-life-newsletter/> accessed 15 December 2013.

Catholic Press and Information Office (Dublin), *The Catholic Church and Abortion* (Dublin: Veritas, 1994).

Commission of the Bishops' Conferences of the European Community, "Risk of Promoting the Destruction of Human Embryos", 26 July 2006 <http://www.zenit.org/english/visualizza.phtml?sid=93173> accessed 6 March 2007.

Congregation for the Doctrine of the Faith, *Instruction on Respect for Human Life in Its Origin and on the Dignity of Procreation [Donum Vitae]* (Dublin: Veritas, 22 February 1987).

— *Instruction Dignitas Personae: On Certain Bioethical Questions*, 8 September 2008 <http://www.vatican.va/roman_curia/congregations/cfaith/documents/rc_con_cfaith_doc_20081208_dignitas-personae_en.html> accessed 24 December 2011.

Connell, Desmond, "Child resents a parentage based on power", *Irish Times*, 8 March 1999 <http://www.irishtimes.com/news/child-resents-a-parentage-based-on-power-1.160394> accessed 9 April 2016.

— "EU Funding for Embryonic Stem-Cell Research: Statement by Cardinal Desmond Connell: Sunday, 23rd November 2003 – immediate", internet document released by the Communications Office, Archdiocese of Dublin <www.dublindiocese.ie>.

Daly, Cahal B. Cardinal, Introduction to *The Bishops and the Law on Public Morality*, July 2005 <http://www.armagharchdiocese.org/2008/05/01/july-the-bishops-and-the-law-on-public-morality/> accessed 2 November 2014.

Daly, Gabriel, "Catholic Ethos and Other Mysteries", Association of Catholic Priests' website, 7 May 2017 <https://www.associationofcatholicpriests.ie/2017/05/catholic-ethos-and-other-mysteries/> accessed 27 February 2018.

Donders, Joseph G. (ed.), *John Paul II: The Encyclicals in Everyday Language* (Maryknoll, NY: Orbis, 1996).

Duffy, Joseph, "The Diocese of Clogher; News: 24 November 2003" <http://www.clogherdiocese.ie/news/news-24november2003-homilystmacartans-stemcellresearch.html> accessed 12 October 2004.

Flannery, Austin (general ed.), *Vatican Council II: More Postconciliar Documents* (Collegeville, Minn.: Liturgical Press, 1982 (1st edn)).

— (general ed.), *Vatican Council II: The Conciliar and Post Conciliar Documents* (Dublin: Dominican Publications, 1992 (revised edn)).

Francis I, Pope, *Amoris Laetitia* <http://www.catholicbishops.ie/wp-content/uploads/2016/04/Amoris-Laetitia.pdf> accessed 9 April 2016.

Haas, John M., "Begotten Not Made: A Catholic View of Reproductive Technology", 1998, United States Conference of Catholic Bishops website <http://www.usccb.org/about/pro-life-activities/respect-life-program/haas-rlp98-begotten-not-made-catholic-view-of-reproductive-technology.cfm> accessed 2 January 2018.

Institute of Obstetricians and Gynaecologists (Ireland), "Statement from the Institute of Obstetricians and Gynaecologists", 10 January 2018 <https://www.rcpi.ie/news/releases/statement-from-the-institute-of-obstetricians-and-gynaecologists/> accessed 30 October 2018.

— "Statement from the Institute of Obstetricians and Gynaecologists", 29 January 2018 <https://www.rcpi.ie/news/releases/statement-from-the-institute-of-obstetricians-and-gynaecologists-2/> accessed 29 January 2018.

— "Repeal of the Eighth Amendment: Information for the public" <https://www.rcpi.ie/faculties/obstetricians-and-gynaecologists/repeal-the-eighth-amendment-info-for-the-public/> accessed 4 April 2018.

Iona Institute, presentation about Article 40.3.3 to the Citizens' Assembly, 5 March 2017 <https://www.citizensassembly.ie/en/Meetings/The-Iona-Institute-s-Paper.pdf> accessed 9 March 2017.

Irish Bishops' Conference, "Publication of Catholic Bishops' Submission to Government Commission on Assisted Human Reproduction", Catholic Communications Office press release, 12 February 2003 <http://www.catholiccommunications.ie/Pressrel/12-february-2003.html> accessed 1 November 2004.

— "News, 13 November 2003: Catholic Bishops' Letter to Taoiseach on Embryonic Stem Cell Research Made Public", Catholic Communications Office <http://www.catholiccommunications.ie/News/news-13november2003-lettertotaoiseach.html> accessed 12 October 2004.

— "Notification on Recent Developments in Moral Theology and Their Implications for the Church and Society", July 2004 <http://www.catholiccommunications.ie/> accessed 25 February 2007.

— "The Sacredness of Human Life", issued after meetings of 9–11 March 1992; *Doctrine and Life*, vol. 42 (May–June 1992), pp. 345–6.

— *Towards a Creative Response to Infertility: A Detailed Response of the Irish Catholic Bishops' Conference to the Report of the Commission on Assisted Human Reproduction* (Dublin: Veritas, 2006).

Irish Catholic Bishops' Conference, *The Cry of the Earth: A Pastoral Reflection on Climate Change by the Irish Catholic Bishops' Conference* (2009).

— "The importance of speaking in the public square – Address by Archbishop Eamon Martin", 25 March 2017 <http://www.catholicbishops.ie/2017/03/25/the-importance-of-speaking-in-the-public-square-address-by-archbishop-eamon-martin/> accessed 29 March 2017.

— *The Meaning of Marriage*, n.d. <http://www.accord.ie/images/uploads/docs/The_Meaning_of_Marriage.pdf> accessed 17 October 2015.

— "Our Common Humanity", 6 March 2018 <https://www.catholicbishops.ie/2018/03/06/our-common-humanity-statement-on-the-second-day-of-the-spring-2018-general-meeting-of-the-irish-catholic-bishops-conference/> accessed 28 May 2018.

— Presentation to the Citizens' Assembly, 5 March 2017 <https://www.citizensassembly.ie/en/Meetings/ICBC-s-Paper.pdf> accessed 9 March 2017.

— "Statement on behalf of Archbishop Dermot Clifford concerning the decision of the UCC Board of Governors regarding facilitating research on embryonic stem cells", press release, 28 October 2008.

— "Statement by Bishop Alphonsus Cullinan on HPV vaccines", 2 October 2017 <http://www.catholicbishops.ie/2017/10/02/statement-by-bishop-alphonsus-cullinan-on-hpv-vaccines/> accessed 7 October 2017.

Irish Episcopal Conference, "Submission to the Government Commission on Assisted Human Reproduction by the Irish Episcopal Conference – December 2001", Catholic Communications Office <http://www.catholiccommunications.ie/Pressrel/ahrsubmission.html> accessed 12 October 2004; and *Doctrine and Life*, vol. 53, no. 3 (March 2003), pp. 181–7.

John Paul II, Pope, *Evangelium Vitae: The Value and Inviolability of Human Life* (London: Catholic Truth Society, 1995).

Klaus, Hanna, "Evaluation and Treatment of Infertility" (Washington, DC: National Conference of Catholic Bishops, 1999) <http://www.njnfp.org/documents/FOCUS-Infertility.pdf> accessed 3 January 2017.

Leshner, Alan I, AAAS Response to the "National Institutes of Health (NIH) Guidelines for Human Stem Cell Research, published in the *Federal Register* on April 23", 20 May 2009 (accessed from the AAAS website, 20 February 2010).

Leshner, Alan I. and James A. Thomson, "Standing in the Way of Stem Cell Research", *Washington Post*, 3 December 2007; sourced from American Association for the Advancement of Science (AAAS) website, 18 February 2010.

Martin, Diarmuid, "The Defence of Human Life", 23 May 2018, Archdiocese of Dublin <http://www.dublindiocese.ie/choose-life-2018/> accessed 28 May 2018.

— "Homily of Archbishop Diarmuid Martin at Mass in Church of Saint Dominick, Dublin, 6 July 2013" <http://www.catholicbishops.ie/2013/07/06/homily-archbishop-diarmuid-martin-mass-church-saint-dominick-dublin/> accessed 14 December 2013.

— Homily notes, "Ordination of Dominican Deacons", at St Saviour's Priory, Dominick Street, 15 March 2015 <http://dublindiocese.ie/2015/03/15/ordination-of-dominican-deacons/> accessed 17 March 2015.

Martin, Eamon, "Pastoral Message for the new year 2018 from Archbishop Eamon Martin: 'To Serve Human Life is to Serve God' (Pope Francis)", Irish Catholic Bishops' Conference <https://www.catholicbishops.ie/2018/01/06/pastoral-message-for-the-new-year-2018-from-archbishop-eamon-martin-to-serve-human-life-is-to-serve-god-pope-francis/> accessed 8 January 2018.

Maternal Death Enquiry Ireland, *Data Brief No. 1* (December 2015) <https://www.ucc.ie/en/media/research/maternaldeathenquiryireland/MDEIrelandDataBriefNo1December2015.pdf> accessed 4 November 2017.

— *Data Brief No. 2* (December 2016) <https://www.ucc.ie/en/media/research/maternaldeathenquiryireland/MDEIrelandDatabriefNo2December2016.pdf> accessed 4 November 2017.

National Centre for Pharmacoeconomics (Ireland), "Cost-effectiveness of Lumacaftor/Ivacaftor (Orkambi) for cystic fibrosis in patients aged 12 years and older who are homozygous for the F508del mutation in the CFTR gene", http://www.ncpe.ie/wp-content/uploads/2015/12/Website-summary-orkambi.pdf, June 2016> accessed 8 August 2016.

O'Hare, M.F., E. Manning, P. Corcoran and R.A. Greene, *Confidential Maternal Death Enquiry in Ireland: Report for 2013–2015* (Cork: December 2017) <https://www.ucc.ie/en/media/research/maternaldeathenquiryireland/ Confidential-Maternal-Death-Enquiry-Report-2013---2015--Web.pdf> accessed 29 October 2018.

Pius XI, Pope, *Casti Connubii* (31 December 1930), commentary by Fr. Vincent McNabb (London: Sheed & Ward, 1933).

Pius XII, Pope, "The Holy Father Condemns Artificial Insemination", translation of an address to the fourth International Convention of Catholic Doctors, 29 September 1949, *Linacre Quarterly*, vol. 16, no. 4 (October 1949), pp. 1–6 <https://epublications.marquette.edu/cgi/viewcontent.cgi?referer=https:// www.google.ie/&httpsredir=1&article=1162&context=lnq> accessed 2 April 2018.

Progressive Democrats, "Tanaiste welcomes publication of Commissions' Report" <http://www.progressivedemocrats.ie/press_room/1403/> accessed 20 May 2005.

Psychological Society of Ireland, "5 Facts on The Eighth Amendment and Mental Health" <https://www.psychologicalsociety.ie/> accessed 12 May 2018.

— "Psychological Society of Ireland releases fact-based position on abortion and mental health, and supports repeal of the Eighth Amendment" <https://www. psychologicalsociety.ie/> accessed 12 May 2018.

Religious Sisters of Charity, "Statement by Sr Mary Christian, Congregational Leader of the Religious Sisters of Charity", 31 May 2017 <https://www. associationofcatholicpriests.ie/2017/05/the-new-national-maternity-hospital-and-the-religious-sisters-of-charity/> accessed 19 February 2018; and <https://static.rasset.ie/documents/news/statement-by-sr-mary-christian. pdf> accessed 24 February 2018.

Save the 8th, "Statement from Psychiatrists", press conference, 16 May 2018 <https://www.save8.ie/statement-from-psychiatrists/> accessed 30 October 2018.University College Cork, "Governing Body Meeting", *UCC News*, October 2008, p. 21.

— "UCC Statement following Governing Body Meeting of 28/10/2008 at which consideration was given to embryonic stem cell research recommendations" <http://www.ucc.ie/en/mandc/news/fullstory,63377,en.html> accessed 28 October 2008.

Secondary Sources

Abbott, Alison, "Italians Sue over Stem Cells", *Nature*, vol. 460, issue no. 7251 (2 July 2009), p. 19.

— "Faster Route to Stem-like Cells", *Nature*, vol. 10 (November 2009) <http://www.nature.com.library.ucc.ie/news/2009/091108/full/news.2009.1070.html> accessed 16 February 2010.

— "Irish Election Raises Questions for Stem Cell Research", *Nature* (28 February 2011) <http://blogs.nature.com/news/2011/02/irish_election_raises_question.html> accessed 20 November 2011.

Agnew, Paddy, "Vatican stands by Cardinal's remarks on referendum", *Irish Times*, 27 May 2015 <http://www.irishtimes.com/news/social-affairs/religion-and-beliefs/vatican-stands-by-cardinal-s-remarks-on-referendum-1.2227805?mode=print&ot=example.AjaxPageLayout.ot> accessed 28 May 2015.

Ahlstrom, Dick, "Gene therapy and stem-cell advances", *Irish Times*, 24 February 2005, p. 15.

— "Over 50% favour embryo research, says poll", *Irish Times*, 17 November 2005.

— "Can stem cells change the world?" *Irish Times*, 30 April 2009.

— "'Retrograde' closure of bioethics body criticised", *Irish Times*, 17 December 2009 <http://www.irishtimes.com/newspaper/ireland/2009/1217/1224260838471_pf.html> accessed 11 January 2010.

Ainsworth, Claire, *et al.* "Human Cloning: If not today, tomorrow", *New Scientist*, vol. 177, no. 2377 (11 January 2003), pp. 8–11.

Allison, Jill, *Motherhood and Infertility in Ireland: Understanding the Presence of Absence* (Cork: Cork University Press, 2013).

— "Enduring Politics: The culture of obstacles in legislating for assisted reproduction technologies in Ireland", *Reproductive Biomedicine and Society Online*, vol. 3 (December 2016), pp. 134–41 <https://www.sciencedirect.com/science/article/pii/S2405661816300399> accessed 18 February 2019.

Asma, Stephen T., "Abortion and the Embarrassing Saint", *The Humanist*, vol. 54, no. 3 (May–June 1994), pp. 30–3.

Bardon, Sarah, "Mullen calls on Kenny to debate in same-sex marriage campaign", *Irish Times*, 28 April 2015 <http://www.irishtimes.com/news/politics/mullen-calls-on-kenny-to-debate-in-same-sex-marriage-campaign-1.2191262?mode=print&ot=example.AjaxPageLayout.ot> accessed 28 April 2015.

— "No surrogacy legislation before election, says Kenny", *Irish Times*, 20 May 2015 <http://www.irishtimes.com/news/politics/oireachtas/no-surrogacy-legislation-before-election-says-kenny-1.2219658?mode=print&ot=example.AjaxPageLayout.ot> accessed 20 May 2015.

— "Varadkar say he will not lobby FG colleagues on abortion law", *Irish Times*, 17 December 2015 <http://www.irishtimes.com/news/politics/varadkar-says-he-will-not-lobby-fg-colleagues-on-abortion-law-1.2469855?mode=print&ot=example.AjaxPageLayout.ot> accessed 19 December 2015.

— "Eighth Amendment Committee comes under tough scrutiny", *Irish*

Times, 20 October 2017 <https://search-proquest-com.ucc.idm.oclc.org/docview/1952920900/8B6789A6B32D480BPQ/36?accountid=14504> accessed 21 October 2017.

— "Focusing on Down syndrome misguided, says Boylan", *Irish Times*, 29 January 2018 <https://search-proquest-com.ucc.idm.oclc.org/docview/1991848056/F8BF870E10D24106PQ/10?accountid=14504> accessed 29 January 2018.

Barry, Ann, *et al.*, letter to the editor, *Irish Times*, 29 May 2013 <https://search-proquest-com.ucc.idm.oclc.org/docview/1355766846/AAEAA021B9644D10PQ/118?accountid=14504> accessed 24 February 2018.

Barry, Aoife, "FactCheck: Are 90% of babies with Down syndrome in Britain aborted?", TheJournal.ie, 4 February 2018 <http://www.thejournal.ie/factcheck-babies-abortion-3823611-Feb2018/> accessed 6 October 2018.

Beesley, Arthur, "At odds on the stem-cell research issue", *Irish Times*, 24 December 2003, p. 6.

— "Taoiseach disputed cardinal's stance on stem cells", *Irish Times*, 24 December 2003, p. 1.

Bonnar, John, *et al.*, letter to the editor, *Irish Times*, 11 May 2018 <https://search-proquest-com.ucc.idm.oclc.org/docview/2036892729/96F336D60BE14F28PQ/110?accountid=14504> accessed 11 May 2018.

Bottone, Angelo, "'Mother', 'father' to be replaced by 'parent 1', 'parent 2'", 12 September 2018, Iona Institute <https://ionainstitute.ie/mother-and-father-to-be-replaced-by-parent-1-and-parent-2/> accessed 23 January 2019.

Boylan, Peter, letter to the editor, *Irish Times*, 2 May 2013 <https://search-proquest-com.ucc.idm.oclc.org/docview/1347389624/802830BBB37144DCPQ/140?accountid=14504> accessed 18 November 2019.

— "Big problems remain over NMH structure", *Irish Times*, 3 June 2017 <http://www.irishtimes.com/opinion/peter-boylan-big-problems-remain-over-new-nmh-structure-1.3105640> accessed 3 June 2017.

— YouTube interview, accessed through "Q&A: The Answers to your Questions about the Eighth Amendment", TheJournal.ie, 16 May 2018 <http://www.thejournal.ie/eighth-amendment-ref-q-a-3999597-May2018/> accessed 10 October 2018.

— *In the Shadow of the Eighth* (Penguin Ireland, 2019).

Burgess, John, "Could a Zygote be a Human Being?", *Bioethics*, vol. 24, issue 2 (February 2010), pp. 61–70.

Byrne, Luke, "Priests told: deny communion to TDs who support abortion", *Irish Independent*, 6 February 2013 <http://www.independent.ie/irish-news/priests-told-deny-communion-to-tds-who-support-abortion-29051662.html> accessed 24 December 2015.

Cahill, Lisa Sowle, "The Embryo and the Fetus: New moral contexts", *Theological*

Studies, vol. 54, no. 1 (March 1993), pp. 124–42.

— "Stem Cells: A bioethical balancing act", *America*, vol. 184, no. 10 (26 March 2001).

Camosy, Charles, "Concern for Our Vulnerable Prenatal and Neonatal Children: A brief reply to Giubilini and Minerva", *Journal of Medical Ethics*, vol. 39, no. 5 (May 2013), pp. 296–8.

Campbell, Louise, "Current Debates about Legislating for Assisted Dying: Ethical concerns", *Medico-Legal Journal of Ireland*, vol. 24, no.1 (2018), pp. 20–7 <https://login-westlaw-ie.ucc.idm.oclc.org/maf/wlie/app/document? src=toce&docguid=ID47A32FC7D524948A7F3527560CE1085&crumb-action=append&context=13> accessed 2 December 2018.

Carey, Sarah, "Maternity hospital row should be over money – not the politics of fertility", *Sunday Independent*, 23 April 2017, p. 29.

Carolan, Mary, "Embryo case 'to raise question' of when life begins", *Irish Times*, 4 July 2006, p. 4.

— "Man wants no more children with his wife", *Irish Times*, 6 July 2006, p. 4.

— "Woman expects husband to maintain any children", *Irish Times*, 6 July 2006, p. 4.

— "Counsel rejects AG's 'dramatic' position in embryos case", *Irish Times*, 7 July 2006, p. 4.

— "Ruling expected soon on frozen embryos consent", *Irish Times*, 7 July 2006, p. 4.

— "Science dictates that embryo is human being, expert tells court", *Irish Times*, 26 July 2006, p. 4.

— "Embryo is beginning of life, says doctor", *Irish Times*, 22 July 2006, p. 4.

— "Expert says inaction by lawmakers unforgivable", *Irish Times*, 22 July 2006, p. 4.

— "Fertility treatment code 'unworkable'", *Irish Times*, 28 July 2006, p. 4.

— "IVF embryos can be adopted, expert tells court", *Irish Times*, 28 July 2006, p. 4.

— "Existence of embryos outside womb 'precarious'", *Irish Times*, 16 November 2006, p. 4.

— "Woman loses bid to have embryos implanted", *Irish Times*, 16 November 2006, p. 4.

— "Gay sperm donor given access to his son", *Irish Times*, 11 December 2009 <http://www.irishtimes.com/newspaper/ireland/2009/1211/1224260512642_pf.html> accessed 3 February 2010.

— "'Disturbing' failure to enact laws on fertility treatment criticised", *Irish Times*, 16 December 2009, p. 4.

— "Embryos are not the 'unborn,' court rules", *Irish Times*, 16 December 2009, p. 4.

— "Irish father wins surrogacy case over child born in India", *Irish Times*, 6 March 2013, p. 2.

— "Agencies urge broad definition of motherhood in Supreme Court surrogacy case", *Irish Times*, 6 February 2014 <http://www.irishtimes.com/news/crime-and-law/courts/agencies-urge-broad-definition-of-motherhood-in-supreme-court-surrogacy-case-1.1681015> accessed 7 February 2014.

— "Judgment reserved in surrogacy case", *Irish Times*, 7 February 2014, p. 6.

Carr, Alan, *et al.*, letters to the editor, *Irish Times*, 21 May 2015 <http://www.irishtimes.com/opinion/letters/marriage-referendum-countdown-to-polling-day-1.2220003?mode=print&ot=example.AjaxPageLayout.ot> accessed 25 May 2015.

Carroll, Áine, "Anti-abortion campaigners dodging the issue: what to do with unwanted pregnancies if Eighth is repealed", *Irish Times*, 18 April 2018 <https://search-proquest-com.ucc.idm.oclc.org/docview/2026045109/806D78EAAF3849D5PQ/85?accountid=14504> accessed 20 April 2018.

Carroll, Rory, "Northern Ireland to legalise abortion and same-sex marriage", *Guardian*, 22 October 2019 <https://www.theguardian.com/uk-news/2019/oct/21/northern-ireland-set-to-legalise-abortion-and-same-sex-marriage> accessed 22 October 2019.

Catholic Herald and Standard, "CAHR recommendations 'extreme and unethical' – PLC", 20 May 2005, no. 6200, p. 6.

— "Stem-cell research could get green light", 16 June 2006, p. 6.

— "Minister backs embryo research in Ireland", 30 June 2006, p. 6.

CBS News, "Husband: Ireland hospital denied Savita Halappanavar life saving abortion because it is a 'Catholic country,'" 14 November 2012 <http://www.cbsnews.com/news/husband-ireland-hospital-denied-savita-halappanavar-life-saving-abortion-because-it-is-a-catholic-country/> accessed 26 January 2014.

Cherry, Mark J., "Pope Francis, Weak Theology, and the Subtle Transformation of Roman Catholic Bioethics", *Christian Bioethics*, vol. 21, no. 1 (2015), pp. 84–8.

Childress, James F., "Reproductive Interventions: Theology, Ethics, and Public Policy" in Charles E. Curran (ed.), *Moral Theology: Challenges for the Future, Essays in Honour of Richard A. McCormick* (New York: Paulist Press, 1990), pp. 285–309.

Clarke, Desmond, *Church and State: Essays in Political Philosophy* (Cork: Cork University Press, 1985).

Clarke, Vivienne, "National Maternity Hospital 'will be completely independent' – Mahony", *Irish Times*, 20 April 2017 <http://www.irishtimes.com/news/health/national-maternity-hospital-will-be-completely-independent-mahony-1.3055036> accessed 4 May 2017.

Clynes, Martin, "Human Embryonic Stem Cells and Cloning: Science and bioethics at a crossroads", *Studies*, vol. 93, no. 371 (Autumn 2004), pp. 261–7.

Coady, C.A.J., "The Common Premise for Uncommon Conclusions", *Journal of Medical Ethics*, vol. 39, no. 5 (May 2013), pp. 284–8.

Cohen, Philip, and David Concar, "The Awful Truth", *New Scientist*, no. 2291 (19 May 2001); pp. 14-15, www.newscientist.com> accessed 29 December 2006.

Collins, Stephen, "Political realities shape party positions on abortion Bill", *Irish Times*, 10 February 2015 <http://www.irishtimes.com/news/politics/political-realities-shape-party-positions-on-abortion-bill-1.2098740> accessed 12 February 2015.

— "Bill will recognise and protect diverse family units", *Irish Times*, 18 February 2015, p. 14.

— "Family law legislation hailed as 'major step'", *Irish Times*, 18 February 2015, p. 1.

— "Majority for repeal of Eighth Amendment, poll shows", *Irish Times*, 23 February 2016 <http://www.irishtimes.com/news/politics/majority-for-repeal-of-eighth-amendment-poll-shows-1.2544564> accessed 23 February 2016.

Conneely, Ailbhe, "Harris seeks availability of second doctor in abortion cases", RTÉ News, 29 November 2018 <https://www.rte.ie/news/politics/2018/1128/1013989-abortion-dail/> accessed 1 January 2019.

Conrad, Kathryn, "Fetal Ireland: National bodies and political agency", Éire-Ireland, vol. 36, no. 3–4 (Fall/Winter 2001), pp. 153–73.

Cope, Heidi, Melanie E. Garrett, Simon G. Gregory and Allison E. Ashley-Koch, "Pregnancy Continuation and Organizational Religious Activity Following Prenatal Diagnosis of a Lethal Fetal Defect is Associated with Improved Psychological Outcome", *Prenatal Diagnosis*, vol. 35, no. 8 (April 2015) <https://www.researchgate.net/publication/274967787_Pregnancy_continuation_and_organizational_religious_activity_following_prenatal_diagnosis_of_a_lethal_fetal_defect_is_associated_with_improved_psychological_outcome_Psychological_outcome_following_pre> accessed 12 June 2016.

Corcoran, Jody, "Abortion landslide down to reluctant, not silent, Yes", *Sunday Independent*, 3 June 2018, p. 3.

Corcoran, Jody, and Daniel McConnell, "A New Beginning: Historic Yes for gay marriage after surge in youth vote", *Sunday Independent*, 24 May 2015, pp. 1, 5.

Corkery, Pádraig, "The Use of Embryonic Stem Cells – Recent Developments", *The Furrow*, vol. 53, no. 1 (January 2002), pp. 24–34.

— "Ferment in Bioethics – How Can the Christian Tradition Help?" *The Furrow*, vol. 53, no. 3 (March 2002), pp. 131–9.

— *Bioethics and the Catholic Moral Tradition* (Dublin: Veritas, 2010).

Cosgrave, William, "Recent Moral Thinking on Human Genetic Engineering", *Doctrine and Life* 34, no. 8 (October 1984), pp. 441–9.

Coulter, Carol, "'Catholic archbishop outlines changes in relationships from family planning: Contraceptive culture' has led to unhappy, resentful children", *Irish Times*, 3 March 1999, p. 6.

— "State now faces EU deadline on fertility regulations", *Irish Times*, 13 May 2005.

— "Parties in frozen embryos row to hear how case will proceed", *Irish Times*, 4 July 2006, p. 1.

— "Foetus may not always be an unborn, argues State", *Irish Times*, 14 July 2006, p. 1.

— "Widening the grounds for abortion", *Irish Times*, 14 July 2006, pp. 16.

— "Case shows IVF consent forms must be clearer and broader", *Irish Times*, 19 July 2006, p. 4.

— "Court again calls for law on assisted human reproduction", *Irish Times*, 16 December 2009, p. 15.

— "Why surrogacy has nothing to do with same-sex marriage", *Irish Times*, 27 April 2015 <http://www.irishtimes.com/opinion/why-surrogacy-has-nothing-to-do-with-same-sex-marriage-1.2189717?mode=print&ot=example.AjaxPageLayout.ot> accessed 28 April 2015.

Coulter, Carol, and Alison Healy, "New court hearing in embryos case opens tomorrow", *Irish Times*, 19 July 2006, p. 1.

Coveney, Simon, "Here's how my thinking shifted on the Eighth Amendment", Independent.ie, 26 March 2018 <https://www.independent.ie/irish-news/simon-coveney-heres-how-my-thinking-shifted-on-the-eighth-amendment-36743798.html> accessed 18 December 2018.

Cullen, Paul, "Fertility treatment law likely to face delay", *Irish Times*, 16 November 2006.

— "Frozen embryos and the Constitution: what was at stake in this case", *Irish Times*, 16 November 2006.

— "Mixed reactions but most agree legislation is needed", *Irish Times*, 16 November 2006.

— "Obstetricians challenge Boylan evidence", *Irish Times*, 1 May 2013 <https://search-proquest-com.ucc.idm.oclc.org/docview/1346974341/A946912076344457PQ/58?accountid=14504> accessed 11 November 2017.

— "Analysis: Leo Varadkar's low-key report on abortion", *Irish Times*, 30 June 2015 <http://www.irishtimes.com/news/health/analysis-leo-varadkar-s-low-key-report-on-abortion-1.2267303?mode=print&ot=example.AjaxPageLayout.ot> accessed 1 July 2015.

— "Abortion legislation should be repealed, says professor", *Irish Times*, 4 January 2016 <http://www.irishtimes.com/news/health/abortion-legislation-should-be-repealed-says-professor-1.2483463> accessed 4 January 2016.

— "Catholic ethos 'a red herring' for maternity hospital, says doctor", *Irish Times*, 10 May 2016 <http://www.irishtimes.com/news/health/catholic-ethos-a-red-herring-for-maternity-hospital-says-doctor-1.2641390> accessed 31 May 2017.

— "Latest criticism ratchets up international pressure for change", *Irish Times*, 10 June 2016, p. 3.

— "Symphysiotomy: the whitewash that never was", *Irish Times*, 23 November 2016 <https://www.irishtimes.com/opinion/symphysiotomy-the-whitewash-that-never-was-1.2878271> accessed 8 February 2018.

— "Nuns should hand over maternity hospital site – Coombe ex-master", *Irish Times*, 26 April 2017 <http://www.irishtimes.com/news/health/nuns-should-hand-over-maternity-hospital-site-coombe-ex-master-1.3061247> accessed 28 April 2017.

— "National Maternity Hospital relocation planner resigns", *Irish Times*, 28 April 2017 <http://www.irishtimes.com/news/health/national-maternity-hospital-relocation-planner-resigns-1.3064217> accessed 28 April 2017.

— "Peter Boylan: 'I've been vilified by a lot of people'", *Irish Times*, 28 April 2017 <http://www.irishtimes.com/news/health/peter-boylan-i-ve-been-vilified-by-a-lot-of-people-1.3064091> accessed 28 April 2017.

— "Decision marks a huge victory for people power", *Irish Times*, 30 May 2017.

— "St Vincent's hospitals to drop Catholic guidelines", *Irish Times*, 30 May 2017.

— "St Vincent's must retain ownership of new maternity hospital, says chairman", *Irish Times*, 30 May 2017.

— "She left Ireland feeling like 'a criminal leaving her country'", *Irish Times*, 14 June 2017, p. 5.

— "Irish abortion law violated woman's human rights, says UN", *Irish Times*, 14 June 2017, p. 5.

— "Catholic bishop claims cervical cancer vaccine 'only 70% safe'", *Irish Times*, 27 September 2017 <https://www.irishtimes.com/news/health/catholic-bishop-claims-cervical-cancer-vaccine-only-70-safe-1.3235705> accessed 30 September 2017.

Cullen, Paul, and Ruadhán Mac Cormaic, "Woman on life support: medics feared legal position", *Irish Times*, 22 December 2014 <http://www.irishtimes.com/news/social-affairs/woman-on-life-support-medics-feared-legal-position-1.2045891?mode=print&ot=example.AjaxPageLayout.ot> accessed 2 January 2015.

Cunningham, Patrick, "Absence of rules on stem-cell research misleading", *Irish Times*, 17 April 2009, p. 7.

— "Advances in stem-cell research may resolve ethical issues", *Irish Times*, 22 April 2009 <http://www.irishtimes.com/newspaper/opinion/2009/0422/1224245127531_pf.html> accessed 28 April 2009.

Curran, Tom, "Helping a person to die – why new compassionate laws are needed", *Irish Times*, 29 April 2015 <http://www.irishtimes.com/opinion/helping-a-person-to-die-why-new-compassionate-laws-are-needed-1.2192306?mode=print&ot=example.AjaxPageLayout.ot> accessed 29 April 2015.

Cyranoski, David, "Japan Relaxes Human Stem-cell Rules: But scientists fear it is too late to regain lost ground", *Nature*, vol. 460, issue no. 7259 (27 August 2009), p. 1068.

Daly, Greg, "Vatican urged to block hospital plan", *Irish Catholic*, 8 June 2017 <http://www.irishcatholic.ie/article/vatican-urged-block-hospital-plan> accessed 8 June 2017.

— "Top obstetricians condemn medical scaremongering around Eighth", *Irish Catholic*, 10 May 2018 <https://www.irishcatholic.com/top-obstetricians-condemn-medical-scaremongering-around-eighth/> accessed 1 November 2018.

— "Archbishop in the dark on nuns' maternity hospital plans", *Irish Catholic*, 6 December 2018 <https://www.irishcatholic.com/archbishop-in-the-dark-on-nuns-maternity-hospital-plans/> accessed 21 November 2019.

D'Arcy, Ciarán, "Abortion policy must be reviewed, groups say", *Irish Times*, 30 June 2015 <http://www.irishtimes.com/news/social-affairs/abortion-policy-must-be-reviewed-groups-say-1.2268295?mode=print&ot=example. AjaxPageLayout.ot> accessed 1 July 2015.

— "Opposing sides clash during abortion rallies in Dublin", *Irish Times*, 4 July 2015 <http://www.irishtimes.com/news/social-affairs/opposing-sides-clash-during-abortion-rallies-in-dublin-1.2273918?mode=print&ot=example. AjaxPageLayout.ot> accessed 10 July 2015.

— "Issue of assisted suicide 'coming down the tracks' for Ireland", *Irish Times*, 16 October 2015, report on Emily O'Reilly's address to the Conference on *Strengthening the Voice of Older People* (Dublin) <http://www.irishtimes.com/news/social-affairs/issue-of-assisted-suicide-coming-down-the-tracks-for-ireland-1.2394640?mode=print&ot=example.AjaxPageLayout.ot> accessed 17 October 2015.

— "Catholic Bishop clarifies weekend comments on National Maternity Hospital", *Irish Times*, 25 April 2017 <http://www.irishtimes.com/news/health/catholic-bishop-clarifies-weekend-comments-on-national-maternity-hospital-1.3060692> accessed 28 April 2017.

— "What is the situation with abortion in Ireland?" *Irish Times*, 17 December 2017 <https://search-proquest-com.ucc.idm.oclc.org/docview/1977074550/98232BC1419B4E49PQ/18?accountid=14504> accessed 17 December 2017.

de Londras, Fiona, "UN move confirms law on abortion is unsustainable", *Irish Times*, 10 June 2016, p. 16.

Delay, Cara, "Pills, Potions, and Purgatives: Women and abortion methods in Ireland, 1900–1950", *Women's History Review*, vol. 28, no. 3 (2019), pp. 479–99.

Dennis, A.R., "Ethical Dilemmas and the Modern Doctor", *Doctrine and Life*, vol. 30, no. 1 (January 1980), pp. 6–15.

Doctrine and Life, "Respect for Human Embryos and Artificial Human Procreation: Summary of the Recent Vatican Document", vol. 37, no. 4

(April 1987), pp. 205–12.

Doerflinger, R.M., "The Problem of Deception in Embryonic Stem Cell Research", *Cell Proliferation*, vol. 41, issue s1 (February 2008), pp. 65–70.

Donnellan, Eithne, "A clash of cultures", *Irish Times*, 8 October 2005 <https://www.irishtimes.com/news/a-clash-of-cultures-1.503193> accessed 14 February 2018.

Donnellan, Eithne, Patsy McGarry and Olivia Kelleher, "UCC governors to consider embryonic stem-cell research", *Irish Times*, 28 October 2008 <http://www.irishtimes.com/newspaper/frontpage/2008/1028/1225061111939_pf.html> accessed 30 October 2008.

Donnelly, Mary and Claire Murray (eds), *Ethical and Legal Debates in Irish Healthcare: Confronting complexities* (Manchester: Manchester University Press, 2016).

Dooley, Dolores, letter to the editor, *Irish Times*, 28 January 2010 <http://www.irishtimes.com/newspaper/letters/2010/0128/1224263288324_pf.html> accessed 28 January 2010.

Doran, Shane, "The world looks on as Irish voters make history", *Sunday Independent*, 24 May 2015, p. 5.

Doyle, Kevin, "Kenny gives ministers free vote on abortion campaign", *Irish Independent*, 9 January 2016 <http://www.msn.com/en-ie/news/national/kenny-gives-ministers-free-vote-on-abortion-campaign/ar-CCjcfS?ocid=spartandhp> accessed 9 January 2016.

Duffy, Rónán, "'God's Plan for Marriage' is being distributed to 1,300 parishes ahead of referendum", TheJournal.ie, 3 December 2014 <http://www.thejournal.ie/same-sex-marriage-bishops-1813682-Dec2014/> accessed 17 October 2015.

— "FactCheck: Is the Bishop of Waterford right to say the HPV vaccine is '70% safe'?", TheJournal.ie <http://www.thejournal.ie/hov-bishop-factcheck-3620053-Sep2017/> accessed 30 September 2017.

Dwyer, Killian, "Artificial Human Reproduction", *Doctrine and Life*, vol. 34, no. 10 (December 1984), pp. 587–90.

Economist, "The gift of life: surrogacy", vol. 423, no. 9040 (13 May 2017) <https://search-proquest-com.ucc.idm.oclc.org/docview/1898478309/12A62D38D6F1454APQ/6?accountid=14504> accessed 23 January 2019.

— "Help wanted; Surrogacy", vol. 423, no. 9040 (13 May 2017) <https://search-proquest-com.ucc.idm.oclc.org/docview/1898476635/12A62D38D6F1454APQ/47?accountid=14504> accessed 23 January 2019.

— "Don't mention the Church", vol. 426, no. 9084 (24 March 2018) <https://search-proquest-com.ucc.idm.oclc.org/docview/2017355779/9F9C8952DC8F4C11PQ/10?accountid=14504> accessed 20 April 2018.

Edmondson, Ricca, "Moral Debate and Social Change", *Doctrine and Life*, vol. 42 (May–June 1992), pp. 233–43.

Edwards, Elaine, "Doctors agree plan in event of repeal", *Irish Times*, 14 April 2018, p. 4.

— "Halappanavar inquiry chairman calls for repeal", *Irish Times*, 23 May, p. 7.

Ekman, Kajsa Ekis, "All surrogacy is exploitation – the world should follow Sweden's ban", *Guardian*, 26 February 2016 <https://www.theguardian.com/commentisfree/2016/feb/25/surrogacy-sweden-ban> accessed 6 March 2019.

Elgot, Jessica, and Henry McDonald, "Northern Irish women win access to free abortions as May averts rebellion", *Guardian*, 29 June 2017 <https://www.theguardian.com/world/2017/jun/29/rebel-tories-could-back-northern-ireland-abortion-amendment> accessed 30 June 2017.

Elkink, Johan A., David M. Farrell, Theresa Reidy and Jane Suiter, "Understanding the 2015 Marriage Referendum in Ireland: Context, campaign, and conservative Ireland", *Irish Political Studies*, vol. 32, issue 3 (2017), pp. 361–81.

Emerson, Newton, "The DUP flexes religious muscle while terminating moves towards liberalism", *Sunday Times*, 27 May 2018, p. 16.

Engelhardt, H. Tristram, Jr, "Confronting Moral Pluralism in Posttraditional Western Societies: Bioethics critically reassessed", *Journal of Medicine and Philosophy*, vol. 36, issue 3 (2011), 243–60. <https://academic.oup.com/jmp/article-abstract/36/3/243/894157> accessed 11 July 2011.

Enright, Mairead, *et al.*, letter to the editor, *Irish Times*, 9 April 2018 <https://search-proquest-com.ucc.idm.oclc.org/docview/2022902932/E7A4FE80CC2E4595PQ/89?accountid=14504> accessed 9 April 2018.

Erwin, Alan, "Legal action taken over guidelines on abortion in North", *Irish Times*, 12 November 2015 <http://www.irishtimes.com/news/crime-and-law/legal-action-taken-over-guidelines-on-abortion-in-north-1.2427242> accessed 2 December 2015.

Fagan, Seán, "Do We Still Need Natural Law?" *Doctrine and Life*, vol. 47, no. 7 (September 1997), pp. 407–16.

— "*Humanae Vitae* 30 Years on", *Doctrine and Life*, vol. 49, no. 1 (January 1999), pp. 51–4.

— *Does Morality Change?* (Dublin: Columba Press, 2003).Farrell, David M., Jane Suiter and Clodagh Harris, "'Systematizing' Constitutional Deliberation: The 2016–18 citizens' assembly in Ireland", *Irish Political Studies*, vol. 34, issue 1 (2019), pp. 113–23.

Fergusson, David M., John Horwood, and Joseph M. Boden, "Abortion and Mental Health Disorders: Evidence from a 30-year longitudinal study", *British Journal of Psychiatry*, vol. 193 (2008), pp. 444–51.

Fergusson, David M., John Horwood, and Elizabeth M. Ridder, "Abortion in Young Women and Subsequent Mental Health", *Journal of Child Psychology and Psychiatry*, vol. 47, no. 1 (2006), pp. 16–24.

Field, Luke, "The Abortion Referendum of 2018 and a Timeline of Abortion Politics in Ireland to Date", *Irish Political Studies*, vol. 33, issue 4 (2018), pp. 608–28.

Fitzgerald, Mary, "The EU gets Tough on Ethics", *Technology Ireland*, vol. 38, issue 1 (March–April 2007), pp. 27–30.

Fitzpatrick, Chris, "In the media everyone is pro-choice or pro-life. I am both", *Irish Times*, 16 September 2017 https://www.irishtimes.com/life-and-style/health-family/in-the-media-everyone-is-pro-choice-or-pro-life-i-am-both-1.3222318> accessed 23 September 2017.

— "Life doesn't fit on anti-abortion posters", *Irish Times*, 23 April 2018 <https://search-proquest-com.ucc.idm.oclc.org/docview/2028721464/FFAF0465A7F14380PQ/80?accountid=14504> accessed 23 April 2018.

Fletcher, Martin, "Focus of abortion reform now moves north of border", *Sunday Times*, 27 May 2018, p. 2.

Flew, Anthony (ed. consultant), *A Dictionary of Philosophy* (London: Pan Books, 1984).

Foster, Angel M., Amanda Dennis and Fiona Smith, "Do Religious Restrictions Influence Ectopic Pregnancy Management? A national qualitative study", *Women's Health Issues*, issues 21–22 (2011), pp. 104–9.

Fox, Maggie, "Scientists develop stem cell harvesting without harming embryo", *Irish Examiner*, 18 October 2005 <http://archives.tcm.ie/irishexaminer/2005/10/18/story142806485.asp> accessed 23 May 2006.

— "Discovery bypasses need for stem cells", *Irish Independent*, 28 January 2010 <http://www.independent.ie/world-news/discovery-bypasses-need-for-stem-cells-2035882.html> accessed 11 February 2010.

Francis, Leslie, and Anita Silvers, "Infanticide, Moral Status and Moral Reasons: The importance of context", *Journal of Medical Ethics*, vol. 39, no. 5 (May 2013), pp. 289–92.

Freedman, Lori R., and Debra B. Stulberg, "The Research Consortium on Religious Healthcare Institutions: Studying the impact of religious restrictions on women's reproductive health", *Contraception*, vol. 94 (2016), pp. 6–10.

Fullam, Lisa, and William R. O'Neill, "Bioethics and Public Policy", *Theological Studies*, vol. 71 (March 2010), pp. 168–89.

Fuller, Louise, *Irish Catholicism Since 1950: The Undoing of a Culture* (Dublin: Gill and Macmillan, 2002).

Galway for Life, "Scientists' Advance Further Renders Embryonic Stem Cell Research Obsolete", 10 February 2010 <http://galwayforlife.blogspot.com/2010/02/scientists-advance-further-renders.html> accessed 23 August 2010.

— "National Vigil for Life a great success", 9 June 2013 <http://galwayforlife.blogspot.ie/2013/06/national-vigil-for-life-great-success.html> accessed 7 March 2014.

Ganiel, Gladys, *Transforming Post-Catholic Ireland: Religious Practice in Late Modernity* (Oxford: Oxford University Press, 2016).

Gartland, Fiona, "Bishops call over adult stem cell research", *Irish Times*, 15 June 2006, p. 7.

— "Calls made for surrogacy legislation", *Irish Times*, 6 March 2013, p. 2.

— "Judgment gives clear guidance for legislation", *Irish Times*, 8 November 2014, p. 4.

Gately, Susan, "Every Life Counts questions UN committee abortion ruling", 10 June 2016 <http://www.catholicireland.net/every-life-counts-questions-un-committee-abortion-ruling/> accessed 12 June 2016.

George, Robert P., "Infanticide and madness", *Journal of Medical Ethics*, vol. 39, no. 5 (May 2013), 299–301.

Gigli, Gian Luigi, and Elio Sgreccia, Editorial, *Cell Proliferation*, vol. 41, issue s1 (February 2008), pp. 1–3.

Girvin, Brian, "An Irish Solution to an Irish Problem: Catholicism, contraception and change, 1922–1979", *Contemporary European History*, vol. 27, no. 1 (2018), pp. 1–22.

Gissler, Mika, Cynthia Berg, Marie-Hélène Bouvier-Colle and Pierre Buekens, "Injury Deaths, Suicides and Homicides Associated with Pregnancy, Finland 1987–2000", *European Journal of Public Health*, vol. 15, no. 5 (2005), pp. 459–63.

Gissler, Mika, Elina Karalis, and Veli-Matti Ulander, "Decreased Suicide Rate after Induced Abortion, after the Current Care Guidelines in Finland 1987–2012", *Scandinavian Journal of Public Health*, vol. 43 (2015), pp. 99–101.

Giubilini, Alberto, "Abortion and the Argument from Potential: What we owe to the ones who might exist", *Journal of Medicine and Philosophy*, vol. 37 (January 2012), pp. 49–59.

Giubilini, Alberto, and Francesca Minerva, "After-birth Abortion: Why should the baby live?" *Journal of Medical Ethics*, vol. 39, no. 5 (May 2013), pp. 261–3.

Glatz, Carol, "Vatican deplores EU's 'thick-headed' cloning vote", *Catholic Herald and Standard*, 23 June 2006, p. 4.

Gleeson, Colin, "Minister responds to bishop on birth control", *Irish Times*, 6 August 2018 <https://search-proquest-com.ucc.idm.oclc.org/docview/2083431635/9FA2DDAD17434F2DPQ/30?accountid=14504> accessed 7 August 2018.

Gray, Freddy, "Embryonic screening breakthrough prompts new 'designer babies' fears", *Catholic Herald and Standard*, 23 June 2006, p. 3.

Griffin, Gráinne, Orla O'Connor, Ailbhe Smyth and Alison O'Connor, *It's a Yes! How Together for Yes Repealed the Eighth and Transformed Irish Society* (Dublin: Orpen Press, 2019).

Griffin, Leslie C., "The Catholic Bishops vs. the Contraceptive Mandate", *Religions*, vol. 6 (2015), pp 1411–32.

Guon, Jennifer, Benjamin S. Wilfond, Barbara Farlow, Tracy Brazg and Annie

Janvier, "Our Children Are Not a Diagnosis: The experience of parents who continue their pregnancy after a prenatal diagnosis of trisomy 13 or 18", *American Journal of Medical Genetics*, Part A 164A (2013), pp. 308–18.

Hallissey, Mary, "Who Do You Think You Are?", *Law Society Gazette*, August–September 2018 <https://www.lawsociety.ie/globalassets/documents/gazette/gazette-pdfs/gazette-2018/sept-2018-gazette.pdf> accessed 23 January 2019.

Halpenny, Orla, Doctors for Life, letter to the editor, *Irish Times*, 24 February 2018 <https://www.irishtimes.com/opinion/letters/the-eighth-amendment-1.3403495> accessed 24 February 2018.

Hanly, Conor, letter to the editor, *Irish Times*, 18 May 2018 <https://search-proquest-com.ucc.idm.oclc.org/docview/2040319173/C545F39D6F2D4E0FPQ/105?accountid=14504> accessed 18 May 2018.

Hannon, Patrick, "*In Vitro* Fertilisation", *The Furrow*, vol. 38, no. 12 (December 1987), pp. 739–746.

— *Church, State, Morality and Law* (Dublin: Gill and Macmillan, 1992)

— "The Conscience of the Voter and Law-maker", *Doctrine and Life*, vol. 42 (May–June 1992), 244–52.

— "Abortion, Law and Morals", *The Furrow*, vol. 64 (July–August 2013), pp. 387–94.

Harrison, Robert F., "The Development of IVF Practice in Ireland – A personal view", *Human Fertility*, vol. 15, no. 1, pp. 3–10.

Hart, John, *What Are They Saying About Environmental Theology?* (New York: Paulist Press, 2004).

Hayden, Chris, letter to the editor, *Irish Times*, 5 April 2018 <https://www.irishtimes.com/opinion/letters/myths-and-lies-about-abortion-must-be-debunked-1.3450548> accessed 6 April 2018.

Healy, Alison, "Sense of a case just beginning, not ending", *Irish Times*, 19 July 2006, p. 4.

— "Diarmuid Martin: Catholic Church needs reality check", *Irish Times*, 23 May 2015 <http://www.irishtimes.com/news/ireland/irish-news/diarmuid-martin-catholic-church-needs-reality-check-1.2223872?mode=print&ot=example.AjaxPageLayout.ot> accessed 29 October 2015).

Henderson, Mark, "Race to find new cures speeds up as Britain clones human embryo", *The Times*, 20 May 2005, pp. 1, 2.

— "Theoretical promise of cloning is fast becoming a real possibility", pp. 6–7, *The Times*, 20 May 2005.

Hildt, Elisabeth, and Dietmar Mieth (eds), *In Vitro Fertilisation in the 1990s: Towards a Medical, Social and Ethical Evaluation* (Aldershot, UK: Ashgate, 1998).

Hilliard, Mark, "Rhona Mahony warns of legal risk to doctors in abortion cases", *Irish Times*, 9 June 2015 <http://www.irishtimes.com/news/social-affairs/rhona-mahony-warns-of-legal-risk-to-doctors-in-abortion-cases-

1.2243014?mode=print&ot=example.AjaxPageLayout.ot> accessed 10 June 2015.

— "Catholic bishops urge Northern politicians to reject abortion law", *Irish Times*, 9 February 2016 <http://www.irishtimes.com/news/social-affairs/catholic-bishops-urge-northern-politicians-to-reject-abortion-law-1.2528805> accessed 13 February 2016.

Hochedlinger, Konrad, "Your Inner Healers", *Scientific American*, vol. 302, no. 5 (May 2010), pp. 28–35.

Hogan, Claire, "Catholic Church's influence over Irish hospital medicine persists", *Irish Times*, 28 April 2016 <http://www.irishtimes.com/opinion/catholic-church-s-influence-over-irish-hospital-medicine-persists-1.2626856> accessed 16 May 2016.

Holland, Kitty, "Case on Irish abortion law 'possible' after Belfast ruling", *Irish Times*, 30 November 2015 <http://www.irishtimes.com/news/social-affairs/case-on-irish-abortion-law-possible-after-belfast-ruling-1.2449303> accessed 2 December 2015.

— "Abortion should be decriminalised 'in all circumstances' – UN committee", *Irish Times*, 4 February 2016 <http://www.irishtimes.com/news/social-affairs/abortion-should-be-decriminalised-in-all-circumstances-un-committee-1.2522911> accessed 7 February 2016.

— "Woman's conviction for buying abortion pills is 'outrageous,'", *Irish Times*, 5 April 2016.

— "State's women face jail for taking abortion pill", *Irish Times*, 5 April 2016 <http://www.irishtimes.com/news/ireland/irish-news/state-s-women-face-jail-for-taking-abortion-pill-1.2598217> accessed 6 April 2016.

— "Women who take abortion pill 'should not be reported'", *Irish Times*, 6 April 2016 <http://www.irishtimes.com/news/social-affairs/women-who-take-abortion-pills-should-not-be-reported-1.2599522> accessed 6 April 2016.

— "Many states question Irish record on abortion at UN", *Irish Times*, 12 May 2016 <http://www.irishtimes.com/news/social-affairs/many-states-question-irish-record-on-abortion-at-un-1.2644354> accessed 12 May 2016.

— "Abortion pills trio: law making women criminals 'absolutely bad'", *Irish Times*, 25 May 2016 <http://www.irishtimes.com/news/social-affairs/abortion-pills-trio-law-making-women-criminals-absolutely-bad-1.2659395> accessed 25 May 2016.

— "Crowds protest religious ownership of new maternity hospital", *Irish Times*, 9 May 2017 <http://www.irishtimes.com/news/social-affairs/crowds-protest-religious-ownership-of-new-maternity-hospital-1.3074668> accessed 9 May 2017.

— "Accessing abortion is a 'lottery' under Irish rules – psychiatrist", *Irish Times*, 12 June 2017 <http://www.irishtimes.com/news/social-affairs/accessing-abortion-is-a-lottery-under-irish-rules-psychiatrist-1.3116997> accessed 16 June 2017.

— "Protection of Life During Pregnancy Act is 'unworkable'", *Irish Times*, 13 June 2017.

Horgan, Peter, "Barry questions cardinal: will government TDs be excommunicated?", *Cork Independent*, 16 May 2013 <http://corkindependent.com/20130516/news/barry-questions-cardinal-will-government-tds-be-excommunicated-S65288.html> accessed 15 December 2013.

Houlihan, Orla A., and Keelin O'Donoghue, "The Natural History of Pregnancies with a Diagnosis of Trisomy 18 or Trisomy 13: A retrospective case series", *BMC Pregnancy and Childbirth*, November 2013 <http://bmcpregnancychildbirth.biomedcentral.com/articles/10.1186/1471-2393-13-209> accessed 25 March 2017.

Houston, Muiris, "Key questions that arise when a pregnant woman is on life support", *Irish Times*, 18 December 2014 <http://www.irishtimes.com/opinion/key-questions-that-arise-when-a-pregnant-woman-is-on-life-support-1.2043081?mode=print&ot=example.AjaxPageLayout.ot> accessed 23 December 2014.

— "Life support case: ethical considerations a crucial part of best medical practice", *Irish Times*, 30 December 2014 <http://www.irishtimes.com/news/health/life-support-case-ethical-considerations-a-crucial-part-of-best-medical-practice-1.2051411?mode=print&ot=example.AjaxPageLayout.ot> accessed 2 January 2015.

— "A doctor writes: Cost of high-tech drugs a bitter pill to swallow", *Irish Times*, 3 June 2016 <http://www.irishtimes.com/news/health/a-doctor-writes-cost-of-high-tech-drugs-a-bitter-pill-to-swallow-1.2670565> accessed 3 June 2016.

Hug, Chrystel, *The Politics of Sexual Morality in Ireland* (London: Macmillan Press, 1999).

Human Life International (Ireland), "Submission to the Oireachtas Joint Committee on Health, on the General Scheme of the Assisted Human Reproduction Bill 2017" <https://humanlife.ie/latest-news/ivf-submission/> accessed 18 February 2019.

Humphreys, Joe, "Is there a right to life? You might not like the answer", *Irish Times*, 24 April 2018 <https://search-proquest-com.ucc.idm.oclc.org/docview/2029223301/7164D45CCCAF4233PQ/65?accountid=14504> accessed 24 April 2018.

Hurley, Dermot, *Billings Ovulation Method: A Pastoral Approach for Priests and Other Parish Workers* (London: Catholic Truth Society, 1994).

Hynes, Karen, "Stem Cell Research", *Technology Ireland*, vol. 37, no. 2 (May–June 2006), pp. 31–33.

Iglesias, Teresa, *IVF and Justice: Moral, Social and Legal Issues Related to Human in vitro Fertilisation* (London: Linacre Centre, 1990).

Independent.ie, "Citizens Assembly will continue to use the 'contentious' term fatal foetal abnormality", 7 January 2017 <http://www.independent.ie/irish-

news/citizens-assembly-will-continue-to-use-the-contentious-term-fatal-foetal-abnormality-35348988.html> accessed 9 January 2017.

Inglis, Tom, *Moral Monopoly: The Rise and Fall of the Catholic Church in Ireland* (University College Dublin Press, 1998).

Iona Institute, "Government must move to prohibit surrogacy in the interests of children: Surrogacy splits motherhood between up to three women: Surrogacy illegal in most European countries", press release, 5 March 2013 <http://www.ionainstitute.ie/index.php?id=2810> accessed 1 January 2014.

— "State must consider why most European countries ban surrogate motherhood", 26 September 2013 <http://www.ionainstitute.ie/index.php?id=3200> accessed 1 January 2014.

— "The Ethical Case Against Surrogate Motherhood: What we can learn from the law of other European countries" (n.d.), Conclusion <http://ionainstitute.org/assets/files/Surrogacy%20final%20PDF.pdf> accessed 1 January 2014.

— "Varadkar attacked over abortion law comments", 17 December 2014 <http://www.ionainstitute.ie/index.php?id=3790> accessed 22 December 2014).

Iona Institute and Dr Joanna Rose, "General Scheme of the 2017/18 Assisted Human Reproduction Bill: Comments and recommendations concerning donor-conceived children", 2018 <https://ionainstitute.ie/submission-to-health-committee-on-assisted-human-reproduction-bill/> accessed 21 January 2019.

Irish Examiner, "Supreme Court Ruling: Decisions put off for too long", Editorial, 16 December 2009, p. 16.

— "Save the 8th: Graphic posters 'wrong and unhelpful'", *Irish Examiner*, 1 May 2018 <https://www.irishexaminer.com/breakingnews/ireland/save-the-8th-graphic-posters-wrong-and-unhelpful-840262.html> accessed 9 December 2018.

Irish Independent, "Surrogacy appeal to Supreme Court underway", 3 February 2014 <http://www.independent.ie/irish-news/courts/surrogacy-appeal-to-supreme-court-underway-29974763.html> accessed 7 February 2014.

Irish Stem Cell Foundation, "Irish public policy and human embryonic stem cell research: A policy document by the Irish Stem Cell Foundation, April 2010" <http://www.irishstemcellfoundation.org/docs/policy.pdf> accessed 24 May 2010.

— "About Us" <http://www.irishstemcellfoundation.org/aboutus.htm> accessed 24 May 2010.

Irish Times, "Husband's case on embryos upheld", 19 July 2006, p. 4.

— "British IVF laws requires both parties' consent at all times", 29 July 2006, p. 4.

— "Court adjourns embryos case", 1 August 2006, p. 4.

— "Political failings and embryo case", Editorial, 16 December 2009, p. 17.

— "Genetic parents win surrogate twins case", 6 March 2013, p. 2.

— "Full text of court ruling on North's abortion laws", 30 November 2015 <http://www.irishtimes.com/news/crime-and-law/full-text-of-court-ruling-

on-north-s-abortion-laws-1.2448877> accessed 2 December 2015.

— "NI Catholic bishops respond to abortion judgment", *Irish Times*, 30 November 2015 <http://www.irishtimes.com/news/social-affairs/religion-and-beliefs/ni-catholic-bishops-respond-to-abortion-judgment-1.2449422> accessed 2 December 2015.

— "Ipsos MRBI poll: abortion, voters and nuance", 27 May 2017 <http://www.irishtimes.com/opinion/editorial/ipsos-mrbi-poll-abortion-voters-and-nuance-1.3097371?mode=print&ot=example.AjaxPageLayout.ot> accessed 26 June 2017.

— "Bishop says wildlife will be protected better: Bishop said if the amendment is repealed the unborn baby will be left with no protection", 21 May 2018 <https://search-proquest-com.ucc.idm.oclc.org/docview/2041434788/A66B53F0A07F4786PQ/22?accountid=14504> accessed 21 May 2018.

Janoff, Abby F., "Rights of the Pregnant Child vs. Rights of the Unborn under the Convention on the Rights of the Child", *Boston University International Law Journal*, vol. 22, no. 1 (2004), pp. 163–88 <http://www.bu.edu/law/journals-archive/international/volume22n1/documents/163-188.pdf> accessed 6 June 2016.

Janvier, Annie, Barbara Farlow and Benjamin S. Wilfond, "The Experience of Families with Children with Trisomy13 and 18 in Social Networks", *Pediatrics*, vol. 130, no. 2 (August 2012), pp. 293–8.

Jaquier, M., A. Klein and E. Boltshauser, "Spontaneous Pregnancy Outcome after Prenatal Diagnosis of Anencephaly", *British Journal of Obstetrics and Gynaecology*, vol. 113, no. 8 (August 2006), pp. 951–3.

Johnson, Mark, "Delayed Hominization: Reflections on some recent Catholic claims for delayed hominization", *Theological Studies*, vol. 56, no. 4 (December 1995), pp. 743–63.

Jowit, Juliette, "Northern Ireland's abortion laws remain restrictive and unclear", *Guardian*, 6 January 2016 <http://www.theguardian.com/world/2016/jan/06/northern-ireland-abortion-laws-restrictive-unclear-legal-women> accessed 13 February 2016.

TheJournal.ie, "Savita inquest: Jury returns verdict of medical misadventure", 19 April 2013 <http://www.thejournal.ie/savita-inquest-jury-returns-verdict-of-medical-misadventure-876458-Apr2013/> accessed 17 March 2016.

— "'I actually struggle with this myself': Taoiseach quizzed on Eighth Amendment on TV3 couch", 25 February 2016 <http://www.msn.com/en-ie/news/national/%e2%80%9ci-actually-struggle-with-this-myself%e2%80%9d-taoiseach-quizzed-on-eighth-amendment-on-tv3-couch/ar-BBpYyaJ?ocid=spartandhp> accessed 25 February 2016.

Keane, Declan, "Maternity hospital must move with the times – so please stop misstating facts", *Irish Times*, 4 June 2017, p. 12.

Keane, Ronan, "Repeal does not mean the unborn have no right to life", *Irish Times*, 16 May 2018 <https://search-proquest-com.ucc.idm.oclc.org/

docview/2038990392/51D67B8B79584ABCPQ/87?accountid=14504> accessed 16 May 2018.

— Letter to the editor, *Irish Times*, 21 May 2018 <https://www.irishtimes.com/opinion/letters/referendum-on-the-eighth-amendment-1.3501920> accessed 21 May 2018.

Keena, Colm, "Religious congregations control health service assets worth hundreds of millions", *Irish Times*, 2 May 2017 <http://0-search.proquest.com.library.ucc.ie/docview/1893721953/fulltext/18EE7F22E2394B63PQ/31?accountid=14504> accessed 15 May 2017.

— "Claims of abortion committee bias rejected", *Irish Times*, 23 November 2017 <https://search-proquest-com.ucc.idm.oclc.org/docview/1967208927/730CF42E2CA64593PQ/54?accountid=14504> accessed 23 November 2017.

Kelly, Fiach, "Joan Burton says abortion laws do not serve women well", *Irish Times*, 19 December 2014 <http://www.irishtimes.com/news/politics/joan-burton-says-abortion-laws-do-not-serve-women-well-1.2044589?mode=print&ot=example.AjaxPageLayout.ot> accessed 22 December 2014.

— "Amendment limiting abortion to rape cases 'unworkable', say former AGs", *Irish Times*, 16 May 2018 <https://search-proquest-com.ucc.idm.oclc.org/docview/2038990025/51D67B8B79584ABCPQ/59?accountid=14504> accessed 16 May 2018.

— "Retain campaign makes bid to shift narrative", *Irish Times*, 23 May 2018, p. 6.

Kelly, Gerald, "The Teaching of Pope Pius XII on Artificial Insemination", *Linacre Quarterly*, vol. 23, no. 1 (February 1956), pp. 5–17 <https://epublications.marquette.edu/cgi/viewcontent.cgi?referer=https://www.google.ie/&httpsredir=1&article=3780&context=lnq> accessed 2 April 2018.

Kelly, Michael, "Church approves most stem cell research: How your MEP voted", *Irish Catholic*, 22 June 2006, p. 6.

— "Church does need a 'reality check' after the referendum", *Irish Catholic*, 27 May 2015 <http://irishcatholic.ie/article/church-does-need-%E2%80%98reality-check%E2%80%99-after-referendum> accessed 28 May 2015.

Kelly, Olivia, "IVF report delayed pending court embryo case outcome", *Irish Times*, 7 July 2006, p. 4.

Kennedy, Donald (editor-in-chief), "Retraction", post date 12 January 2006, *Science* <www.sciencemag.org>.

Keogh, Dermot, *Twentieth-Century Ireland: Nation and State* (Dublin: Gill and Macmillan, 1994).

Kersting, Anette, and Birgit Wagner, "Complicated Grief after Perinatal Loss", *Dialogues in Clinical Neuroscience*, vol. 14, no. 2 (June 2012), pp. 187–94

<http://www.ncbi.nlm.nih.gov/pmc/articles/PMC3384447/> accessed 20 August 2016.

Kilfeather, Vivion, "'Unborn' refers to child within the womb, rules court", *Irish Examiner*, 16 December 2009, p. 6.

— "'Science will not wait for us to update our laws'", *Irish Examiner*, 16 December 2009, p. 6.

Kirwan, Liam, *An Unholy Trinity: Medicine, Politics and Religion in Ireland* (Dublin: Liffey Press, 2016).

Krizhanovsky, Valery, and Scott W. Lowe, "The Promises and Perils of p53", *Nature*, vol. 460, issue no. 7259 (27 August 2009), pp. 1085–6.

Kuhse, Helga, "Some Comments on the Paper 'After-birth Abortion: Why should the baby live?'", *Journal of Medical Ethics*, vol. 39, no. 5 (May 2013), pp. 323–4.

Laing, Jacqueline A., "Infanticide: A reply to Giubilini and Minerva", *Journal of Medical Ethics*, vol. 39, no. 5 (May 2013), pp. 336–40.

Leahy, Pat, "Middle ground has shifted on abortion, but will politicians shift with it?", *Irish Times*, 15 June 2016, p. 4.

— "Kenny says UN abortion ruling not binding", *Irish Times*, 15 June 2016, p. 1.

— "Majority support repeal of Eighth Amendment, poll shows", *Irish Times*, 8 July 2016 <http://www.irishtimes.com/news/politics/majority-support-repeal-of-eighth-amendment-poll-shows-1.2714191> accessed 8 July 2016.

— "Irish Times/Ipsos MRBI poll: Replace constitutional control on abortion", *Irish Times*, 3 March 2017 <http://www.irishtimes.com/news/social-affairs/irish-times-ipsos-mrbi-poll-replace-constitutional-control-on-abortion-1.2995968> accessed 3 March 2017.

— "Poll shows public support for abortion is cautious and conditional", *Irish Times*, 3 March 2017 <http://www.irishtimes.com/news/social-affairs/poll-shows-public-support-for-abortion-is-cautious-and-conditional-1.2995696> accessed 3 March 2017.

— "Bitter abortion ballot campaign on the horizon: Dáil must decide if they should frame a workable abortion referendum", *Irish Times*, 30 June 2017 <http://0-search.proquest.com.library.ucc.ie/docview/1914683154/2E43CE9A9A6E41A0PQ/96?accountid=14504> accessed 30 June 2017.

— "Reconciling positions on abortion is a political debate", *Irish Times*, 21 October 2017 <https://search-proquest-com.ucc.idm.oclc.org/docview/1953294531/4E0D4C9BF246E0PQ/88?accountid=14504> accessed 21 October 2017.

— "National Women's Council targets middle ground with abortion campaign", *Irish Times*, 13 November 2017 <https://search-proquest-com.ucc.idm.oclc.org/docview/1963034940/41897DB437EC4D54PQ/35?accountid=14504> accessed 13 November 2017.

— "Opinion polls suggest middle ground will be decisive", *Irish Times*, 14 December 2017.

— "Repeal side well ahead despite dip in support", *Irish Times*, 20 April 2018 <https://search-proquest-com.ucc.idm.oclc.org/docview/2027380697/16E3869566784158PQ/5?accountid=14504> accessed 20 April 2018.

— "Social media group's move reflects repeal nerves", *Irish Times*, 9 May 2018 <https://search-proquest-com.ucc.idm.oclc.org/docview/2035909708/F760F3456B25418CPQ/65?accountid=14504> accessed 9 May 2018.

— "Google ban is unprecedented, so why did they do it?", *Irish Times*, 10 May 2018 <https://search-proquest-com.ucc.idm.oclc.org/docview/2036541119/F245D3E7582421CPQ/44?accountid=14504> accessed 10 May 2018.

— "Save the Eighth group defends booklet design", *Irish Times*, 16 May 2018.

— "Many anti-repeal TDs will back legislation", *Irish Times*, 28 May 2018 <https://search-proquest-com.ucc.idm.oclc.org/docview/2044967023/74D30A4F40924292PQ/8?accountid=14504> accessed 31 December 2018.

— "Yes campaign's outreach to middle ground delivered the landslide", *Irish Times*, 28 May 2018 <https://search-proquest-com.ucc.idm.oclc.org/docview/2044967711/C9B12D887BEA42ABPQ/12?accountid=14504> accessed 28 May 2018.

Leahy, Pat, and Sarah Bardon, "FG Ministers believe only restrictive abortion law will pass: cabinet members reluctant to put forward referendum on changes they do not endorse", *Irish Times*, 28 September 2017 <https://search-proquest-com.ucc.idm.oclc.org/docview/1943388380/8469DAF548564E09PQ/2?accountid=14504> accessed 28 September 2017.

— "Varadkar rejects idea from No side of laws for 'hard cases'", *Irish Times*, 23 May 2018, p. 1.

— "Harris pledges swift action on abortion laws", *Irish Times*, 28 May 2018 <https://search-proquest-com.ucc.idm.oclc.org/docview/2044967575/74D30A4F40924292PQ/1?accountid=14504> accessed 31 December 2018.

Lee, Simon, "Abortion Law: The tragic choices", *Doctrine and Life*, vol. 42 (May–June 1992), pp. 282–97.

Lehrman, Sally, "Undifferentiated Ethics: Stem cells from adult skin are as morally fraught as the embryonic kind", *Scientific American*, vol. 303, no. 3 (September 2010), pp. 11–12.

Linehan, Hugh, "Will Eighth Amendment referendum campaign be manipulated online?", *Irish Times*, 20 November 2017 <https://search-proquest-com.ucc.idm.oclc.org/docview/1965941130/2777F748E12B4619PQ/42?accountid=14504> accessed 20 November 2017.

Little, Joe, "Archbishop says he is deeply saddened over referendum result", RTÉ News, 28 May 2018 <https://www.rte.ie/news/2018/0527/966293-

diarmuid-martin/> accessed 28 May 2018.

Leon, Sharon M., *An Image of God: The Catholic Struggle with Eugenics* (Chicago: University of Chicago Press, 2013).

Levy, Neil, "The Moral Significance of Being Born", *Journal of Medical Ethics*, vol. 39, no. 5 (May 2013), pp. 326–9.

Life Institute, "Vote for Life GE 2016" <http://www.thelifeinstitute.net/current-projects/vote-for-life-2016/vote-for-life-2016--parties-position/> accessed 12 March 2016.

Lord, Miriam, "The day 32 TDs voted against democracy", *Irish Times*, 22 March 2018 <https://search-proquest-com.ucc.idm.oclc.org/docview/2016155084/F67A979856DD449DPQ/54?accountid=14504> accessed 26 April 2018.

— "Stony silence as absolutist bluff called", *Irish Times*, 23 May 2018, p. 5.

Loughlin, Elaine, "Cross-party event cut short as heckler targets Harris", *Irish Examiner*, 23 May 2018, p. 6.

Loughlin, Elaine, and Fiachra Ó Cionnaith, "No canvassers 'ridiculing mental health': Harris", *Irish Examiner*, 22 May 2018, p. 1.

Love Both, "Three mothers that faced pressure to terminate their pregnancies", 10 May 2018 <https://loveboth.ie/three-mothers-pressure-abortion/> accessed 5 October 2018.

— "Should abortion be decriminalised?" <https://loveboth.ie/should-abortion-be-decriminalised/> accessed 24 May 2018.

Lynch, Colum, "Can Pope Francis Get the Catholic Church's Mind Off of Sex?", *Foreign Policy*, 11 May 2015 <https://foreignpolicy.com/2015/05/11/can-pope-francis-get-the-catholic-churchs-mind-off-of-sex/> accessed 1 May 2019.

Lynch, Suzanne, Elaine Edwards and Sarah Bardon, "Fitzgerald promises to address highly critical UN report on Irish abortion law", *Irish Times*, 10 June 2016, p. 3.

Mac Cormaic, Ruadhán, "State's message on surrogacy: 'Leave it to the Oireachtas'", 4 February 2014 <http://www.irishtimes.com/news/crime-and-law/courts/state-s-message-on-surrogacy-leave-it-to-the-oireachtas-1.1678316> accessed 7 February 2014.

— "Medics called for guidelines after two previous cases", *Irish Times*, 22 December 2014 <http://www.irishtimes.com/news/crime-and-law/medics-called-for-guidelines-after-two-previous-cases-1.2046848?mode=print&ot=example.AjaxPageLayout.ot> accessed 23 December 2014.

— "Life support for brain-dead pregnant woman withdrawn", *Irish Times*, 28 December 2014 <http://www.irishtimes.com/news/crime-and-law/life-support-for-brain-dead-pregnant-woman-withdrawn-1.2049636?mode=print&ot=example.AjaxPageLayout.ot> accessed 2 January 2015.

— "Legal conundrum hinges on the definition of the 'unborn'", *Irish Times*, 6

February 2015 <http://www.irishtimes.com/news/crime-and-law/legal-conundrum-hinges-on-the-definition-of-the-unborn-1.2094793> accessed 10 September 2016.

— "State to introduce parts of Children and Family Relationships Act", *Irish Times*, 20 May 2015 <https://www.irishtimes.com/news/politics/state-to-introduce-parts-of-children-and-family-relationships-act-1.2218743?mode=print&ot=example.AjaxPageLayout.ot> accessed 20 May 2015.

— "Citizens' Assembly leans towards change in Ireland's abortion laws", *Irish Times*, 8 January 2017 <http://www.irishtimes.com/news/social-affairs/citizens-assembly-leans-towards-change-in-ireland-s-abortion-laws-1.2929372?mode=print&ot=example.AjaxPageLayout.ot> accessed 9 January 2017.

McCann, Joseph (ed.), *Religion and Science: Education, Ethics and Public Policy* (Drumcondra, Dublin: St Patrick's College, 2003).

McCárthaigh, Seán, "Number of couples divorcing rises 2% to more than 3,400", *Irish Examiner*, 19 July 2006, p. 8.

McCarthy, Alice, "Will Human Embryonic Stem Cell Therapies Finally Grow Up?" *Chemistry & Biology*, vol. 16, issue 5 (29 May 2009), pp. 471–2.

McCarthy, Denis, letter to the editor, *Irish Times*, 26 June 2017 <http://www.irishtimes.com/opinion/letters/the-eighth-amendment-1.3131441?mode=print&ot=example.AjaxPageLayout.ot> accessed 26 June 2017.

McCarthy, Joan, Mary Donnelly, Dolores Dooley, Louise Campbell and David Smith, *End-of-Life Care: Ethics and Law* (Cork: Cork University Press, 2011).

McCarthy, Justine, "Bishop says new hospital must obey the Church", *Sunday Times*, 23 April 2017 <https://search-proquest-com.ucc.idm.oclc.org/docview/1890741404/170D4D30DC054ACFPQ/2?accountid=14504> accessed 22 April 2018.

— "Activists celebrate majority to repeal eighth", *Sunday Times*, 27 May 2018, p. 1.

McCarthy, Justine, and Colin Coyle, "Third master raises NMH fears", *Sunday Times*, 30 April 2017, p. 4.

McCarthy, Michelle, "Revolutionary stem cell research will benefit UCC", *UCC Express*, vol. 12, issue 3 (4 November 2008), p. 10.

McCarthy, Pádraig, "Caring for Mother and Child", *The Furrow*, vol. 64, no. 1 (January 2013), pp. 3–9.

— "Caring for Mother and Child – Legislating for the X Case", *The Furrow*, vol. 64, no. 2 (February 2013), pp. 115–17.

McCarthy, Tommie, letter to the editor, *Irish Times*, 3 February 2010 <http://www.irishtimes.com/newspaper/letters/2010/0203/1224263647755_pf.html> accessed 3 February 2010.

McCormack, Brendan, *et al.*, letter to the editor, *Irish Times*, 21 May 2015 <http://www.irishtimes.com/opinion/letters/marriage-referendum-countdown-

to-polling-day-1.2220003?mode=print&ot=example.AjaxPageLayout.ot>
accessed 25 May 2015.

McDonagh, Enda, and Vincent MacNamara (eds), *An Irish Reader in Moral Theology: The Legacy of the Last Fifty Years* (Dublin: Columba Press, 2013).

McDonagh, Michelle, "Stem cells", *UCC News*, issue 37 (February 2008), pp. 12–13.

— "UCC approves use of embryonic stem cells by single vote", *Irish Independent*, 29 October 2008 <http://www.independent.ie/health/latest-news/ucc-approves-use-of-embryonic-stem-cells-by-single-vote-1511912.html> accessed 1 November 2008.

McDonald, Brian, "Cardinal keeps excommunication threat hanging over abortion TDs", Independent.ie, 5 May 2013 <http://www.independent.ie/irish-news/cardinal-keeps-excommunication-threat-hanging-over-abortion-tds-29242992.html> accessed 15 February 2014.

McDonald, Dearbhail, "'Justice done' as jury acquits carer Gail O'Rorke of assisting sick woman's suicide", Independent.ie, 29 April 2015 <http://www.independent.ie/irish-news/courts/justice-done-as-jury-acquits-carer-gail-ororke-of-assisting-sick-womans-suicide-31180940.html> accessed 30 July 2016).

— "In the name of God, we cannot let this maternity deal collapse", *Sunday Independent*, 23 April 2017, p. 29.

— "Don't throw baby out with the bathwater", *Sunday Independent*, 4 June 2017, p. 12.

McDonald, Henry, "Northern Irish appeal court refuses limited lifting of abortion ban", *Guardian*, 29 June 2017 <https://www.theguardian.com/world/2017/jun/29/northern-irish-appeal-court-refuses-limited-lifting-of-abortion-ban> accessed 30 June 2017.

McDonnell, Orla, and Jill Allison, "From Biopolitics to Bioethics: Church, state, medicine and assisted reproductive technology in Ireland", *Sociology of Health & Illness*, vol. 28, no. 6 (2006), pp. 817–37.

McGarry, Patsy, "Bishops warn of crisis over sanctity of life", *Irish Times*, 8 October 2007, p. 1 <http://www.ireland.com/newspaper/frontpage/2007/1008/1191668714883.html> accessed 8 October 2007.

— "Pro Life Campaign to question parties on abortion stances", *Irish Times*, 15 May 2009 <http://www.irishtimes.com/newspaper/ireland/2009/0515/1224246568320_pf.html> accessed 21 January 2010.

— "Bishop of Elphin expresses regret over comments about gay parents", *Irish Times*, 16 March 2015 <http://www.irishtimes.com/news/social-affairs/religion-and-beliefs/bishop-of-elphin-expresses-regret-over-comments-about-gay-parents-1.2140902?mode=print&ot=example.AjaxPageLayout.ot> accessed 16 March 2015.

— "All churches in Ireland in need of 'reality check'", *Irish Times*, 24 May 2015 <http://www.irishtimes.com/news/social-affairs/religion-

and-beliefs/all-churches-in-ireland-in-need-of-reality-check-
1.2224081?mode=print&ot=example.AjaxPageLayout.ot> accessed 25 May
2015.

— "Same-sex marriage vote an 'unmitigated disaster' for Church", *Irish Times*,
25 May 2015 <http://www.irishtimes.com/news/social-affairs/religion-
and-beliefs/same-sex-marriage-vote-an-unmitigated-disaster-for-church-
1.2225680?mode=print&ot=example.AjaxPageLayout.ot> accessed 25 May
2015.

— "Archbishop Martin seeks removal from chair at Holles Street", *Irish Times*, 27
April 2017, p. 2.

— "IVF, sterilisation and morning-after pill banned by Sisters of Charity", *Irish
Times*, 28 April 2017 <http://www.irishtimes.com/news/social-affairs/
religion-and-beliefs/ivf-sterilisation-and-morning-after-pill-banned-by-
sisters-of-charity-1.3064123> accessed 28 April 2017.

— "Leading priest supports Dr Peter Boylan on new maternity hospital", *Irish
Times*, 29 May 2017 <http://www.irishtimes.com/news/social-affairs/
religion-and-beliefs/leading-priest-supports-dr-peter-boylan-on-new-
maternity-hospital-1.3099455?mode=print&ot=example.AjaxPageLayout.ot>
accessed 29 May 2017.

— "Surprise move recognises more diverse Ireland", *Irish Times*, 30 May 2017, p.
3.

— "Catholic archbishop has no wish to be chair of National Maternity Hospital",
Irish Times, 1 June 2017 <http://www.irishtimes.com/news/social-affairs/
religion-and-beliefs/catholic-archbishop-has-no-wish-to-be-chair-of-
national-maternity-hospital-1.3104383> accessed 2 June 2017.

— "Oireachtas Committee 'appears' to have made up mind, says bishop", *Irish
Times*, 21 October 2017 <https://search-proquest-com.ucc.idm.oclc.org/
docview/1953295123/4E0D4C9BF246E0PQ/31?accountid=14504>
accessed 21 October 2017.

— "Repealing Eighth Amendment 'removes' constitutional protection for
unborn", *Irish Times*, 21 October 2017 <https://search-proquest-com.ucc.idm.
oclc.org/docview/1953294526/4E0D4C9BF246E0PQ/32?accountid=14504>
accessed 21 October 2017.

— "Child with Down Syndrome to feature in anti-abortion billboard campaign",
Irish Times, 29 January 2018 <https://www.irishtimes.com/news/social-
affairs/religion-and-beliefs/child-with-down-syndrome-to-feature-in-anti-
abortion-billboard-campaign-1.3372867> accessed 31 January 2018.

— "Love Both challenges Minister on claim about
abortion on disability grounds", *Irish Times*, 11 May
2018 <https://search-proquest-com.ucc.idm.oclc.org/
docview/2036892082/96F336D60BE14F28PQ/46?accountid=14504>
accessed 11 May 2018.

— "Pope's message on fake news welcomed", *Irish Times*, 14

May 2018 <https://search-proquest-com.ucc.idm.oclc.org/docview/2038137921/7B7D35945F184915PQ/54?accountid=14504> accessed 14 May 2018.

— "Psychiatrist says to suggest abortion a solution to mental illness 'naive in the extreme'", *Irish Times*, 1 May 2018 <https://www.irishtimes.com/news/social-affairs/psychiatrist-says-to-suggest-abortion-a-solution-to-mental-illness-naive-in-the-extreme-1.3480660> accessed 4 November 2018.

— "Anti-abortion group targets hospitals", *Irish Times*, 2 May 2018 <https://search-proquest-com.ucc.idm.oclc.org/docview/2033122916/FF2DB3D6F5C2462FPQ/41?accountid=14504> accessed 3 May 2018.

— "Ireland 'obliterated' right to life of the unborn, says Catholic primate", *Irish Times*, 28 May 2018.

— "Mixed reaction to announcement of Rome assent to transfer of site at St Vincent's", *The Irish Times*, 8 May 2020 <https://www.irishtimes.com/news/social-affairs/religion-and-beliefs/mixed-reaction-to-announcement-of-rome-assent-to-transfer-of-site-at-st-vincent-s-1.4248635> accessed 8 May 2020.

McGarry, Patsy, Mark Brennock and Barry Roche, "Aherne elaborates on his defence of Church", *Irish Times*, 12 November 2005.

McGee, Andrew, "The Moral Status of Babies", *Journal of Medical Ethics*, vol. 39, no. 5 (May 2013), pp. 345–8.

McGee, Harry, "Nuclear Deterrence: Fools' Paradise", *Doctrine and Life*, vol. 31, no. 9 (November 1981), pp. 565–75.

— "Major proposals may be vulnerable to Supreme Court challenge", *Irish Examiner*, 13 May 2005.

— "Boylan stands over claim majority of institute's members support repeal", *Irish Times*, 16 May 2018 <https://search-proquest-com.ucc.idm.oclc.org/docview/2038985449/51D67B8B79584ABCPQ/60?accountid=14504> accessed 16 May 2018.

— "How the tide turned against the Eighth", *Irish Times*, 28 May 2018 <https://search-proquest-com.ucc.idm.oclc.org/docview/2044968134/C9B12D887BEA42ABPQ/15?accountid=14504> accessed 28 May 2018.

McGreevy, Ronan, "Committee 'couldn't find' any anti-abortion medical experts to argue for Eighth", *Irish Times*, 20 February 2018 <https://www.irishtimes.com/news/ireland/irish-news/committee-couldn-t-find-any-anti-abortion-medical-experts-to-argue-for-eighth-1.3397941> accessed 20 February 2018.

— "Assembly selection defended: Chairwoman of Citizens' Assembly says abortion outcome unaffected by audit", *Irish Times*, 23 February 2018 <https://search-proquest-com.ucc.idm.oclc.org/docview/2007254403/65364351C711406FPQ/47?accountid=14504> accessed 25 February 2018.

McGreevy, Ronan, and Paul Cullen, "Board of National Maternity Hospital reaffirms move to St Vincent's campus", *Irish Times*, 27 April 2017, p. 2.

McGuinness, Eamon, "Medical myths about Eighth Amendment must be challenged", *Irish Times*, 6 April 2018 <https://www.irishtimes.com/opinion/medical-myths-about-eighth-amendment-must-be-challenged-1.3451748> accessed 6 April 2018.

McLaughlin, P.J., *The Church and Modern Science* (Dublin: Clonmore and Reynolds, 1957).

McMahan, Jeff, "Infanticide and Moral Consistency", *Journal of Medical Ethics*, vol. 39, no. 5 (May 2013), pp. 273–80.

McMahon, Áine, "Catholic Church 'bereavement' after same-sex marriage vote", *Irish Times*, 2 June 2015 <http://www.irishtimes.com/news/social-affairs/religion-and-beliefs/catholic-church-bereavement-after-same-sex-marriage-vote-1.2234500?mode=print&ot=example.AjaxPageLayout.ot> accessed 29 October 2015.

— "Irish doctors call for decriminalisation of abortion", *Irish Times*, 20 November 2015 <http://www.irishtimes.com/news/social-affairs/irish-doctors-call-for-decriminalisation-of-abortion-1.2437846> accessed 8 October 2016.

— "Eighth Amendment has caused death of cancer patients, says obstetrician", *Irish Times*, 9 April 2018 <https://search-proquest-com.ucc.idm.oclc.org/docview/2022902451/E7A4FE80CC2E4595PQ/9?accountid=14504> accessed 9 April 2018.

McManus, John, "Vincent's should be split up while there is a chance: The maternity hospital row was never about nuns or their Catholic ethos", *Irish Times*, 31 May 2017 <http://0-search.proquest.com.library.ucc.ie/docview/1903657551/1AD98059EE834B2DPQ/80?accountid=14504> accessed 31 May 2017.

McSweeney, P.L.H., letter to the editor, *Irish Times*, 29 January 2010 <http://www.irishtimes.com/newspaper/letters/2010/0129/1224263355254_pf.html> accessed 29 January 2010.

Madden, Deirdre, "In Vitro Fertilisation: The moral and legal status of the human pre-embryo", *Medico-Legal Journal of Ireland*, vol. 3 (1), 1997, pp. 12–20.

— "Is there a Right to a Child of One's Own?", *Medico-Legal Journal of Ireland*, vol. 5, no. 1 (1999), pp. 8–13.

— "Recent Developments in Assisted Human Reproduction: Legal and ethical issues", *Medico-Legal Journal of Ireland*, vol. 7, no. 2 (2001), pp. 53–62.

— "Assisted Reproduction in Ireland – Time to Legislate", Guest Editorial, *Medico-Legal Journal of Ireland*, vol. 17, no. 1 (2011), pp. 3–5.

— "Is there a Right to a 'Good Death'?", *Medico-Legal Journal of Ireland*, vol. 19, no. 2 (2013), pp. 60–7.

— *Medicine, Ethics and the Law* (Haywards Heath, UK: Bloomsbury Professional, 2016 (3rd edn)).

Maguire, Siobhan, and Dearbhail McDonald, "Playing with time", *Sunday Times*, 9 July 2006, p. 12.

Major, Brenda, *et al.*, "Abortion and Mental Health: Evaluating the Evidence",

American Psychologist, vol. 64, issue 9 (2009) <http://web.a.ebscohost.com.
ucc.idm.oclc.org/ehost/detail/detail?vid=3&sid=79664021-f9b0-4e81-87a5-
2972aa6ae1bd%40sessionmgr4007&bdata=JnNpdGU9ZWhvc3QtbGl2ZQ
%3d%3d#AN=2009-23092-001&db=pdh> accessed 5 May 2018.

Malcolm, Elizabeth, and Greta Jones (eds), *Medicine, Disease and the State in
Ireland, 1650–1940* (Cork: Cork University Press, 1999).

Manninen, Bertha Alvarez, "Yes, the Baby Should Live: A pro-choice response to
Giubilini and Minerva", *Journal of Medical Ethics*, vol. 39, no. 5 (May 2013),
pp. 330–5.

Marks, Joel, "Confessions of an ex-moralist", *New York Times*, 21 August 2011
<http://opinionator.blogs.nytimes.com/2011/08/21/confessions-of-an-ex-
moralist/?hp> accessed 29 August 2011.

— "An Amoral Manifesto (1)", *Philosophy Now*, issue 80 (August–September
2011) <http://www.philosophynow.org/issue80/An_Amoral_Manifesto_
Part_I> accessed 29 August 2011.

Marks, Lara V., *Sexual Chemistry: A History of the Contraceptive Pill* (New Haven:
Yale University Press, 2001).

Meredith, Finola, "Abortion referendum aftermath: is Northern Ireland next?",
Irish Times, 9 June 2018 <https://www.irishtimes.com/news/social-affairs/
abortion-referendum-aftermath-is-northern-ireland-next-1.3522667>
accessed 23 June 2018.

Minihan, Mary, "Lack of legislation puts judiciary in 'unenviable' position, says
FG", *Irish Times*, 16 December 2009, p. 4.

Minihan, Mary, and Carol Coulter, "Harney to propose law on assisted human
reproduction: Supreme Court finds failure to legislate 'disturbing'", *Irish
Times*, 16 December 2009, p. 1.

Mitchell, Susan, "Warning over stem cell research in Ireland", ThePost.ie (*Sunday
Business Post* online), 6 March 2011 <http://www.thepost.ie/story/text/
ojeysnojmh/> accessed 31 March 2011.

Momigliano, Anna, "When Left-Wing Feminists and Conservative Catholics
Unite", *The Atlantic*, 28 March 2017 <https://www.theatlantic.com/
international/archive/2017/03/left-wing-feminists-conservative-catholics-
unite/520968/> accessed 8 March 2019.

Monaghan, John, *et al.*, letter to the editor, *Irish Times*, 1 May
2013 <https://search-proquest-com.ucc.idm.oclc.org/
docview/1346974835/8E07E88C521D44EAPQ/153?accountid=14504>
accessed 1 May 2013.

Moore, Tom, and Tom Cotter, "Choosing sides", *UCC News*, issue 41 (September
2008), pp. 1–2.

Moriarty, Gerry, "Catholic bishops 'shocked and disturbed' by abortion
ruling", *Irish Times*, 1 December 2015 <http://www.irishtimes.com/news/
social-affairs/catholic-bishops-shocked-and-disturbed-by-abortion-
ruling-1.2449437> accessed 2 December 2015.

— "Women – aged 69, 68 and 71 – tell PSNI they bought abortion pills", *Irish Times*, 24 May 2016 <http://www.irishtimes.com/news/ireland/irish-news/women-aged-69-68-and-71-tell-psni-they-bought-abortion-pills-1.2658862> accessed 25 May 2016.

Moriarty, Gerry, and Freya McClements, "Abortion decriminalised in NI despite unionist opposition", *Irish Times*, 22 October 2019 <https://search-proquest-com.ucc.idm.oclc.org/docview/2307239589/B1F6A6273B634695PQ/1?accountid=14504> accessed 22 October 2019.

Mothers and Fathers Matter, *Don't Deny a Child the Right to a Mother and a Father: Vote No on 22 May* [2015].

Mudiwa, Lloyd, "Barbed exchange between medics", *Irish Medical Times*, 18 January 2013 <https://www.imt.ie/news/barbed-exchanges-between-medics-18-01-2013/> accessed 6 November 2018.

Muir, Hazel (ed.), *Larousse Dictionary of Scientists* (New York: Larousse, 1994).

Mullally, Una, "Election result is not a victory for anti-abortion lobby", *Irish Times*, 2 March 2016 <http://www.irishtimes.com/opinion/una-mullally-election-result-is-not-a-victory-for-anti-abortion-lobby-1.2557019?__vfz=c_pages%3D11000002670848> accessed 3 March 2016.

Murphy, Byron, "Stem cell research policy is noted by UCC Governing Body", *UCC Express*, vol. 12, issue 3 (4 November 2008), p. 3.

Murphy, Séamus, "Stem Cell Research: Science and philosophy", *Studies*, vol. 93, no. 371 (Autumn 2004), pp. 269–79.

Murray, Donal, *Christian Morality and In Vitro Fertilisation: A Question of Morality* (Dublin: Veritas Publications, 1985).

— "Some Thoughts on the Abortion Debate", *Doctrine and Life*, vol. 63 (February 2013), pp. 5–21.

Murtagh, Peter, "Twitter rejects restriction accusation from Irish anti-abortion campaigners", *Irish Times*, 14 April 2018, p. 4.

Nelson, Katherine E., Laura C. Rosella, Sanjay Mahant and Astrid Guttmann, "Survival and Surgical Interventions for Children with Trisomy 13 and 18", *Journal of the American Medical Association*, vol. 316, no. 4 (2016), pp. 420–8.

New Scientist, Editorial, "Still the gold standard: Halting embryonic stem cell research now would be nothing short of rash", vol. 198, no. 2654 (3 May 2008), p. 3.

Newman, Christine, "Court hears case for embryo protection", *Irish Times*, 21 July 2006, p. 4.

Ní Aodha, Gráinne, "Most Irish people think referendum posters should be banned", TheJournal.ie, 26 May 2018 <https://www.thejournal.ie/referendum-posters-ban-4034334-May2018/> accessed 11 December 2018.

— "Bishop says Catholics who voted Yes have sinned and should go to confession", TheJournal.ie, 28 May 2018 <http://www.thejournal.ie/bishop-catholics-who-voted-yes-sinned-4039904-May2018/> accessed 28 May 2018.

Nicholas, Cory R., and Arnold R. Kriegstein, "Cell Reprogramming gets Direct", *Nature*, vol. 463, no. 7284 (25 February 2010), pp. 1031–2.

Nolan, Ann, and Shane Butler, "AIDS, Sexual Health, and the Catholic Church in 1980s Ireland: A public health paradox?", *American Journal of Public Health*, vol. 108, no. 7 (2018), pp. 908–13.

Nugent, Ryan, "Catholics who voted Yes must repent to be worthy of communion: bishop", Independent.ie, 2 June 2018 <https://www.independent.ie/irish-news/politics/catholics-who-voted-yes-must-repent-to-be-worthy-of-communion-bishop-36970575.html> accessed 3 June 2018.

Oakley, Justin, "'After-birth Abortion' and Arguments from Potential", *Journal of Medical Ethics*, vol. 39, no. 5 (May 2013), pp. 324–5.

Oakley, Richard, "Options for treating infertility", *Sunday Tribune*, 11 July 1999, p. 5.

O'Brien, Breda, "Abortion – we can do better than women in prison and dead babies in bins", *Irish Times*, 9 April 2016 <http://www.irishtimes.com/opinion/breda-o-brien-abortion-we-can-do-better-than-women-in-prison-and-dead-babies-in-bins-1.2603648> accessed 17 May 2016.

— "Amnesty abandons values of Seán MacBride", *Irish Times*, 23 April 2016 <http://www.irishtimes.com/opinion/amnesty-abandons-values-of-se%C3%A1n-macbride-1.2621162> accessed 16 May 2016.

— "Why terminology matters when it comes to pregnancy loss", *Irish Times*, 20 August 2016 <http://www.irishtimes.com/opinion/breda-o-brien-why-terminology-matters-when-it-comes-to-pregnancy-loss-1.2761949> accessed 20 August 2016.

— "Signs are not good from Citizens' Assembly", *Irish Times*, 11 February 2017, p. 14.

— "If you vote for choice you are facilitating abortions", *Irish Times*, 24 May 2018, p. 16.

O'Brien, Carl, "Majority of women want abortion legalised", *Irish Times*, 29 September 2007, p. 1 <http://www.ireland.com/newspaper/frontpage/2007/0929/1191014902496.html> accessed 8 October 2007.

— "The reproduction revolution", *Irish Times*, 19 November 2011 <https://search-proquest-com.ucc.idm.oclc.org/docview/904689669/fulltext/238C39D788CB4D01PQ/6?accountid=14504> accessed 28 March 2018.

— "Updating family law for the needs of the 21st century", 18 November 2013 <http://www.irishtimes.com/news/social-affairs/updating-family-law-for-the-needs-of-the-21st-century-1.1598175> accessed 19 November 2013.

O'Brien, Stephen, "Varadkar hails quiet revolution", *Sunday Times*, 27 May 2018, p. 1.

— "Pro-life TDs seek disability clause in abortion bill", *Sunday Times*, 3 June 2018, p. 1.

— "How the 'No' Campaign fell apart", *Sunday Times*, 3 June 2018, p. 17.

O'Carroll, J.P., "Bishops, Knights – and Pawns? Traditional thought and the Irish abortion referendum debate of 1983", *Irish Political Studies*, vol. 6 (1991), pp. 53–71.

Ó Cionnaith, Fiachra, "Call to use no vote as starting point", *Irish Examiner*, 23 May 2018, p. 6.

Ó Cionnaith, Fiachra, and Eoin English, "Professor: Savita would be alive today if not for 8th", *Irish Examiner*, 22 May, p. 6.

O'Connor, Fergal, "The Church, Society and Abortion: A comment", *Doctrine and Life*, vol. 30, no. 3 (March 1980), pp. 156–60.

O'Connor, Marie, "Mutilated by brutal 'surgery of last resort'", *Sunday Independent*, 7 September 2008 <https://www.pressreader.com/ireland/sunday-independent-ireland/20080907/282071977702278> accessed 7 February 2018.

O'Connor, Niall, "Referendum on repealing the Eighth Amendment will be Labour Party priority – Tanaiste", 26 September 2015 <http://www.independent.ie/irish-news/politics/referendum-on-repealing-eighth-amendment-will-be-labour-party-priority-tanaiste-31560276.html> accessed 27 September 2015.

O'Connor, Niall, and Philip Ryan, "Act of defiance", *Sunday Independent*, 29 November 2015, p. 1.

O'Doherty, Cahir, "Irish religious orders confirm they will not pay Magdalene Laundry victims", *Irish Central* <https://www.irishcentral.com/news/irish-nuns-orders-confirm-they-will-not-pay-magdalene-laundry-victims> accessed 5 February 2017.

O'Doherty, Caroline, "Now the big question: should a frozen embryo be protected by the Constitution?", *Irish Examiner*, 19 July 2006, p. 1.

O'Donoghue, Emma, "Embryonic Stem Cell Research is a Pointless Development", *UCC Express*, vol. 12, issue 3 (4 November 2008), p. 10.

O Faolain, Aodhan, "Sipo's order that Amnesty should return €137,000 grant is quashed after High Court appeal", TheJournal.ie, 31 July 2018 <https://www.thejournal.ie/sipo-amnesty-decision-4156736-Jul2018/> accessed 15 December 2018.

Ó Fátharta, Conall, "Flanagan: €25.7m paid out to 682 Magdalene Laundry survivors", *Irish Examiner*, 13 November 2017 <https://www.irishexaminer.com/ireland/flanagan-257m-paid-out-to-682-magdalene-laundry-survivors-462711.html> accessed 6 February 2018.

O'Grady, Peadar, Maeve Ferriter and Tiernan Murray, on behalf of Doctors for Choice, letter to the editor, *Irish Times*, 5 July 2016 <http://www.irishtimes.com/opinion/letters/the-eighth-amendment-1.2710201> accessed 5 July 2016.

O'Halloran, Marie, "Taoiseach pledges citizens' assembly on abortion issue", *Irish Times*, 17 December 2015 <http://www.irishtimes.com/news/politics/oireachtas/taoiseach-pledges-citizens-assembly-on-abortion-issue-

1.2469135?mode=print&ot=example.AjaxPageLayout.ot> accessed 19 December 2015.

O'Hanlon, Eilis, "Embryo case raises born-again question on the origins of life", *Sunday Independent*, 23 July 2006, p. 27.

O'Hanlon, Gerry, "Catholic Church needs to empower the laity", *Irish Times*, 1 June 2015

O'Leary, Cornelius, and Tom Hesketh, "The Irish Abortion and Divorce Referendum Campaigns", *Irish Political Studies*, vol. 3 (1988), pp. 43–62.

O'Leary, Don, *Roman Catholicism and Modern Science: A History* (New York: Continuum, 2006).

— *Irish Catholicism and Science: From "Godless Colleges" to the "Celtic Tiger"* (Cork: Cork University Press, 2012).

O'Loughlin, Ed, "As Irish abortion vote nears, fears of foreign influence rise", *New York Times*, 26 March 2018 <https://search-proquest-com.ucc.idm.oclc.org/docview/2019741852/70F07B3255C44BFBPQ/2?accountid=14504> accessed 20 April 2018.

O'Mahony, Conor, "The Constitution, the Right to Procreate and the Marriage Referendum", Constitution Project @UCC <http://constitutionproject.ie/?p=503> accessed 24 April 2015.

O'Mahony, T.P., "Status of the unborn has yet to be determined by Supreme Court", *Irish Examiner*, 19 July 2006, p. 7.

O'Regan, Eilish, "Mater does U-turn on cancer trial", Independent.ie, 19 October 2005 <https://www.independent.ie/irish-news/mater-does-uturn-on-cancer-trial-25962301.html> accessed 14 February 2018.

O'Regan, Michael, "Broader embryo debate urged by Dr Martin", *Irish Times*, 21 July 2006, p. 5.

O'Reilly, Kevin E., "Sisters of Charity must reject any NMH deal that will destroy innocent life", *Irish Times*, 13 June 2017 <http://www.irishtimes.com/opinion/sisters-of-charity-must-reject-any-nmh-deal-that-will-destroy-innocent-life-1.3117120> accessed 13 June 2017.

O'Riordan, Billy, "Anti-abortion group seeks to defend graphic imagery on posters", *Irish Examiner*, 30 May 2018 <https://www.irishexaminer.com/breakingnews/views/analysis/anti-abortion-group-seeks-to-defend-graphic-imagery-on-posters-845795.html> accessed 14 December 2018.

O'Riordan, Conor (ed.), *Debating the Eighth: Repeal or Retain?* (Dublin: Orpen Press, 2018).

O'Sullivan, Claire, "Supreme Court ruling: meaning of life", *Irish Examiner*, 16 December 2009, p. 1.

— "Lack of enthusiasm blocked report on law", *Irish Examiner*, 16 December 2009, p. 6.

— "TD assured he will not be excommunicated for backing abortion laws", *Irish Examiner*, 22 June 2013 <http://www.irishexaminer.com/ireland/

td-assured-he-will-not-be-excommunicated-for-backing-abortion-laws-234822.html> accessed 15 February 2014.

O'Toole, Fintan, "Down syndrome will be central issue in abortion referendum", *Irish Times*, 23 January 2018 <https://search-proquest-com.ucc.idm.oclc.org/docview/1992712965/1F34273BEAC942C6PQ/58?accountid=14504> accessed 16 February 2018.

— "Eighth demands punishment for women", *Irish Times*, 1 May 2018 <https://search-proquest-com.ucc.idm.oclc.org/docview/2032559721/EBB4E07422794B5FPQ/63?accountid=14504> accessed 1 May 2018.

Ó Tuathail, Séamas, *et al.*, letter to the editor, *Irish Times*, 23 April 2018 <https://search-proquest-com.ucc.idm.oclc.org/docview/2028721567/2480E698EBBF447CPQ/82?accountid=14504> accessed 23 April 2018.

Owens, Gary, letter to the editor, *Irish Times*, 25 January 2018 <https://www.irishtimes.com/opinion/letters/eighth-amendment-and-disability-1.3367321> accessed 25 January 2018).

Oxford Concise Science Dictionary (Oxford: Oxford University Press, 1996 (3rd edn)).

Penet, Jean-Christophe, "Closer to Brussels than to Rome? The EU as the new external referent for a secularised Irish society and a redefined Catholic identity", Études Irlandaises, vol. 34, no. 1 (2009), pp. 53–66.

Penner, Paul S., and Richard T. Hull, "The Beginning of Individual Personhood", *Journal of Medicine and Philosophy*, vol. 33 (2008), 174–82.

Pollak, Andy, "78% of Catholics follow own consciences in making moral decisions, survey shows", *Irish Times*, 16 December 1996, p. 1.

— "Poll shows church's moral authority in decline", *Irish Times*, 16 December 1996, p. 5.

Pollak, Sorcha, "More than 1,000 doctors call for Yes vote", *Irish Times*, 14 May 2018 <https://search-proquest-com.ucc.idm.oclc.org/docview/2038137870/7B7D35945F184915PQ/53?accountid=14504> accessed14 May 2018.

Pollak, Sorcha, and Carl O'Brien, "March for Choice hears call for abortion referendum", *Irish Times*, 26 September 2015 <http://www.irishtimes.com/news/social-affairs/march-for-choice-hears-call-for-abortion-referendum-1.2366549?mode=print&ot=example.AjaxPageLayout.ot> accessed 26 September 2015.

Popkin, Richard H., and Avrum Stroll, *Philosophy* (Oxford: Made Simple Books, 1993 (3rd edn)).

Porter, Jean, "Individuality, Personal Identity, and the Moral Status of the Preembryo: A response to Mark Johnson", *Theological Studies*, vol. 56, no. 4 (December 1995), pp. 763–70.

Porter, Lindsey, "Abortion, Infanticide and Moral Context", *Journal of Medical Ethics*, vol. 39, no. 5 (May 2013), pp. 350–2.

Precious Life, "Victory! Nationalists and Unionists Unite to Protect Northern Ireland's Unborn Children" <http://preciouslife.com/news/262/victory-nationalists-and-unionists-unite-to-protect-northern-irelands-unborn-children/> accessed 4 March 2016.

Prinz, Jesse, "Morality is a Culturally Conditioned Response", *Philosophy Now*, issue 82 (November–December 2011) <http://www.philosophynow.org/issue82/Morality_is_a_Culturally_Conditioned_Response> accessed 10 December 2011.

Pro Life Campaign, press release, "Ireland's largest pro-life gathering ever!" http://prolifecampaign.ie/main/well-over-40000-people-attend-national-vigil-for-life/> accessed 7 March 2014).

— "Pro Life Campaign 'will now devote its energies to the repeal of unjust law' as president signs abortion bill into law", 30 July 2013 <http://prolifecampaign.ie/main/portfolio/detail/30th-july-2013-pro-life-campaign-will-now-devote-energies-repeal-unjust-law-president-signs-abortion-bill-law/> accessed 9 March 2014.

— "Over 600 attend Pro Life Campaign national conference in the RDS", 14 October 2013 <http://prolifecampaign.ie/main/portfolio/detail/3723/> accessed 7 March 2014.

— "Babies diagnosed with life-limiting conditions", 2015 <http://prolifecampaign.ie/main/portfolio/detail/the-hard-cases-explained/> accessed 14 September 2016.

— *General Election 2016: Ireland's pro-life laws hang in the balance* (Dublin: Pro Life Campaign).

— "UN committee has become a de facto lobby group for abortion" <http://prolifecampaign.ie/main/portfolio/detail/09-06-16-un-committee-become-de-facto-lobby-group-abortion-plc/> accessed 12 June 2016.

— "Misinformation at heart of Wallace abortion bill, says PLC", 1 July 2016 <http://prolifecampaign.ie/main/portfolio/detail/01-07-16-misinformation-heart-wallace-abortion-bill-says-plc/> accessed 14 September 2016.

— "PLC will mount reasoned and robust defence of 8th Amendment" <http://prolifecampaign.ie/main/portfolio/detail/15-10-16-plc-will-mount-reasoned-robust-defence-8th-amendment/> accessed 19 February 2017.

— "PLC submission highlights lives saved by the Eighth Amendment" <http://prolifecampaign.ie/main/portfolio/detail/16-12-16-plc-submission-highlights-lives-saved-eighth-amendment/> accessed 19 February 2017.

— "PLC challenges Citizens' Assembly to redress 'unacceptable imbalance' in speakers" <http://prolifecampaign.ie/main/portfolio/detail/04-11-17-plc-challenges-citizens-assembly-redress-unacceptable-imbalance-speakers/> accessed 19 February 2017.

— "PLC accuses Noone of making 'highly misleading' statements about committee", 13 November 2017 <http://prolifecampaign.ie/main/portfolio/detail/13-11-17-plc-accuses-noone-making-highly-misleading-statements-

committee/> accessed 15 November 2017.

Quann, Jack, "Disability group Inclusion Ireland to join campaign to repeal Eighth Amendment", 13 April 2018, newstalk.com <https://www.newstalk.com/Disability-group-Inclusion-Ireland-to-join-campaign-to-repeal-Eighth-Amendment> accessed 8 October 2018.

Quilty, Aideen, Sinéad Kennedy and Catherine Conlon (eds), *The Abortion Papers Ireland*: Volume 2 (Cork: Attic Press, 2015).

Quinlan, Ronald, "Letters reveal Taoiseach's efforts to defer to bishops", *Sunday Independent*, 4 February 2007, p. 6.

Quinn, David, "Minister in stem cell funding row", *Irish Catholic*, 22 June 2006, p. 1.

— "'Spare' embryos are human. The courts must protect them", *Sunday Times*, 9 July 2006, p. 16.

— "A very modern tale of sperm donors and their children", *Irish Catholic*, 17 December 2009, p. 19.

— "Shatter's Brave New World attacks children's rights: The Government is trying to set aside nature and replace it with choice", *Irish Catholic*, 6 February 2014 <http://www.irishcatholic.ie/article/shatter%E2%80%99s-brave-new-world-attacks-children%E2%80%99s-rights> accessed 9 February 2014.

— "Less doctrinal emphasis does not equate to radical change", *Irish Catholic*, 12 March 2015.

— "'Yes Equality' family values leaflet is deeply hypocritical", *Irish Catholic*, 14 May 2015 <http://irishcatholic.ie/article/%E2%80%98yes-equality%E2%80%99-family-values-leaflet-deeply-hypocritical> accessed 20 May 2015).

— "Repeal vote is a rubber stamp for eugenics", *Sunday Times*, 10 December 2017, p. 13.

— "The more things change …", *Irish Catholic*, 22 February 2018 <https://www.irishcatholic.com/the-more-things-change/> accessed 18 February 2019.

— "Unborn have no voice, so how could they win?", *Sunday Times*, 27 May 2018, p. 15.

Radkowska-Walkowicz, Magdalena, "How the Political Becomes Private: In vitro fertilization and the Catholic Church in Poland", *Journal of Religion and Health*, vol. 57 (2018), pp. 979–93.

Reichhardt, Tony, "Studies of Faith", *Nature*, vol. 432, no. 7018 (9 December 2004), pp. 666–9 <www.nature.com/nature>.

Reichlin, Massimo, "The Argument from Potential: A reappraisal", *Bioethics*, vol. 11, no. 1 (1997), pp. 1–23.

Reid, Liam, "Government undecided on embryo law", *Irish Times*, 16 November 2006, p. 4.

Religious Sisters of Charity, "Religious Sisters of Charity to Gift to People of Ireland Lands at St Vincent's Healthcare Group to the Value of €200 million" /https://rsccaritas.com/index.php/rscnews/1112-gift-to-people-of-ireland/ accessed 9 May 2020.

Reville, William, "Is it time to ensure that ethics match the science?" *Irish Times*, 9 February 2006, p. 15.

— "If the embryo is fully human, we are obliged to keep it from harm", *Irish Times*, 18 May 2006, p. 15.

— "Life Continuum", *UCC News*, issue 40 (May 2008), pp. 1–2.

— "Killing of embryos in human stem-cell research is wrong", *Irish Times*, 21 January 2010 <http://www.irishtimes.com/newspaper/sciencetoday/2010/0121/1224262767052_pf.html> accessed 21 January 2010.

Ring, Evelyn, "Calls for legislation to protect embryos", *Irish Examiner*, 16 December 2009, p. 6.

— "Eighth 'has led to dangerous abortions'", *Irish Examiner*, 22 May 2018, p. 6.

Rini, Regina A., "Of Course the Baby should Live: Against 'after-birth abortion'", *Journal of Medical Ethics*, vol. 39, no. 5 (May 2013), pp. 353–6.

Roche, Barry, "UCC gives go-ahead for embryonic stem-cell research", *Irish Times*, 28 October 2008 <http://www.irishtimes.com/newspaper/breaking/2008/1028/breaking67_pf.html> accessed 9 November 2008.

— "Repealing Eighth 'could lead to euthanasia and eugenics'", *Irish Times*, 16 April 2018.

— "Bishop says culture of abortion would be 'horrendous'", *Irish Times*, 8 May 2018 <https://search-proquest-com.ucc.idm.oclc.org/docview/2035453235/ABC7884B2DEA435EPQ/38?accountid=14504> accessed 8 May 2018.

— "Mother might still be alive but for Eighth Amendment – gynaecologist", *Irish Times*, 13 May 2018 <https://www.irishtimes.com/news/ireland/irish-news/mother-might-still-be-alive-but-for-eighth-amendment-gynaecologist-1.3493958> accessed 11 November 2018.

RTE.ie, "Site for new maternity hospital still under religious control – Boylan", 9 November 2019 <https://www.rte.ie/news/ireland/2019/1109/1089729-national-maternity-hospital/> accessed 9 November 2019.

RTÉ News, "Midwife confirms she told Savita Halappanavar Ireland is a 'Catholic country'", 11 April 2013 <http://www.rte.ie/news/health/2013/0410/380613-savita-halappanavar-inquest/> accessed 28 January 2014.

— "UN criticises religious orders over refusal to contribute to Magdalene redress fund", 23 May 2014 <https://www.rte.ie/news/2014/0523/619228-magdalene-redress/> accessed 5 February 2018.

— "Senior doctor calls for absolute separation of church and medicine", 2 May 2017 <https://www.rte.ie/news/2017/0428/871017-national-maternity-hospital/> accessed 17 February 2018.

— "Catholic bishop warns about arguments for abortion", 27 January 2018 <https://www.rte.ie/news/ireland/2018/0127/936344-catholic-bishop-warns-about-arguments-for-abortion/> accessed 27 January 2018.

RTÉ Radio 1, "Dr Mahony about abortion of babies with Down Syndrome", transcript of interview of Dr Rhona Mahony by Claire Byrne, *News at 1*, 9 May 2018, Love Both website <https://loveboth.ie/rhona-mahony-down-syndrome-test/> accessed 5 October 2018.

Ryan, Áine, and Michael Commins, "Taoiseach refers Cardinal Brady to Constitution", 7 May 2013 <http://www.mayonews.ie/index. php?option=com_content&view=article&id=17734:taoiseach-refers-cardinal-brady-to-constitution&catid=23:news&Itemid=46> accessed 16 February 2014.

Ryan, Órla, "Bishop says new maternity hospital should obey rules of Catholic Church", TheJournal.ie, 23 April 2017 <http://www.thejournal.ie/new-maternity-hospital-3354182-Apr2017/> accessed 28 April 2017.

— "Pro-life doctor says no woman has died because of the Eighth Amendment", TheJournal.ie, 10 April 2018 <https://www.thejournal.ie/eamon-mcguinness-eighth-amendment-3949918-Apr2018/> accessed 29 October 2018.

Ryan, Thomas, letter to the editor, *Irish Times*, 23 February 2017 <https://www. irishtimes.com/opinion/letters/the-eighth-amendment-1.3402287> accessed 23 February 2018.

Ryan-Sheridan, Susan, *Women and the New Reproductive Technologies in Ireland* (Cork: Cork University Press, 1994).

Save the 8th, "Abortion Until 6 Months", April 2018 <https://www.save8.ie/did-you-know-this-is-abortion-up-to-6-months/> accessed 10 May 2018.

— "Statement On Pro-Life Speakers at Catholic Masses", 5 May 2018 <https:// www.save8.ie/save-the-8th-statement-on-pro-life-speakers-at-catholic-masses/> accessed 8 May 2018.

— "Disability Voices for Life" <https://www.save8.ie/abortion-disability/disability-voices-for-life/> accessed 9 May 2018.

— "Our Posters" <https://www.save8.ie/posters/> accessed 23 May 2015.

Savulescu, Julian, "Abortion, Infanticide and Allowing Babies to Die, 40 Years On", *Journal of Medical Ethics*, vol. 39, no. 5 (May 2013), pp. 257–9.

Selgelid, Michael J., "Moral Uncertainty and the Moral Status of Early Human Life", *Journal of Medical Ethics*, vol. 39, no. 5 (May 2013), p. 324.

Shanahan, Catherine, "Warning over lack of laws on stem cell research", *Irish Examiner*, 27 April 2010 <http://www.examiner.ie/ireland/warning-over-lack-of-laws-on-stem-cell-research-118297.html> accessed 24 May 2010.

— "Parents angered by referendum posters", *Irish Examiner*, 7 May 2018 <https://www.irishexaminer.com/ireland/parents-angered-by-referendum-posters-470336.html> accessed 11 December 2018.

Shannon, Thomas A., "Delayed Hominization: A response to Mark Johnson", *Theological Studies*, vol. 57, no. 4 (December 1996), pp. 731–4.

— "Delayed Hominization: A further postscript to Mark Johnson", *Theological Studies*, vol. 58, no. 4 (December 1997), pp. 715–17.

Sheehan, Maeve, "Hospital deal hanging in the balance as row rages about

Church and State", *Sunday Independent*, 23 April 2017, p. 16.

Sheehan, Maeve, and Philip Ryan, "Revealed: the deal to curb nuns' role", *Sunday Independent*, 23 April 2017, pp. 1, 4.

Sheehy, Clodagh, "Abortion row priest blocked cancer trials", Herald.ie, 8 August 2013 <https://www.herald.ie/news/abortion-row-priest-blocked-cancer-trials-29484085.html> accessed 14 February 2018.

Sheldon, Sally, *et al.*, letters to the editor, *Irish Times*, 23 April 2018 <https://search-proquest-com.ucc.idm.oclc.org/docview/2028721567/2480E698EBBF447CPQ/82?accountid=14504> accessed 23 April 2018.

Sherley, J.L., "The Importance of Valid Disclosures in the Human Embryonic Stem Cell Research Debate", *Cell Proliferation*, vol. 41, issue s1 (February 2008), pp. 57–64.

Sherlock, Cora, "Say no to abortion on demand", *Irish Times*, 24 May 2018, p. 4.

Shipman, Tim, and Caroline Wheeler, "Northern Irish flock to Britain weekly for abortions: abortion law reform demanded [Ulster Region]", *Sunday Times* (London), 22 July 2018 <https://search-proquest-com.ucc.idm.oclc.org/docview/2072972929/8AD109881E574741PQ/40?accountid=14504> accessed 26 July 2018.

Sixsmith, Martin, "The Catholic church sold my child", *Guardian*, 19 September 2009 <https://www.theguardian.com/lifeandstyle/2009/sep/19/catholic-church-sold-child> accessed 20 February 2019.

Skene, L., and M. Parker, "The Role of the Church in Developing the Law", *Journal of Medical Ethics*, vol. 28 (2002), pp. 215–18.

Smith, David, *Life and Morality: Contemporary Medico-Moral Issues* (Dublin: Gill and Macmillan, 1996).

Smyth, Patrick, and Dick Ahlstrom, "Controversy as company clone human embryo", *Irish Times*, 26 November 2001 <http://www.ireland.com/newspaper/font/2001/1126/fro3.htm> accessed 12 October 2004.

Soldner, Frank, Dirk Hockemeyer *et al.*, "Parkinson's Disease Patient-Derived Induced Pluripotent Stem Cells Free of Viral Reprogramming Factors", *Cell*, vol. 136 (6 March 2009), pp. 964–77.

Spadaro, Antonio, SJ, "A Big Heart Open to God: An interview with Pope Francis", *America: The Jesuit Review*, 30 September 2013 <https://www.americamagazine.org/faith/2013/09/30/big-heart-open-god-interview-pope-francis> accessed 1 May 2019.

Stanton, David, "Child-centred Bill will improve lives of many families", *Irish Times*, 18 February 2015, p. 14.

Staunton, Denis, "Bush blocks federal funds for embryonic stem cell research", *Irish Times*, 20 July 2006, p. 11.

Steinfels, Peter, "Bishops and Abortion Law: Learning from the American experience", *Doctrine and Life*, vol. 63, no. 7 (September 2013), pp. 4–20.

Sullivan, Stephen, and Martin Codyre, "A Legal Limbo", *Irish Examiner*, 17 December 2009.

Sullivan, Stephen, and Fionnuala Gough, "Crux of the unborn", *Irish Examiner*, 15 December 2009.

Swedish Women's Lobby, "Feminist No to Surrogacy Motherhood" <http://sverigeskvinnolobby.se/en/project/feminist-no-to-surrogacy-motherhood/> accessed 23 January 2019.

Takahashi, Kazutoshi, and Shinya Yamanaka, "Induction of Pluripotent Stem Cells from Mouse Embryonic and Adult Fibroblast Cultures by Defined Factors", *Cell*, vol. 126 (25 August 2006), pp. 663–76.

Takahashi, Kazutoshi, *et al.*, "Induction of Pluripotent Stem Cells from Adult Human Fibroblasts by Defined Factors", *Cell*, vol. 131 (30 November 2007), pp. 1–12.

Taylor, Charlie, "UCC gives go-ahead for embryonic stem-cell research", *Irish Times*, 28 October 2008 <http://www.irishtimes.com/newspaper/breaking/2008/1028/breaking67_pf.html> accessed 30 October 2008.

Together for Yes, "As Doctors we make difficult decisions every day: 1,642 of us are agreed on this one" <http://www.togetherforyes.ie/doctors/> accessed 13 November 2018.

Tollefsen, Christopher, "The Future of Roman Catholic Bioethics", *Journal of Medicine and Philosophy*, vol. 43 (2018), pp. 667–85.

Tooley, Michael, "Philosophy, Critical Thinking and 'After-birth Abortion: Why should the baby live'?", *Journal of Medical Ethics*, vol. 39, no. 5 (May 2013), pp. 266–72.

Torjesen, Ingrid, "Five Minutes with ... Joanna Rose", *British Medical Journal*, vol. 351 (4 November 2015) <https://www-bmj-com.ucc.idm.oclc.org/content/351/bmj.h5864> accessed 13 February 2019.

Uttley, Lois, Sheila Reynertson, Lorraine Kenny and Louise Melling, *Miscarriage of Medicine: The Growth of Catholic Hospitals and the Threat to Reproductive Health Care* (New York: American Civil Liberties Union, and MergerWatch, 2013) <https://www.aclu.org/report/miscarriage-medicine> accessed 30 September 2019.

Verhagen, A.A. Eduard, "The Groningen Protocol for Newborn Euthanasia: Which way did the slippery slope tilt?", *Journal of Medical Ethics*, vol. 39, no. 5 (May 2013), pp. 293–95.

Vierbuchen, Thomas, Austin Ostermeier *et al.*, "Direct Conversion of Fibroblasts to Functional Neurons by Defined Factors", *Nature*, vol. 463, no. 7284 (25 February 2010), pp. 1035–41.

Vogel, Gretchen, "Ireland: Embryo ruling keeps stem cell research legal", *Science*, vol. 327, issue no. 5961 (1 January 2010), p. 25.

— "Reprogrammed Cells Come Up Short, for Now", *Science*, vol. 327 (5 March 2010), p. 119.

Vogel, Gretchen, and Constance Holden, "Field Leaps Forward with New Stem

Cell Advances", *Science*, vol. 318, no. 5854 (23 November 2007), pp. 1224–5 <http://www.sciencemag.org/cgi/content/full/318/5854/1224> accessed 23 November 2007.

Wall, Martin, "'Informed discussion' of embryo rights urged", *Irish Times*, 21 July 2006, p. 5.

— "EU divided on stem-cell research funds", *Irish Times*, 24 July 2006, p. 7.

— "Court may decide on right of foetus in life support case", *Irish Times*, 19 December 2014 <http://www.irishtimes.com/news/ireland/irish-news/court-may-decide-on-right-of-foetus-in-life-support-case-1.2043125> accessed 22 December 2014.

Walsh, David J., E. Scott Sills, Gary S. Collins, Christine A. Hawrylyshyn, Piotr Sokol and Anthony P.H. Walsh, "Irish Public Opinion on Assisted Human Reproduction Services: Contemporary assessments from a national sample", *Clinical and Experimental Reproductive Medicine*, vol. 40, no. 4 (December 2013), pp. 169–73 <https://www.ncbi.nlm.nih.gov/pmc/articles/PMC3913896/> accessed 17 March 2019.

Walsh, Jimmy, "'Cowardice' being shown on reproduction issue: Seanad Report", *Irish Times*, 16 December 2009, p. 8.

Weiss, Rick, "Scientists claim advance in stem cell research", *Irish Times*, 18 October 2005 <http://www.ireland.com/newspaper/world/2005/1018/4065415237FR18STEM.html> accessed 23 May 2006.

Westphal, Sylvia Pagán, and Philip Cohen, "Cloned Cells Today. Where tomorrow?", *New Scientist*, vol. 181, no. 2435 (21 February 2004), pp. 6–7.

Whelan, Christopher T., *Values and Social Change in Ireland* (Dublin: Gill and Macmillan, 1994).

Whelan, Noel, "Why was a court ruling required to decide fate of pregnant woman on life support?", *Irish Times*, 2 January 2015 <http://www.irishtimes.com/opinion/why-was-a-court-ruling-required-to-decide-fate-of-pregnant-woman-on-life-support-1.2052877?mode=print&ot=example.AjaxPageLayout.ot> accessed 2 January 2015.

— "No side posters may prove counterproductive", *Irish Times*, 24 April 2015 <http://www.irishtimes.com/opinion/noel-whelan-no-side-posters-may-prove-counterproductive-1.2186624?mode=print&ot=example.AjaxPageLayout.ot> accessed 24 April 2015.

— "Simple repeal of Eighth Amendment carries risks", *Irish Times*, 19 January 2018 <https://search-proquest-com.ucc.idm.oclc.org/docview/1988763759/47009D2C03FA4A7EPQ/86?accountid=14504> accessed 19 January 2018.

White, Alex, "Government Publishes General Scheme of the Protection of Life during Pregnancy Bill 2013", 1 May 2013 <http://alexwhitetd.wordpress.com/2013/05/01/government-publishes-general-scheme-of-the-protection-of-life-during-pregnancy-bill-2013/> accessed 15 February 2014.

Whyte, Fiona, and Seán Malone, *Without a Doubt: An Irish Couple's Journey through IVF, Adoption and Surrogacy* (Dublin: Merrion Press, 2017).

Whyte, Gerry, "High Court had to determine what word unborn meant", *Irish Times*, 16 November 2006, p. 18.

— "Repeal or Replace? The legal implications of amending Article 40.3.3", conference paper at "Abortion, Disability and the Law" conference, jointly hosted by Anscombe Bioethics Centre and Consultative Group on Bioethics of the Irish Catholic Bishops' Conference, 20 October 2017, Irish Catholic Bishops' Conference website <https://www.catholicbishops.ie/2017/10/20/papers-delivered-at-the-conference-abortion-disability-and-the-law/> accessed 5 July 2018.

Whyte, J.H., *Church and State in Modern Ireland 1923–1979* (Dublin: Gill and Macmillan, 1984 (2nd edn)).

Wilkinson, D.J.C., P. Thiele, A. Watkins and L. De Crespigny, "Fatally Flawed? A review and ethical analysis of lethal congenital malformations", *British Journal of Obstetrics and Gynaecology*, vol. 119, issue 11 (October 2012), pages 1302–8 (online, accessed 16 December 2015).

Wilmut, Ian, "The Moral Imperative of Human Cloning", *New Scientist*, vol. 181, no. 2435 (21 February 2004), pp. 16–17.

Yamanaka, S., "Induction of Pluripotent Stem Cells from Mouse Fibroblasts by Four Transcription Factors", *Cell Proliferation*, vol. 41, s1 (February 2008), pp. 51–6.

Yamanaka, Shinya, "A Fresh Look at iPS Cells", *Cell*, vol. 137 (3 April 2009), pp. 13–17.

— "Elite and Stochastic Models for Induced Pluripotent Stem Cell Regeneration", *Nature*, vol. 460, issue no. 7251 (2 July 2009), pp. 49–52.

Yes Equality, *Marriage and Family Matter: Vote Yes on May 22nd* [2015].

YesEqualityCork, *Vote Yes for Equality on May 22nd* [2015].

Your Guide to the Referendum – Information on the Government's Proposals, published by, and sponsors included: Family & Life, Life Institute, www.save8.ie, www.protectthe8th.ie, and Coalition Against Abortion on Demand (May 2018).